The Auditory Processing of Speech

Speech Research 10

Editors

Vincent J. van Heuven
Louis C. W. Pols

Mouton de Gruyter
Berlin · New York

The Auditory Processing of Speech

From Sounds to Words

Edited by

M. E. H. Schouten

Mouton de Gruyter
Berlin · New York 1992

Mouton de Gruyter (formerly Mouton, The Hague)
is a division of Walter de Gruyter & Co., Berlin.

⊗ Printed on acid-free paper which falls within the guidelines of the ANSI to ensure permanence and durability.

Library of Congress Cataloging-in-Publication Data

The Auditory processing of speech : from sounds to words /
edited by M. E. H. Schouten.
p. cm. – (Speech research 10)
Includes bibliographical references
ISBN 3-11-013589-2 (acid-free paper)
1. Speech perception. 2. Hearing. I. Schouten, Marten Egbertus Hendrik, 1946– . II. Series.
BF463.S64A9 1992
401′.9–dc20 92-35685
CIP

Die Deutsche Bibliothek – Cataloging-in-Publication Data

The **auditory processing of speech** : from sounds to words / ed. by M. E. H. Schouten. – Berlin ; New York : Mouton de Gruyter, 1992
(Speech research ; 10)
ISBN 3-11-013589-2
NE: Schouten, Marten E. H. [Hrsg.]; GT

Printing: Gerike GmbH, Berlin. – Binding: Lüderitz & Bauer, Berlin. – Printed in Germany.

Preface

This book, and the workshop on which it is based, was made possible by generous funding from the Research Institute for Language and Speech, the Department of Linguistics, the Faculty of Arts, and, as part of the 1991 lustrum activities, the Board of Governors of the University of Utrecht.
Special thanks are due to H. Duifhuis, R. Pastore, L. Pols, G. Smoorenburg, and Q. Summerfield for their help in putting together this volume.
Blue Cat (Utrecht, The Netherlands) solved all post-editorial and lay-out problems.

Table of Contents

Chapter 6. *Word Perception and beyond*

Editor's Introduction

Bert Schouten
Research Institute for Language and Speech
University of Utrecht
Trans 10
3512 JK Utrecht
The Netherlands

A message from a speaker to a listener has to travel a very long way, from an intention on the part of the former, via an acoustic signal, through the transducer stages of the peripheral auditory system, to an understanding on the part of the latter. Research into these enormously complicated processes has always assumed that it is useful to divide them up into a number of partly consecutive, partly simultaneous processing stages, which can be investigated separately. Speaking involves the formulation of a message into an utterance with the help of syntax, semantics, morphology, phonology, phonetics, and the physiology of the speech organs, while listening means decoding the resulting acoustic signal by means of peripheral auditory analysis, feature extraction, phoneme perception, word perception, and so on, up the linguistic chain. The names of all these stages, or "levels", designate just as many separate research areas, some of which grew up together so that they speak more or less the same language, whereas other ones evolved separately, developing terminologies which are so far apart that it is hard to realize that they are actually part of the same enterprise.

Although not all these separate "modules" have been investigated to the same extent, it is undeniable that a great deal of knowledge has been built up, and continues to be built up, about the workings of each one of them. Relatively little is known, however, about how they interrelate, cooperate, overlap, or even interfere with each other in order to enable speaker and listener to communicate in real time. Levelt (1989) represents the first attempt to obtain an integrated view of the speaker; no such attempt has so far been made in relation to the listener. The present book is about the listener, but it is neither as wide-ranging nor as integrated as Levelt's book; moreover, its emphasis is on peripheral at the expense of central processes, whereas Levelt's book about the speaker tends to favour central processes at the expense of the more peripheral ones.

The reason why the present book is less integrated is that it does not present one person's point of view, but consists of 35 papers by researchers from a limited number of related fields between the auditory periphery and word recognition, who came together one week in July 1991 to inform each other about the state of knowledge and about current research in their respective areas. This was the second meeting under the title "The Psychophysics of Speech Perception", held at the Research Institute for Language and Speech in Utrecht. The first meeting, in 1986, had helped to bring about an exchange of ideas between the areas of psychoacoustics, auditory physiology, and phoneme perception (see Schouten, 1987); in the second one in 1991 a cautious step was taken in a more central direction by inviting contributions from experts on word perception. This extension of the subject matter was a relatively small one: it did not go much beyond the perception of single words, without any wider syntactic or semantic context, but it was quite large enough for some participants, who saw themselves confronted with unfamiliar methods and ways of thinking. There appears to be a very wide gulf between the fields of signal processing and of the representation of linguistic knowledge; this gulf will have to be bridged if we are one day to achieve a unified view of how a message gets to be understood by a listener. Clearly, this book does not even begin to build such a bridge; all it does in this respect is put out a few feelers from the auditory periphery towards the centre. At the first meeting in 1986, the divide between physiologists and phoneme perception researchers turned out to be bridgeable because both sides had a strong interest in signal processing; higher-level units than phonemes, however, are much further removed from the signal, and tend to be investigated in a far more symbolic and abstract way, with the word as a unit sitting on the fence: some word perception researchers have a phonetic orientation, whereas others are linguistic in outlook. This book mainly contains contributions from the first type.

The book moves from the periphery towards the centre in a small number of discrete but inevitably overlapping steps. Chapter 1 deals with models of (aspects of) the auditory system, in relation to the perception of speech sounds. Chapter 2 is both physiological and psychophysical in outlook; it presents research into one of the most intriguing questions about human communication performance: how do we succeed in separating the message we wish to attend to from all the competing sounds (such as other messages) that are simultaneously present? Chapter 3 is about the perception of signals that are more complex, and therefore more speech-like, than the types of signal that are customary in psychoacoustics. Chapter 4 asks what various types of auditory handicap mean for the perception of complex signals such as speech signals. In Chapter 5 we move away from the auditory periphery and bring cognitive entities into play by asking how speech sounds are represented in long-term memory and how this representation influences their perception. Finally, Chapter 6 examines the interface between the auditory input and the mental lexicon: how does a listener gain access to his internal dictionary? At this point the book ends: it does not look at the information available in each entry, once it has been found - it only looks at the nature of the access code (the alphabet, so to speak).

In what follows, a brief summary of all 35 papers will be given; this summary is intended as a guide through the book and as an introduction for the reader who is interested in the the perception of spoken language, but does not have a background in psychology or physics.

Chapter 1. The Auditory System in Relation to Speech Perception.

In his keynote paper, **Duifhuis** summarises recent work on modelling the cochlea (the ear's frequency analyser). Some of this work is based on the assumption that the cochlea is a linear system whose frequency analysis derives from the stiffness of the basilar membrane, which varies through about four orders of magnitude along the length of the cochlea (roughly speaking, greater stiffness leads to a higher resonance frequency). The linear models are set off against more realistic, but also far more complicated, non-linear models in which the cochlea, presumably by means of the outer hair cells, selectively adds energy to the input signal, thus sharpening frequency selectivity and increasing dynamic range. If we want to account for the processing of speech sounds at the level of the cochlea, more complicated non-linear modelling will have to be used: linear models, which give an adequate description of the processing of simple, stationary tones, break down as soon as two tones are presented simultaneously. It is not surprising, therefore, that non-linear modelling plays an important part in a number of other contributions to this chapter, notably those by Horst et al., Oomens et al., Patterson et al., and Kohlrausch et al.

Horst, Javel, and Farley present physiological data bearing on the fact that frequency resolution is considerably better than would be predicted by a linear model of the cochlea. They investigate the hypothesis that this enhanced resolution could be due to timing information extracted from the firing patterns in the auditory nerve. Previous research had shown that such information is indeed available in stimuli with flat phase spectra and at moderate intensities. The new data indicate, however, that other, less regular phase spectra yield much less timing information; the authors conclude that in everyday speech perception, where phase spectra are usually seriously distorted, very little synchronisation will occur between the periodicity of the stimulus and the auditory-nerve firing moments, and that the enhanced frequency resolution is therefore probably due to something else.

Delgutte and Cariani, nevertheless, show that the perceived pitch of various types of complex tones follows the most frequently occurring inter-spike interval very closely (the inter-spike interval is the time between successive firings of a nerve fibre). Although it cannot be said that the most frequent interval really stands out strongly among the less frequent intervals, the correlation is striking.

Sachs, Blackburn, Banks, and Wang move to one level above the cochlea and the auditory nerve, the cochlear nucleus in the brain stem, where the auditory nerve terminates. In their keynote paper they establish a relationship between the morphological properties of two types of cell in the auditory cochlear nucleus and the measured responses of those cells to vowel stimuli. One type of cell, the bushy cell (which has a "primarylike" response), turns out to exhibit the same phase-locking to the stimulus as is found in auditory-nerve fibres, whereas another type, the stellate cell (which has a "chopper" response), maintains a very good rate-place profile, i.e. a topological representation of the frequency-specific stimulation pattern along the basilar membrane. A stellate cell apparently achieves this by "selectively listening" to two different types of auditory-nerve fibres: at low stimulus levels it "listens" to the sensitive but easily saturated fibres that have a high spontaneous firing rate, whereas at high stimulus levels it "listens" to the much less numerous and less sensitive fibres that have a low spontaneous rate. As a result, two spectral representations of the signal are, in principle, available to higher levels of processing: a temporal one and a rate-place one.

Oomens, Breed, De Boer, and Schouten investigate another non-linearity (lateral suppression) that may be of interest in speech perception. Their research focusses on the question of how a gap in the spectrum of a stimulus is represented in the auditory nerve.

The idea behind their experiment is that a spectral gap is often regarded as an important cue for the perception of nasality. They find that a gap in an otherwise flat noise spectrum is rather poorly reflected in the response, but that increasing the level of spectral components at the edge of the gap by 10 dB suppresses the response of fibres tuned to frequencies inside the gap, thus improving its representation in the response.

In the third keynote paper of this chapter, **Patterson, Holdsworth, and Allerhand** present a speech recognition system that is based on a model of the auditory periphery, and includes such non-linear aspects as compression, adaptation, and suppression in the cochlea. By including a form of temporal integration across the spectrum that is triggered by large pulses in the input signal, the authors manage to produce a stable auditory "image", which can be visualised in a motion picture. The movements within this picture are a convincing equivalent of perceptual changes in the (speech) signal; it would appear, therefore, that this type of modelling should work very well for automatic speech recognition and achieve performance levels comparable to what humans can do. Unfortunately, such a performance would require data rates far in excess of what is at present feasible in speech recognisers; an attempt to reduce data rates to more manageable proportions produced results that were not altogether satisfactory. Whether auditory modelling leads to better recognition performance than other methods should become clear by the end of the decade, when much higher data rates will be available on all sides.

Kohlrausch, Püschel, and Alphei present a non-linear model of temporal resolution in the auditory system, in order to give a good account of forward masking by white noise of the perception of a short tone burst, and of the segregation of differently modulated tonal complexes. The non-linear element in their model is a compressive type of feedback, which results in a reduction of the dynamic range of the input signal. It is shown that sound segregation, to the extent that it is based on differences in modulation, is best at modulation differences of 5 Hz, and that this can be modelled satisfactorily by assuming dynamic compression. This paper therefore forms a link with the next chapter; it is included in this chapter because it is mainly about auditory modelling.

Ehret deals with the problem of whether models that are based on physiological measurements performed on animals are relevant for human perception. His answer is affirmative: a great deal of behavioural evidence shows that biologically relevant, species-specific sounds are processed by animals in very much the same way as human beings process speech sounds. This applies up to quite high processing levels, such as categorical perception and hemispheric dominance.

Chapter 2. Separation of Simultaneous Signals

Palmer examines the information, available in the timing of the impulses of auditory-nerve fibres responding to a pair of simultaneously presented vowels, which could provide a basis for their segregation. He does this by calculating autocorrelation functions for each of a large number of frequency channels. By separating the channels into those which do, and those which do not show more than a threshold amount of activity synchronised to the period of one of the two fundamentals, it is possible to segregate the two vowels. This procedure does not require knowledge of the fundamentals and the spectra, except that there are two of each and that they are different.

Cooke, on the other hand, uses a rather different approach to sound source separation, one which does not depend exclusively on pitch estimation, and which therefore seems more suitable for everyday speech perception, where stable pitch information is usually not available. The outputs of the channels of an auditory filter bank are first combined into groups, on the basis of a very simple grouping principle; the groups are then examined for continuity, and temporally successive and spectrally contiguous groups are assumed to form a strand (see Fig. 1 in Cooke's paper, where the F1 strand clearly consists of 6 or 7 successive groups of filters). Then a second-order grouping is applied to the strands to determine which ones belong together; the regularities observed within these second-order groups are ploughed back into the original filter outputs, enabling the system to determine which filters contain information on which signal. The model is not based on physiological data, but it attempts to account for psychophysical data such as those presented by Darwin (see below).

From a perceptual rather than a physiological perspective, **Darwin**'s keynote paper explicitly addresses the same issue as Palmer and Cooke: whether sound source separation is achieved on the basis of pitch differences or on the basis of auditory grouping, involving such cues as onset differences, spatial separation, and disjoint allocation. His conclusion is that both kinds of mechanism play important roles.

Carlyon goes one step further by investigating the separation of formant-like tone complexes which are rather far apart in frequency, but which consist of harmonics of the same fundamental, so that first-order pitch differences cannot supply cues about different sources. Carlyon asked his subjects to distinguish these two-"formant" stimuli from stimuli in which the harmonics in one "formant" were delayed in phase relative to the harmonics in the other one, and from stimuli in which the two sets of harmonics were slightly mistuned in relation to one another. His findings are that such cues are most useful at very low fundamental frequencies.

Summerfield investigates another possible grouping principle for separating different sound sources: coherent frequency modulation. The fundamental frequency of a voice changes continually, taking its harmonics with it; when two voices are present simultaneously, their different coherences could be used to tell them apart. The experiments show, however, that listeners do not really use this cue for sound source separation - the reason may be that harmonicity is such a powerful cue for grouping that there has been no need for additional mechanisms to evolve to register and exploit FM coherence.

Moore's keynote paper looks at aspects of coherent modulation at a more basic level. It presents an overview of recent work on two masking phenomena which seem to be related to auditory grouping: Comodulation Masking Release (CMR) and Modulation Detection Interference (MDI). In both cases, similarly modulated carriers (usually noise bands) that are far apart in frequency seem to be combined by the listener, resulting in better detection of a signal that is masked by one of these noise bands (CMR), and in reduced detection of the modulation itself (MDI). However, the relevance of these phenomena for speech perception is doubtful: attempts to extend CMR to the perception of speech-like sounds have so far yielded little evidence of, for example, a role for CMR in the identification of speech in noise.

Fantini and Moore cast an interesting sidelight on CMR by showing very convincingly that level increment detection (i.e. hearing small differences in loudness) in a modulated noise band is enhanced when coherently modulated noise bands are presented simultaneously. Moreover, at modulation frequencies which the ear can no longer follow (more than 32 Hz), it did not matter whether there was any coherence in the modulations of the various noise bands or not: the addition of any noise bands yielded the same improvement in level detection as the addition of a coherently modulated ("correlated") noise band. This paper establishes a connection between CMR and another research paradigm that is often regarded as being of importance for speech perception: Profile Analysis (Green, 1988). The basic finding in profile analysis is that it is easier to detect an increment in the level of a tone when that tone is part of a wideband tone complex than when it is presented by itself; apparently, listeners find it easier to concentrate on spectral shape than on a single frequency.

Van den Brink, Houtgast, and Smoorenburg present data which show that CMR is at its most effective in situations where detection would otherwise be poor: a short signal placed in a modulation dip, and a long signal masked by a narrow noise band. These results raise questions about the importance of CMR and other modulation effects (see also the discussion of Summerfield's paper above) for the perception of speech sounds.

Festen investigates modulation masking by modulating the same pink noise band (1-4 kHz) with both a sinusoidal probe modulation and a low-frequency noise band masker modulation. He observes very poor frequency selectivity in modulation detection and concludes that there are unlikely to be specialised modulation-rate channels in the auditory system; however, masking is strongly dependent on similarity in modulation rate.

Chapter 3. Perception of Spectral Change and Timbre

In his keynote paper, Houtsma reviews the links between psychoacoustic research and speech perception - the ones relating to pitch and timbre perception. He comes to the conclusion that the relationships are usually not very simple. For example, the perception of prominence in speech, which is cued to a large extent by excursions of the fundamental frequency, is best described in terms of the number of critical bands, rather than the number of semitones, traversed by the excursion. This finding runs counter to expectations based on pure-tone pitch perception, which is a function of log Hz. Another example is the concept of timbre, which does not include spectral change, whereas many speech sounds (and musical instruments) are characterised mainly by transients. An appropriate perceptual concept on which research can be focussed is not available.

Versfeld compares the discrimination of rising and falling spectral envelopes in steady-state noise bands and two-tone complexes, by varying the overall bandwidths and the centre frequencies of the bands and the two-tone complexes. Discrimination performance is expressed in terms of the slope of the spectral envelope (in decibels) that was needed to achieve 75% correct responses. The pattern of results is equivalent for the noise bands and the two-tone complexes: at small bandwidths, involving only one frequency channel, performance is poor. Bandwidths exceeding one semitone, however, result in much better performance, although thresholds increase again as bandwidths are increased further. These results indicate that discrimination is based on a comparison of the spectral edges of the stimulus, and that this is less successful as the edges are farther apart.

Lacerda investigates discrimination by infants of timbre and spectral change in, respectively, synthetic vowels and stop consonants varying only in F2 (steady state or initial or final transition). The results are difficult to interpret, but it seems that the infants are rather insensitive to timbre differences (vowels), but quite sensitive to differences in spectral change (stop consonants), at least as compared to adults. Older infants, however (over 3 months of age), appear to have lost their sensitivity to transitions: they perform poorly in stop consonant discrimination.

Schwartz, Beautemps, Arrouas, and Escudier posit separate systems for the processing of spectral change and of timbre, each of which is related to aspects of articulation, namely "timing" and "targets", respectively. Their aim is to interpret speech perception as "recovery of speech gestures", which links them quite closely with Fowler's (1990) direct-realist theory and with more recent versions of the motor theory (Repp, 1987). Schwartz et al. go one step further, however: they want to find out how the perceptual system recovers the articulatory gestures from the speech signal. What they propose is that the listener uses the acoustic information, in particular the duration of a "plateau" in relation to the transition to that plateau, to calculate the targets that the speaker aims for but often does not reach.

Espinoza-Varas investigates whether psychoacoustic thresholds for stimulus components are affected by the stimuli being speech. Specifically, he tests the hypothesis that two well-known psychoacoustic thresholds are unchanged, regardless of whether they are measured in white noise bursts, or in plosive or fricative noise bursts as they occur in natural speech. The thresholds measured are level increment detection and gap detection. The results show that thresholds are slightly higher in isolated speech noise bursts than they are in white noise bursts, and that they are slightly higher still when the speech bursts are presented in their original syllable context, but the differences are so small that one may draw the conclusion that speech stimuli do not affect general psychoacoustic abilities.

Chapter 4. Loss of Spectral and Temporal Resolution

In a keynote paper, **Shannon, Zeng, and Wygonski** wonder how much speech recognition is still possible when only temporal cues are available. Patients with little or no hearing left do not have any spectral resolution, but experiments have shown that they often have relatively normal temporal resolution, so that in principle they should be able to follow the amplitude modulations that occur in speech, and which provide at least some cues to the identitity of the speech sounds. By the same token, such patients may also benefit from some low-frequency rate-pitch information useful for the voiced-voiceless distinction. Apparently, the mechanism for modulation and rate-pitch detection is situated at a higher level than the auditory periphery: temporal resolution is relatively normal in patients who do not have an auditory nerve, provided the right signals are made available to the cochlear nucleus. This can be done electrically, by means of auditory brainstem implants or, if the auditory nerve is intact, cochlear implants. These same implants are also used to convey temporal information from speech signals. Results from amplitude information fed to a brainstem-implant patient show that very high consonant recognition may be achieved on the basis of this very limited type of information. Performance was comparable to that of patients with multi-electrode cochlear implants, who also received some spectral (frequency-place) information. It is much better than performance obtained with single-channel implants conveying primarily fundamental frequency information. The authors conclude that speech perception is a very special skill that is able to operate on very crude information and does not need all the sophisticated analysing power that is present in the hearing system.

Van Son, Bosman, Lamoré, and Smoorenburg, in a complementary fashion, are interested in how much information can still be conveyed to profoundly impaired or deaf people by making use of what frequency resolution remains. They presented profoundly hearing-impaired subjects with tone patterns consisting of selected harmonics of a 125 Hz fundamental. Subjects had to rate these patterns for similarity. The results, presented as INDSCAL plots, are not very clear, but indicate that subjects base their ratings mainly on a weighting of high versus low frequencies (above or below 800-1000 Hz). However, the authors indicate that the most important cue used by their subjects may have been beats between successive harmonics; this seems to lend support to the conclusions drawn by Shannon et al. above.

Ter Keurs, Festen, and Plomp address a similar question by asking how important frequency resolution is for speech perception. They do this by simulating varying degrees of loss in the form of progressively wider auditory filters (1/8, 1/2, and 2 octaves). It seems that vowel identification suffers more than consonant identification from reduced spectral resolution; this again confirms the findings of Shannon et al.

Chapter 5. Phoneme Perception

Uchanski, Millier, Reed, and Braida, in their keynote paper, investigate the effects of the number of different vowel tokens in an experiment (1, 4, or 16 per phoneme) on vowel identification. One speaker produced 16 repetitions of 10 different vowels in 6 different CVC contexts; the 16 repetitions, or a subset of them, were used as stimuli. It turned out that very little psychoacoustic learning takes place when each phoneme category is represented by multiple tokens: performance improved with practice only in the 1-token condition, but hardly or not at all in the 4- and 16-token conditions.

The decision process in an identification task is modelled as a comparison of cue vectors (as many as there are relevant cues in the signal, but in practice two or three) with prototypes of all possible categories. The resulting d'-values, which reflect listeners' sensitivity to differences between vowel types, were subjected to a separate multi-dimensional scaling analysis for each condition (1, 4, or 16 tokens). The configurations of the ten vowel points (see Fig. 4) are very similar in the three conditions, but two of the three listeners show considerably reduced sensitivity when more than one token per vowel is used.

The results suggest that, if we want to investigate phoneme perception in such a way that training or lengthy experimentation does not reduce the task to a purely psychoacoustic one, in which the normal way of processing speech sounds is no longer used, it is probably sufficient to present four tokens of each of the phoneme categories employed in the experiment.

Li and Pastore are also concerned with prototypes, this time of voiced stop consonants, synthesised by varying F2- and F3-onsets. In two preliminary experiments they first narrowed down the stimulus set to the 13 "best" members of the /b/- and /d/-categories (fastest reaction times and highest unanimity in a classification task). In the main experiment, subjects had to rate the similarity of each of these 13 remaining stimuli to each other and to itself by assigning it a value on a 5-point scale. The results were submitted to a multi-dimensional scaling analysis, which produced a two-dimensional solution which was able to account for 96% of total variance. The onsets loaded highly onto the two dimensions: F2-onsets onto the dimension defining category membership, and F3-onsets onto the dimension defining categorical "goodness". Although to some readers this might suggest that subjects had been able to attend to the two cues in these synthetic stimuli independently in order to estimate the similarity between the two stimuli in a trial, the authors prefer an interpretation in terms of prototypes or exemplars. They find support for this interpretation in the fact that both a prototype- and an exemplar-based model result in predictions of stimulus classification that are 97% accurate.

Schouten and Van Hessen's paper constitutes a warning against the use of 2IFC for evaluating categorical perception. (In a 2IFC experiment subjects have to decide which of the two stimulus intervals contains the signal, or the louder stimulus, or, as in the present case, the more /t/-like stimulus.) The authors found that this type of task compels listeners to refer each stimulus to their internal phoneme prototypes, so that "categorical perception" becomes almost inevitable, at least for stop consonants. As a result, 2IFC discrimination of stop consonants produces d'-values that are almost identical to those obtained in phoneme identification, whereas AX (same-different) discrimination is considerably higher. This is an anomalous finding, which leads the authors to propose a different decision model for 2IFC-discrimination of stop consonants, which explicitly incorporates comparison of stimuli with phoneme prototypes. An important difference with the Li and Pastore data discussed above is that Schouten and Van Hessen used natural stimuli, which did not contain any explicit cues that subjects could concentrate on. What this may mean is that the warning against 2IFC does not apply to synthetic stimuli such as those used by Li and Pastore, where subjects can actually avoid prototype comparison by paying attention to the separate formant onsets.

Sawusch uses the word-recognition tasks of naming (repeating what has been heard) and lexical decision (deciding whether a word or a non-word has been presented) in order to determine the nature of the prototypes, which in the papers above have generally been assumed to be phonemes, but which could just as well be allophones, syllables, or even words. He collected naming and lexical decision data for CVC words as a function of priming: the target stimulus was preceded by a "prime", which overlapped to varying degrees with the target. The pattern of reaction times was closest to that predicted by the hypothesis that the prototypes used for recognising stop consonants in CVC syllables are different for initial and final stops - they represent position-specific phonemes.

CHAPTER 6. WORD PERCEPTION AND BEYOND

Frauenfelder's keynote paper describes an experiment that appears to confirm Sawusch's conclusion: in a syllable detection task, when there is a mismatch between the target syllable and the syllabic structure of the carrier presented to the listener (for example, subjects have to detect the French syllable "pal" in the carrier "palace"), this leads to longer reaction times than when there is no mismatch, but only if the "ambisyllabic" consonant (/l/ in the example) is a liquid. Liquids are the consonants that have the most clearly different initial and final allophones; the results therefore indicate that the basic speech prototypes may be position-specific allophones.

Frauenfelder's paper contains much more, however: it is a very clear overview of the various theories concerning the interface between phonetic analysis of the speech signal and access to the lexicon, i.e. of the question of what kind of alphabet is used for the organisation of the mental lexicon: an acoustic, phonetic, or phonological one (or perhaps a combination of these).

Nusbaum and Henley, in the second keynote paper of this chapter, present an overview of the various accounts of the "window of analysis" used in speech perception. Many researchers have wondered whether there is a fixed time interval over which a listener integrates information; if the duration of such an interval corresponded to the duration of a phoneme, or a syllable, or even a word, then we would know which of these should be regarded as the unit of perception. Nusbaum and Henley show convincingly that there is no fixed window: decisions about speech sounds are based on information from other speech sounds, other syllables, and even other words.

Quené addresses a problem that has often been ignored in the word-perception literature. The assumption usually seems to be that the beginnings and endings of words are detected as a matter of course. In running speech this is rarely the case, however; it is Quené's aim to discover the segmentation cues that are contained in the signal, and to investigate their perceptual relevance. In his paper he looks at two temporal word boundary cues, namely word-initial consonant lengthening and the lengthening of the onsets of word-initial vowels. He does this by creating ambiguous natural stimuli which may be segmented in two ways, and by manipulating the two temporal cues. The results indicate that the manipulations have some effect on the perceived word boundary, but that these effects are small compared to the effect of what the speaker intended. The speaker must therefore have used other, more powerful, cues; presumably, these cues are spectral rather than temporal.

Bosman, Smoorenburg, and Bronkhorst present a simple model for calculating the number of independent elements on a particular level of representation, by comparing e.g. phoneme scores, syllable scores, and sentence scores on the same material. If the three phonemes in a CVC syllable occur independently from each other, the syllable score is simply the product of the three phoneme scores (expressed as proportions or probabilities). The exponent in the power-law relationship between them is 3; if it is less than 3, this means that the phonemes are not completely independent from each other. The data bear this out: nonsense syllables lead to an exponent of 3, whereas it is 2.6 for meaningful syllables. The authors' hypothesis that for hearing-impaired listeners the exponent should be even smaller, since these listeners have to rely much more on context, is not confirmed for the syllable scores compared to the phoneme scores, but receives some support from a comparison of syllable and sentence scores.

The message in **Terhardt's** keynote paper is, at least in part, that it is not useful to split perception (or, as he calls it, "information processing") into peripheral and central segments: it is a continuous hierarchy of knowledge-driven and irreversible decisions, all the way from the cochlea to the interpretation of the speaker's message. The outputs of all these decision processes can be observed, but not influenced, by the "self". Although Terhardt's illustrations of this idea are mainly confined to his views on pitch perception at various levels, his intentions in this paper are more wide-ranging: he steps back from pitch perception in order to obtain a wider perspective on the perceptual process as a whole. As a result, he says a lot of things that were regarded as controversial at the conference, at least to those who disagree with his views on spectral pitches, especially of components that are regarded as unresolvable, but I feel strongly that it was good to have at least one contribution that did not have the rather narrow focus of straightforward experimental data.

References

Fowler, C. (1990). Sound-producing sources as objects of perception: rate-normalization and nonspeech perception, *J. Acoust. Soc. Am. 88*, 1236-1249.

Green, D.M. (1988). *Profile analysis*, Oxford University Press.

Levelt, W.J.M. (1989). *Speaking. From intention to articulation*, MIT Press.

Repp, B.H. (1987). The role of psychophysics in understanding speech perception, in: *Schouten (1987)*.

Schouten, M.E.H. (1987) (editor). *The psychophysics of speech perception*, Martinus Nijhoff Publishers.

Chapter 1
The Auditory System in Relation to Speech Perception

Cochlear Modelling and Physiology

H. Duifhuis
Biophysics Department and Centre for Behavioural,
Cognitive and Neuro-sciences (BCN-Groningen)
Rijksuniversiteit Groningen
the Netherlands

1. Introduction

The auditory sensor is a crucial element in the auditory information flow. More precisely, the cochlea embodies a complex sensory system, where considerable preprocessing takes place before the actual sensory cells transduce acoustic vibrations into electrical responses. This presentation of auditory modelling and of the underlying physiological expertise emphasizes the cochlear steps in auditory processing.

Essential preprocessing takes place at three different levels[1]: outer ear, middle ear, and inner ear (cochlea). Outer ear transmission and middle ear transmission are often considered to be relatively simple, viz. linear, with bandpass characteristics. In reality they are more complex. On the one hand, the precise properties of actual shapes are still under study and provide new results. On the other hand it has become obvious — and could have been much earlier — that the nonlinear inner ear 'feeds back' into the periphery and invalidates, at least partly, a linear analysis.

In this paper I will concentrate on the peripheral cochlear processes, and pay little attention to outer and middle ear. I want to emphasize, however, that the connection plays a crucial role in the 'coupling' mentioned above.

2. Historical Development of Cochlear Macromechanics

Studies of cochlear macromechanics evolved during the first half of this century, after Békésy had provided the first experimental data about cochlear mechanics (compiled in Békésy, 1960). Recall that the optical technique he used provided a resolution of the order of 0.5 μm, and that stimulus levels of 120 — 160 dB SPL were required for his observations of cochlear partition motion[2].

Békésy's work was the basis for theoretical studies. Around 1950 two 1-dimensional theories describing cochlear transmission and analysis were published: the so-called short-wave model by Ranke, and the long-wave model by Zwislocki. The latter became the more popular for a considerable period, until it became clear that in fact the characteristic changes from long-wave at the cochlea entrance to short-wave near the point of resonance (e.g. Siebert, 1974; and several other more recent papers).

Around the same time it became feasible to analyse 2-dimensional cochlea models (Lesser and Berkeley, 1972), and a little later 3-dimensional cochlea models were attacked (Steele and Taber, 1979; Lighthill, 1981; de Boer, 1984). The initial studies all used linear analysis, and investigated cochlear transmission with increasing mathematical rigour, or increasing hardware complexity in electrical or physical models. The mathematical analysis of the more-dimensional models still has to rely on numerical evaluation.

Most studies attempt to estimate basilar membrane deflection or velocity in response to an acoustic stimulus, arguing that the sensory receptor cell is driven by a quantity that is simply proportional to membrane deflection (ter Kuile, 1900). Some other studies also consider the trans-membrane pressure explicitly, and in the linear case there is a straightforward impedance relation between these quantities. A more general biophysical approach was introduced by Lighthill (1981) when he analysed the energy flow in the cochlea (see also Neely, 1981). I consider this a fruitful approach because it concentrates on general biophysical concepts which apply to linear as well as nonlinear cochleae (Duifhuis, 1988). In short, this approach shows that a narrow-band acoustic energy influx into the cochlea focuses on the cochlear partition 'just' before the point of resonance (i.e., the point of which the local resonance frequency equals the stimulus frequency). Biophysically this is a logical principle: the energy flow focuses on those sensory cells which respond most strongly. There it is expended in the local damping. In concurrent hair cell research and modelling this point is sometimes underrated by proposing that the basic mechano-sensory property of the hair cell is its stiffness. Stiffness is involved in energy flow and temporary energy storage; damping, on the other hand, determines net energy absorption. In the following section the basic properties of linear analysis of cochlear mechanisms are presented. The fact that the intact auditory system, however, is nonlinear is based on experience that has been accumulated over several centuries. The earliest reports on aural combination tones are from around 1750 by Sorge (Germany), Romieu (France), and Tartini (Italy) [see, e.g., the description by Helmholtz, 1885, p. 152]. Two-tone suppression effects, shown physiologically (e.g., Sachs and Kiang, 1968) as well as psychophysically (e.g., Houtgast, 1972) also turned out to be the result of cochlear nonlinearity. Even though the database is enormous, not all theoreticians assume that cochlear nonlinearity is 'essential' (i.e. exists down to threshold levels; e.g. de Boer, 1989; Zweig, 1991). A major problem with the study of nonlinear properties of the ear is that the mathematical tools are less developed. This implies that numerical techniques have to be used which, despite the rapid increase of computation power over the last 10 years, remain cumbersome.

Description of the system is even more complex if the possibility of active behaviour is also taken into account. Active behaviour implies production of acoustic energy by the ear rather than absorption. Production is particularly apparent in spontaneous oto-acoustic emissions, first observed in 1978 (Kemp), and now a well established phenomenon.

These two points are taken into account in the section on nonlinear and active cochlear mechanics. The developments of theoretical analysis and experimental data have evolved in parallel over the last decade, which in some cases led to reconsideration of established interpretation. Current experimental research at the sensor level presents a large amount of new data, insights, and speculation about the cochlear mechanism, in particular about outer hair cells. I will give a personal estimate of the relevance of some of the most recent findings, but also stress that several crucial questions are still unanswered. In other words, the biophysical understanding of important hearing properties such as level, frequency, and time sensitivity, even at the level before neural information processing, has still a considerable way to go. These points are presented in the section on cochlear physiology, which, for 'historical' reasons, is given toward the end of this paper.

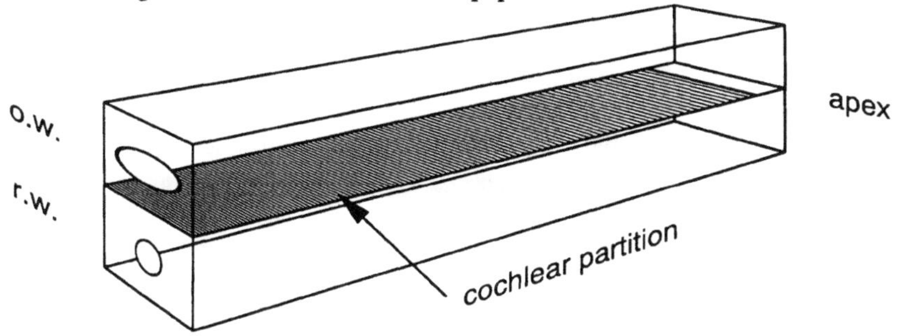

Fig. 1 Right angular box model of the cochlea (see text points 1 - 7); o.w.: oval window, r.w.: round window.

3. Linear Passive Cochlear Macromechanics

This section presents a summary of the basics of contemporary work on linear passive cochlear mechanics. A more detailed treatment is given in Duifhuis, 1988. Recently some intriguing new points have been put forward by Shera and Zweig (1991), and those are incorporated. Nonlinearity and active behaviour are addressed in the next subsequent section.

In general the following geometrical and mechanical simplifications are made in cochlea models (see Fig. 1):

1. The cochlea is an isolated cavity with rigid walls, and it communicates only through its oval and round windows.
2. The cochlear fluid is inviscid and linear; there is no fluid-mechanical difference between perilymph and endolymph.
3. The spiral coiling is ignored.
4. The scala media and scala vestibuli are considered as one duct, i.e., the presence of Reissner's membrane is considered mechanically irrelevant.
5. All mechanical properties of the sensory structure in the organ of Corti are modelled by a net cochlear partition impedance function (second order).
6. Up to recently (Shera and Zweig, 1991) the cross-sectional areas of the ducts were assumed to be constant over the length of the cochlea (which is certainly not true for all mammals). The cross-sections are usually approximated by rectangles.
7. The impedance of the round window is neglected.

The last two points will be addressed in more detail at the end of this section, for the other points I refer to previous publications (e.g., Viergever, 1980).

The combined presence of oval and round window allows cochlear fluid displacement in response to an acoustic stimulus. This fluid displacement is to be distinguished from acoustic responses in the cochlear fluid. I mention this point again because several textbooks miss it.

Sound waves propagate in cochlear fluid, as in water, at a velocity of approx. 1.5 km/s. This implies that sound waves in the mid-frequency range have a wavelength which is much larger than the largest dimension of the cochlea, its length of about 35 mm. Therefore one often assumes that the cochlear fluid behaves as if it is incompressible. At the highest audio-frequencies this is no longer true. This point is relevant for echolocating mammals. A simple mechanical representation of a 1-dimensional cochlea model is presented in Fig. 2.

To us the fluid displacement is the most relevant. The displacement, which propagates practically instantaneously, excites the cochlear partition. The resulting excitation pattern is — somewhat misleadingly — called the cochlear travelling wave. This excitation of the cochlear partition is determined by local mechanical properties, described by mass, damping, and stiffness. Using these properties in units per surface area, one assumes mass to be constant. The frequency map is then determined primarily by a stiffness parameter which has to change about 4 orders of magnitude over the length of the cochlea. Damping is adjusted to match the frequency sensitivity. The fluid mass in the ducts combined with the partition stiffness provides the energy transmission line. Transmission decreases as energy is absorbed by the damping term, and all energy appears to be expended just before the point of resonance.

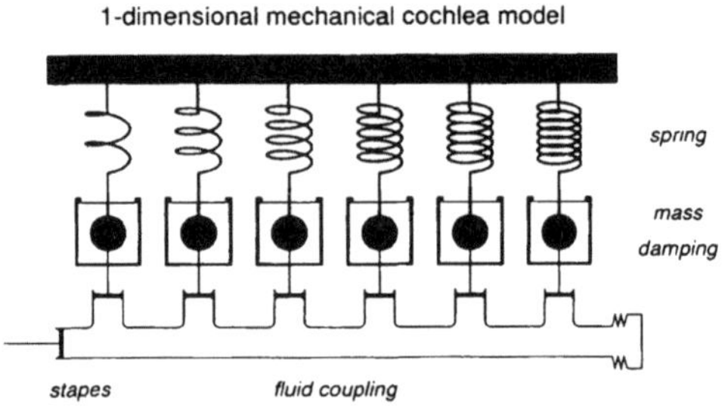

Fig. 2 A mechanical cochlea model. The cochlear fluid is driven by a piston at the stapes. This drives [masses also coupled to the fluid by a piston] all mass - spring - damping elements, representing elements of the cochlear partition, simultaneously. Mass is constant, stiffness of the spring decreases - as does the fluid resistance - with increasing distance from the stapes. Thus, resonance frequency decreases. Due to these varying response properties, resulting vibrations of the masses suggest a travelling wave entering the cochlea. [In this mechanical model the drum at the right end represents the round window. Note that in this picture the fluid balance is incomplete because of omission of the scala tympani.]

The traditional assumption about the physiological basis for the varying stiffness parameter relates it to local basilar membrane properties. Ideas about damping were less clear. I have proposed previously that the acoustic energy influx is dissipated in the subtectorial space, and that in a cochlea with intact hair cells the dissipation is partly compensated for by mechanical energy produced by the hair cells (Duifhuis, 1988). More specifically we propose now that the auditory sensor optimally transmits the acoustic energy to its sensory cells, the hair cells, losing as little as possible in viscosity or other mechanical resistance in the subtectorial space.

Recently Shera and Zweig (1991) have pointed out that the rectangular duct model with exponentially varying stiffness has to lead to what they call the *cochlear catastrophe*. The gradient in the cochlear partition impedance causes a gradient in the transmission line property as long as longitudinal fluid coupling is independent of place. Near the stapes this leads to a discontinuity which causes reflections of retrograde waves, and in general it predicts a low-frequency input impedance which rolls off in amplitude (between 3 and 6 dB/oct) and correspondingly in phase. This is in disagreement with experimental data. Shera and Zweig point out that toward the basal end the cochlear ducts taper considerably. In a first estimate, this tapering, which determines the longitudinal fluid mass coupling, may well match the partition stiffness gradient, so that the gradient in transmission line impedance vanishes. In that case first the reflection of retrograde waves disappears, and so far these have only been computed but not observed, and secondly, the sensitivity for low-frequency signals increases. Study of cochlea shape suggests that this tapering might hold for roughly the first 15% of the distance along the organ of Corti. The authors conclude that following this interpretation the efficiency of the middle ear at transferring acoustic power into the cochlea remains roughly constant below 700 Hz.

If one computes the acoustic power flow that enters the cochlea, then one finds that the input through the stapes immediately splits up into two parallel apical flows into the two cochlear ducts. This is due to the assumption that no energy is lost at the round window. This does not necessarily imply that for all practical purposes the impedance of the round window should be put to zero. It only implies that the real part of the impedance should be negligible, but it implies nothing for the imaginary part. It is rather plausible that a finite stiffness component is involved. At the moment we still have to evaluate the quantitative implications of this possibility.

4. Nonlinear and Active Cochlear Mechanics

This section presents theoretical considerations based largely on interpretation of data that have been available for a decade or more. Interpretation in terms of underlying macroscopic properties, to which this section is limited, is fairly robust over time. New data, to be presented in the next section, indicate the demand for adjustments of the microscopical interpretation.

A general remark concerning the study of nonlinear systems is in order. Such a study cannot build on a well-developed set of systems analysis tools. It is no longer valid to build up a complex block using one-way-coupled elements. If there is a single nonlinear element at some point its presence may be detectable everywhere. All coupling is now two-way-interaction. Frequency domain analysis loses much of its power, and time domain analysis is required. This demands considerable computation power.

Over the last decade it has become clear that active and nonlinear behaviour of the cochlea has a possible similarity to that of a classical Van der Pol-oscillator. This was first proposed by Johannesma (1980). It was worked out in more detail in several groups (e.g., van Netten and Duifhuis, 1983, Duifhuis et al., 1985, Jones et al., 1986, Diependaal et al., 1987, van Dijk and Wit, 1988). We have been working on a cochlea model with many active components. Initially this was set up with spatial parameters that varied smoothly. Our major emphasis, however, shifted toward potentially more realistic biophysical models. First, for the nonlinear damping term we no longer use the classical parabolic shape, but a function that can be thought of in two parts. A passive part with exponential 'tails', which provides response behaviour with a log-like characteristic. Then there is an additional active part that can produce net active behaviour if it is strong enough.

Active, oscillatory behaviour of adjacent points over a wide range in a cochlea is only meaningful on a discrete grid, because the points can have opposite amplitudes, which is impossible for arbitrarily close points[3]. The physiological structure of the organ of Corti yields a grid size of about 10 µm. The computational grid that we use is still one order of magnitude coarser. This provides one reason why we cannot yet take all fine structural properties into account. The other is that up to now data sufficiently accurate to do so, were lacking. The computational task provided by the coarser grid is manageable. Our primary aim is to investigate the effect of the shape of the damping term in the Van der Pol-oscillator. For the time being we have restricted ourselves to a further analysis of the 1-dimensional cochlea model.

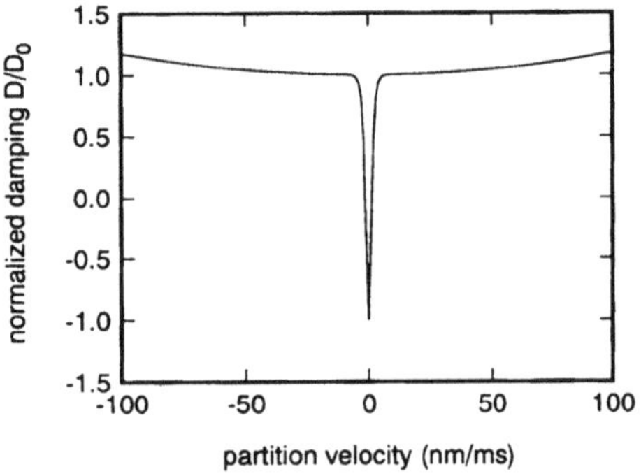

Fig. 3 The physical equation is transformed to a dimensionless version:

$$(y_{tt} + Dy_t + S_y)_{xx} - a^2 y_{tt} = 0$$

This uses the scales x_0 = 35 mm, y_0 = 1 nm, and t_0 = 1 ms. The remaining constants are $s_0 x = 10^{10}$ Pa/m, λ = 300 m^{-1}, a = 70, so that $S = 2.10^4 exp(-10.5x)$. The amplitude independent factor $D_0(x) = 5\sqrt{2}\ exp(-5.25x)$ scales the dependent part of D to the order 1.
The complete form that we use for D, which is given in this Figure, is:

$$D(x,t) = D_0(x)\left(\frac{\chi \sinh(\alpha y_t)}{\alpha y_t} - \frac{2\gamma}{\cosh(\beta y_t)}\right)$$

where the positive part provides the log-like behaviour and the negative part accounts for the active properties.

A mathematical formulation of a coupled Van der Pol-oscillator cochlea model is:

$$(my_{tt} + dy_t + sy)_{xx} - \frac{2\rho}{h} y_{tt} = 0 \qquad (1)$$

where m=0.5 kg/m², d, and s = s_0 exp(-λx) represent cochlear partition mass, damping and stiffness per unit area. ρ is the fluid density, h the scala height, and y the partition amplitude. The cochlea is modelled with 400 elements that follow from Eq. 1. One element is added to act as a simple middle ear, thus giving a physical coupling with the atmosphere. The helicotrema point lacks one neighbour, but sees a fluid environment. The nonlinearity is put into the damping d, as indicated in Fig. 2.

Van den Raadt and Duifhuis (1990) have presented results of the analysis of parameter sensitivity of this form. The results can be summarized as follows: The increment of both width and depth of the active term increases the limit cycle amplitude. Increasing the depth, however, yields fairly soon a limit cycle behaviour similar to that of the parabolic oscillator with an increasing value of the classical ε. This means that the nonlinear behaviour becomes obvious. Increment of width, on the other hand, yields a smoother oscillation with an increasing onset part, similar to the response of a filter with increasing selectivity (decreasing bandwidth).

It has been apparent for some time that the behaviour of coupled oscillators is unpredictable in detail. Recently Van den Raadt has shown (unpublished) that this is a form of mathematical chaos. (Coupling of a few oscillators already can, but does not have to lead to chaotic behaviour.) In practice such a chaotic behaviour is barely, if at all, distinguishable from stochastic behaviour. Thus, formally this could provide the lower sensitivity limit, just like Brownian motion.

5. Cochlear physiology

Skipping a proper account of the development of basilar membrane response measurements in general over the past 25 years, in this context it is justified to mention the work by Rhode (1971), who was the first to point out the distinct nonlinear response near resonance. During the past decade the measuring techniques have improved considerably. This has led to the suggestion that basilar membrane tuning and auditory nerve fiber tuning are in principle identical (e.g., Khanna and Leonard, 1982; Sellick et al., 1983; Robles et al., 1986). Basilar membrane tuning, as well as neural tuning, depend on level, i.e., are nonlinear. The tip of the neural tuning curve is strongly dependent on IHC and OHC[4] - integrity (e.g., Kiang et al., 1986). Similarity of basilar membrane tuning and auditory nerve fiber tuning then suggests that the sharp tuning is determined by properties of the (intact) hair cells, and, in terms of a second order mechanical system, that the macromechanical stiffness and damping are predominated by hair cell (body and hair bundle) stiffness and damping. In fact this conclusion is at variance with the idea that the basilar membrane properties completely determine tuning. The intermediate sensory structure, the hair cells, play a prevalent part in two directions: affecting input as well as output. This suggestion is in agreement with more recent results from Khanna et al. (1989), who reported that in the apical region of the guinea-pig cochlea the motion near the stereocilia may be 40 dB greater than that of the local basilar membrane (see also Wilson, 1991).

This tentative conclusion confirms the point that the second order mechanical system is an oversimplification. For a better understanding a thorough analysis of the micromechanics within the organ of Corti has to be incorporated, and several groups are now working in this direction. The problem thus far has been that the database for such an approach was too small, leaving too many free theoretical parameters, but this database is now increasing rapidly, as will be indicated in the following paragraphs.

Evidence that the hair bundle morphology is correlated with tuning frequency has been available for some time for several species. Lim (1980) presented data for the chinchilla, where ciliary height increases smoothly from about 1 µm at the base to about 5 µm at the apex (Fig. 4). Similar results have been reported for the bird (e.g., Tilney and Saunders, 1983; Gleich and Manley, 1988), the alligator lizard (Holton and Hudspeth, 1983) and the bobtail lizard (Köppl, 1988). Hair bundle morphology, of which cilia length is one relevant parameter, is thought to influence bundle stiffness (Strelioff and Flock, 1984), and hence, in combination with the proper mass term, the resonance frequency of the hair cell (see also Freeman and Weiss, e.g., 1990).

In order to obtain such information directly, measurements of hair bundle responses have been set up on single isolated hair cells, or on hair cells in experimentally accessible structures. A relevant point is that bundle deflection at threshold is of the order of 1 nm at most, and probably almost one order of magnitude less. This implies that over a large dynamic range bundle deflection is extremely small compared to bundle size: e.g., height of

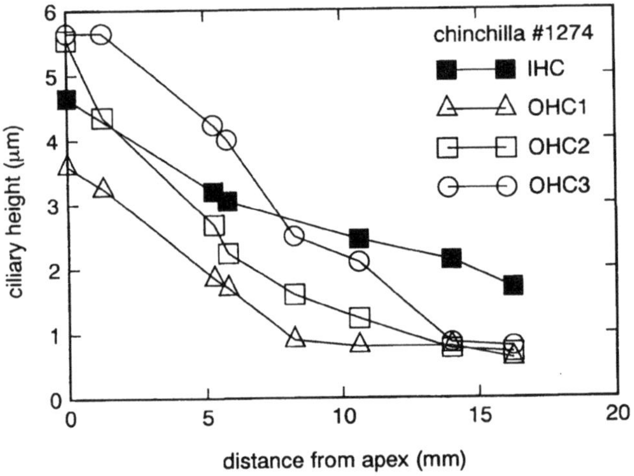

Fig. 4 Length of the tallest cilia in IHC and OHC bundles at different positions in the cochlea in the chinchilla (after Lim, 1980).

the order of several µm. One experimental approach has been to measure bundle deflection in response to a driving force. The stationary relation between the two is determined by bundle stiffness. Estimates of bundle stiffness are of the order of a few mN/m. Stiffness data also demonstrate clear nonlinear effects (Howard and Hudspeth, 1988).

As pointed out in the 'historical development'-section, stiffness alone does not give information about the sensitivity of the sensor in terms of energy transduction. Energy transduction is determined by the damping property of the cell. So far very few studies address this point (Howard and Hudspeth, 1987; Van Netten and Kroese, 1989; Russell, Richardson and Kössl, 1989). One reason is that it is technically more difficult to measure damping than to measure stiffness. Estimates of bundle damping are of the order of a few µNs/m per hair cell. A close look at the nonlinear effects reported by Howard and Hudspeth (1988) to me appears to imply that, in addition to stiffness nonlinearity mentioned above, damping nonlinearity is involved. This means that the Van der Pol-oscillator description (only nonlinear damping), despite the fact that it describes some interesting aspects of the data (e.g., Long et al., 1991), cannot tell the full story. One well-established phenomenon, viz. the difference between nonlinear behaviour above and below local resonance frequency, I am convinced, cannot be accounted for by a damping nonlinearity.

Another finding is that the shape of outer hair cells depends on stimulus level and environmental conditions[5]. In electrophysiological experiments it has been possible to demonstrate a mechanical response of the hair cell to electrical, biochemical, or acoustical stimulation: the cell body length can change. Data on the motility of isolated hair cells under such stimulation are currently classified as fast motility (e.g., Brownell, 1985; Ashmore, 1987) where hair cell length follows electrical stimulation up to several 10s of kHz, or as slow motility, measured under modified biochemical environment (e.g., Flock et al., 1986; Zenner, 1986) and under acoustical stimulation (Canlon et al., 1988).

Recently a direct correlation has been reported between OHC body length and tuning frequency, within as well as across mammals (Pujol et al., 1991; see Fig. 5). As the length increases linearly from 10 µm to 75 µm the tuning frequency decreases logarithmically from 160 kHz to 20 Hz, i.e., 1 octave per 5µm. OHC diameter remains roughly constant (6 to 7µm), except near the extreme apex, where in most of the species the diameter increases to 10µm.

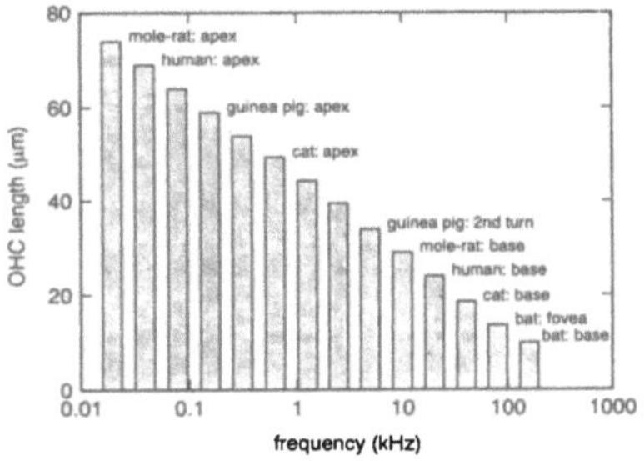

Fig. 5 Relation between OHC body length and tuning frequency for mammals (after Pujol et al., 1991).

These new results lead to speculations about the role of outer hair cells: e.g., electromechanical oscillatory behaviour to improve sensitivity or to improve frequency selectivity. This could be the source of the active behaviour. Also, intact outer hair cells demonstrate nonlinearity which is helpful in stabilizing active elements (limit cycle 'stability' of an oscillator), and which has to be present anyway to account for the generation of aural distortion products (in particular combination tones).

The next step is to analyse the biochemistry of the hair cell in more detail. So far little is known about the receptor channels. The current idea is that these are directly mechanically engaged by cilia tip links, (e.g., Pickles et al., 1984) and are not very cation specific (e.g., Hudspeth, 1986).

In all, we appear to approach the situation where modelling the organ of Corti no longer has to be hampered by too many free (unknown) parameters, but where micromechanical study can build on really testable assumptions.

6. SUMMARY

Cochlear modelling and physiology are approaching a state where most of the macromechanical issues appear to become solvable. For instance, the role of the outer hair cells, which has been mysterious for decades, is beginning to be understood. It now leads to testable speculations. The function of the basilar membrane is under reconsideration. In the intact cochlea the hair cells appear to play the predominant macromechanical role. This applies probably to linear as well as nonlinear properties.

Let me end with a note on the relevance of all this for speech sounds. Probably our auditory system is optimized to a great extent for speech processing. That implies dealing with short sounds at levels of the order of 60 dB SPL. Neither absolute threshold experiments, nor experiments with stationary stimuli provide the most relevant information. The extrapolation of such data to the relevant range is still hampered by nonlinear difficulties. The major goal of the nonlinearity is to allow coverage of a large dynamic range, and to do this fast. The actual auditory nonlinearity does this in a way that leaves spectral as well as temporal information of relatively broadband signals largely intact. In other words, technically speaking, the nonlinearity apparently provides an very fast automatic gain control. Active behaviour in the cochlea improves sensitivity at very low levels. At the moment it is not clear whether its role at normal speech levels — if speech in an auditorium is more normal than in a very quiet room — is significant.

Acknowledgements

The author gratefully acknowledges the contributions of several colleagues in the BCN - Groningen. In particular the critical discussions with and the many suggestions made by S. M. van Netten were very valuable.

Notes

1. It will be pointed out later that this separation stems from linear considerations, and has to be used with caution.

2. Linear extrapolation of his observation yields 0.5 nm at 60 dB and 0.5 pm at 0 dB.

3. If activity occurs over a narrow range, then the strongest oscillator will entrain (synchronize) its neighbours. The relevant range width is, a.o., determined by the strength of the 'leader'.

4. IHC: inner hair cell, OHC: outer hair cell

5. In fact this has only been proved for isolated hair cells.

References

Ashmore, J. F. (1987). A fast motile response in guinea-pig outer hair cells: the cellular basis of the cochlear amplifier. *J. Physiol.* 388, 323-347.

von Békésy, G. (1960). *Experiments in Hearing*. McGraw-Hill, New York.

de Boer, E. (1984). Auditory physics. *Physical principles in hearing theory* II, *Physics Reports* 105, 141-226.

de Boer, E. (1989). On the nature of cochlear resonance, in: *Cochlear Mechanisms*, edited by J. P. Wilson and D. T. Kemp (Plenum, New York), pp. 465-474.

Brownell, W. E., Bader, C. R., Bertrand, D., and de Ribaupierre, Y. (1985). Evoked mechanical responses of isolated cochlear outer hair cells. *Science* 227, 194-196.

Canlon, B., Brundin, L., and Flock, Å. (1988). Acoustic stimulation causes tonotopic alterations in the length of isolated outer hair cells from the guinea pig hearing organ. *Proc. Natl. Acad. Sci.* USA 85, 7033-7035.

Diependaal, R. J., Duifhuis, H., Hoogstraten, H. W., and Viergever, M. A. (1987). Numerical methods for solving one-dimensional cochlear models in the time domain. *J. Acoust. Soc. Am.* 82, 1655-1666.

van Dijk, P., and Wit, H. P. (1988). Phase-lock of spontaneous oto-acoustic emissions to a cubic difference tone, in: *Basic Issues in Hearing*, edited by H. Duifhuis, J. W. Horst, and H. P. Wit (Academic, London), pp. 101-105.

Duifhuis, H. (1988). Cochlear macromechanics, in: *Auditory Function. Neurobiological basis of hearing*, edited by G. M. Edelman, W. E. Gall, and W. M. Cowan, chapter 6, pp. 189-211 (A Neurosciences Institute Publication, Wiley, New York).

Duifhuis, H., Hoogstraten, H. W., van Netten, S. M., Diependaal, R. J., and Bialek, W. (1985). Modelling the cochlear partition with coupled Van der Pol oscillators, in: *Peripheral Auditory Mechanisms*, edited by J. B. Allen, J. L. Hall, A. E. Hubbard, S. T. Neely, and A. Tubis (Springer, New York), pp. 290-297.

Flock, Å., Flock, B., and Ulfendahl, M. (1986). Mechanisms of movement in outer hair cells and a possible structural basis. *Arch. Otorhinolaryngol.* 243, 83-90.

Freeman, D. M., and Weiss, T. F. (1990). Superposition of hydrodynamic forces on a hair bundle. *Hear. Res.* 48, 1-16.

Gleich, O., and Manley, G. A. (1988). Quantitative morphological analysis of the sensory epithelium of the starling and pigeon basilar papilla. *Hear. Res.* 34, 69-85.

Helmholtz, H. L. F. (1885). *On the Sensation of Tone.* 2nd edition, (Longman & Co., reproduced by Dover, New York, 1954).

Holton, T., and Hudspeth, A. J. (1983). A micromechanical contribution to cochlear tuning and tonotopic organization. *Science* 222, 508-510.

Houtgast, T. (1972). Psychophysical evidence for lateral inhibition in hearing. *J. Acoust. Soc. Am.* 51, 1885-1894.

Howard, J., and Hudspeth, A. J. (1987). Mechanical relaxation of the hair bundle mediates adaptation in mechanoelectrical transduction by the bullfrog's saccular hair cell. *Proc. Natl. Acad. Sci. USA* 84, 3063-3068.

Howard, J., and Hudspeth, A. J. (1988). Compliance of the hair bundle associated with gating of mechanoelectrical transduction channels in the bullfrog's saccular hair cells. *Neuron* 1, 189-199.

Hudspeth, A. J. (1986). The ionic channels of a vertebrate hair cell. *Hear. Res.* 22, 21-27.

Johannesma, P. I. M. (1980). Narrow band filters and active resonators. Comments on papers by D. T. Kemp & R. A. Chum, and H. P. Wit & R. J. Ritsma, in: *Psychophysical, physiological, and behavioural studies in hearing*, edited by G. van den Brink and F. A. Bilsen (Delft University Press, Delft), pp. 62-63.

Jones, K., Tubis, A., Long, G. R., Burns, E. M., and Strickland, E. A. (1986). Interactions among multiple spontaneous otoacoustic emissions, in: *Peripheral Auditory Mechanisms*, edited by J. B. Allen, J. L. Hall, A. Hubbard, S. T. Neely, and A. Tubis (Springer-Verlag, Berlin), pp. 266-273.

Kemp, D. T. (1978). Stimulated acoustic emissions from within the human auditory system. *J. Acoust. Soc. Am.* 64, 1386-1391.

Khanna, S. M., Ulfendahl, M., and Flock, Å. (1989). Comparison of tuning of outer hair cells and the basilar membrane in the isolated cochlea. *Acta Otolaryngol. Suppl.* 467, 151-156.

Khanna, S. M., and Leonard, D. G. B. (1982). Basilar membrane tuning in the cat cochlea. *Science* 215, 305-306.

Kiang, N. Y. S., Liberman, M. C., and Sewell, W. F. (1986). Single unit clues to cochlear mechanisms. *Hear. Res.* 22, 171-182.

ter Kuile, E. (1900). *Die Uebertragung der Energie von der Grundmembran auf die Haarzellen*, Pflügers Archiv 79, 146-157.

Köppl, C. (1988). Morphology of the basilar papilla of the bobtail lizard *Tiliqua rugosa*. *Hear. Res.* 35, 209-228.

Lesser, M. B., and Berkeley, D. A. (1972). Fluid mechanics of the cochlea. Part 1. *J. Fluid Mech.* 51, 497-512.

Lighthill, J. (1981). Energy flow in the cochlea. *J. Fluid Mech.* 106, 149-213.

Lim, D. J. (1980). Cochlear anatomy related to cochlear micromechanics. A review. *J. Acoust. Soc. Am.* 67, 1686-1695.

Long, G. R., Tubis, A., and Jones, K. L. (1991). Modeling synchronization and suppression of spontaneous oto-acoustic emissions using Van der Pol oscillators: Effects of aspirin administration. *J. Acoust. Soc. Am.* 89, 1201-1212.

Neely, S. T. (1981). Fourth-Order Partition Dynamics for a Two-Dimensional Model of the Cochlea. *PhD thesis*, Washington University, St. Louis, Missouri.

van Netten, S. M., and Duifhuis, H. (1983). Modelling an active, nonlinear cochlea, in: *Mechanics of Hearing*, edited by E. de Boer and M. A. Viergever (Nijhoff/Delft Univ. Press, Netherlands), pp. 143-151.

van Netten, S. M., and Kroese, A. B. A. (1989). Hair cell mechanics controls the dynamic behaviour of the lateral line cupula, in: *Cochlear Mechanisms: Structure, Function and Models*, edited by J. P. Wilson and D. T. Kemp (Plenum, New York), pp. 47-55.

Pickles, J. O., Comis, S. D., and Osborne, M. P. (1984). Cross-links between stereocilia in the guinea pig organ of Corti, and their possible relation to sensory transduction. *Hear. Res.* 15, 103-112.

Pujol, R., Lenoir, M., Ladrech, S., Tribillac, F., and Rebillard, G. (1991). Correlation between the length of outer hair cells and the frequency coding of the cochlea, in: *Auditory Physiology and Perception*, edited by Y. Cazals, L. Demany, and K. Horner (Plenum, New York), in press.

van den Raadt, M. P. M. G., and Duifhuis, H. (1990). A generalized Van der Pol-oscillator cochlea model, in: *The Mechanics and Biophysics of Hearing*, edited by P. Dallos, C. D. Geisler, J. W. Matthews, M. Ruggero, and C. R. Steele (Springer, Berlin), pp. 227-234.

Ranke, O. F. (1950). Theory of operation of the cochlea: A contribution to the hydrodynamics of the cochlea. *J. Acoust. Soc. Am.* 22, 772-777.

Rhode, W. S. (1971). Observation of vibration of the basilar membrane in squirrel monkeys using the Mössbauer technique. *J. Acoust. Soc. Am.* 49, 1218-1231.

Robles, L., Ruggero, M. A., and Rich, N. C. (1986). Basilar membrane mechanics at the base of the chinchilla cochlea, I. Input-output functions, tuining curves, and response phases. *J. Acoust. Soc. Am.* 80, 1364-1374.

Russell, I. J., Richardson, G. P., and Kössl, M. (1989). The responses of cochlear hair cells to tonic displacements of the sensory hair bundle. *Hear. Res.* 43, 55-70.

Sachs, M. B., and Kiang, N. Y. S. (1968). Two-tone inhibition in auditory-nerve fibers. *J. Acoust. Soc. Am.* 43, 1120-1128.

Sellick, P. M., Patuzzi, R., and Johnstone, B. M. (1983). Comparison between the tuning properties of inner hair cells and basilar membrane motion. *Hear. Res.* 10, 93-100.

Shera, C. A., and Zweig, G. (1991). A symmetry suppresses the cochlear catastrophe. *J. Acoust. Soc. Am.* 89, 1276-1289.

Siebert, W. M. (1974). Ranke revisited - a simple short-wave cochlea model. *J. Acoust. Soc. Am.* 56, 595-600.

Steele, C. R., and Taber, L. A. (1979). Comparison of WKB calculations and experimental results for three-dimensional cochlear models. *J. Acoust. Soc. Am.* 65, 1007-1018.

Strelioff, D., and Flock, Å. (1984). Stiffness of sensory-cell hair bundles in the isolated guinea pig cochlea. *Hear. Res.* 15, 19-28.

Tilney, L. G., and Saunders, J. C. (1983). Actin filaments, stereocilia, and hair cells of the bird cochlea I. Length, number, width, and distribution of stereocilia of each hair cell are related to the position of the hair cell on the cochlea. *J. Cell Biol.* 96, 807-821.

Viergever, M. A. (1980). Mechanics of the inner ear. *PhD thesis*, Delft University of Technology, Netherlands.

Wilson, J. P. (1991). Cochlear mechanics: present status, in: *Auditory Physiology and Perception*, edited by Y. Cazals, L. Demany, and K. Horner (Plenum, New York), in press.

Zenner, H. P. (1986). Motile responses in outer hair cells. *Hear. Res.* 22, 83-90.

Zweig, G. (1991). Finding the impedance of the organ of Corti. *J. Acoust. Soc. Am.* 89, 1229-1254.

Zwislocki, J. (1950). Theory of the acoustical action of the cochlea. *J. Acoust. Soc. Am.* 22, 778-784.

Coding of Fundamental Frequency in Auditory Nerve Fibers: Effects of Signal Level and Phase Spectrum.

J. Wiebe Horst
Institute of Audiology
University Hospital Groningen
Groningen, The Netherlands

Eric Javel
Division of Otolaryngology
Duke University Medical Center
Durham, NC 27710, USA

Glenn R. Farley
Boys Town National Institute
Omaha, NE 68131, USA

1. INTRODUCTION

It is becoming more and more clear that the auditory system is able to process detailed information on stimuli that are not resolved by the mechanical filtering in the cochlea. Ritsma and Hoekstra (1974) and Hoekstra (1979) have shown that frequency discrimination of complex harmonic stimuli with lowest harmonic numbers of about 10 is comparable to frequency discrimination of pure tones. In agreement with this, Houtsma and Smurzynski (1990) have shown that pitch perception is available for harmonic numbers of the same order. Several authors have suggested that this type of information is conveyed by temporal information in the auditory nerve as represented by the moments of occurrence of action potentials. It is likely that this temporal information plays a role in the perception of speech. Sachs and Young (1980) have demonstrated how well spectra of speech signals are retained in such aspects of temporal coding as period histograms (PHs) and interspike interval histograms (ISIHs). The detail in which complex stimuli are coded in ISIHs was studied by Horst et al. (1986a), who showed that very high degrees of resolution of stimulus harmonics of high order ($n>30$) could be found in the spectra of these ISIHs. However, the degree of resolution turned out to be very dependent on spike rate and stimulus level. Nevertheless, if the system makes efficient use of nerve fibers with low and intermediate spike rates, stimulus components with $n \approx 20$ can be easily resolved in the spectra of the ISIHs. This type of analysis was presented for stimuli with flat phase spectra and, as a consequence, having waveforms with nicely modulated temporal envelopes. In the daily practice of listening to speech this condition will often not be fulfilled. In this paper we will show response spectra for stimuli with various phase spectra and temporal envelopes.

2. RESULTS

The data were collected from single auditory nerve fibers from anaesthetized adult cats. Methods are described in detail by Horst et al. (1986a, 1990). Fig. 1a shows period histograms and their spectra in response to modulated stimuli. These are data from a nerve fiber with a characteristic frequency CF of 576 Hz. The center frequency FC of the stimulus was taken equal to CF. The modulation depth was 100 percent. The phase of the center component (FC) was varied in steps, so that the stimulus ranged from the QFM case (0 degrees) via mixed AM-QFM cases to the AM case (90 degrees) and again to a mixed AM-QFM case (112.5 degrees). In agreement with the stimulus, the PHs show maximal

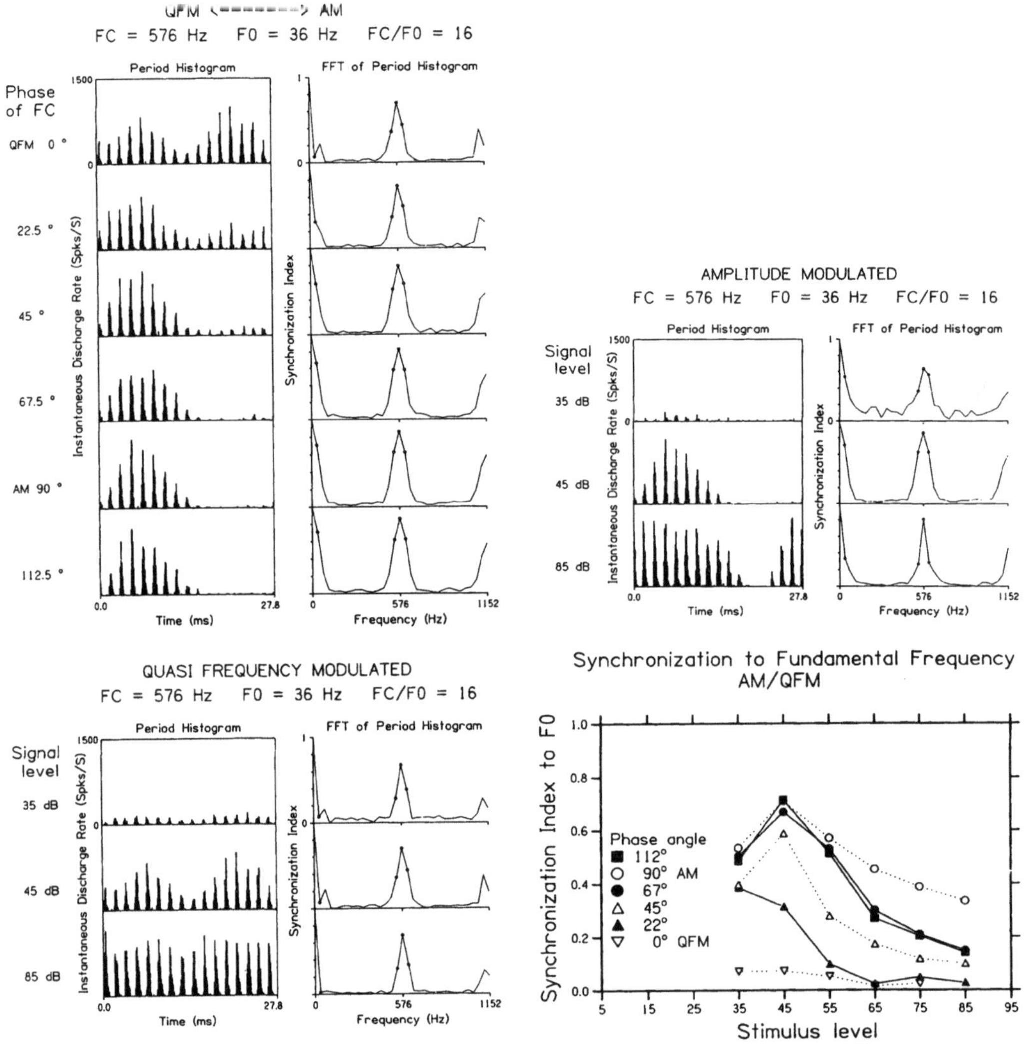

Fig. 1a Responses to three-tone complexes. By changing the phase of the center component, the stimulus was varied from a QFM tone (0o) to an AM tone (90o). The left column shows period histograms. One period of the fundamental frequency was 27.8 ms. The right column shows the spectra of the period histograms expressed as synchronization indices.

Fig. 1b Responses to an AM stimulus for various stimulus levels.

Fig. 1c Responses to a QFM stimulus for various stimulus levels.

Fig. 1d Synchronization to the fundamental frequency as a function of stimulus level and the phase of the center component.

amplitude modulation when the phase of CF was about 90 degrees. There the synchronization to F_0 shown in the response spectra is also maximal. Increase of the stimulus level results in Fig. 1b in flattening of the temporal envelope of the PH and thus in decrease of the synchronization index at F_0. For the QFM stimulus, it is small and increasing the stimulus level forces it to practically zero (Fig. 1c). The influence of the phase of FC and of stimulus level is summarized in Fig. 1d. Clearly, the response at F_0 is strongest for the AM stimulus, and generally the response at F_0 is not very robust.

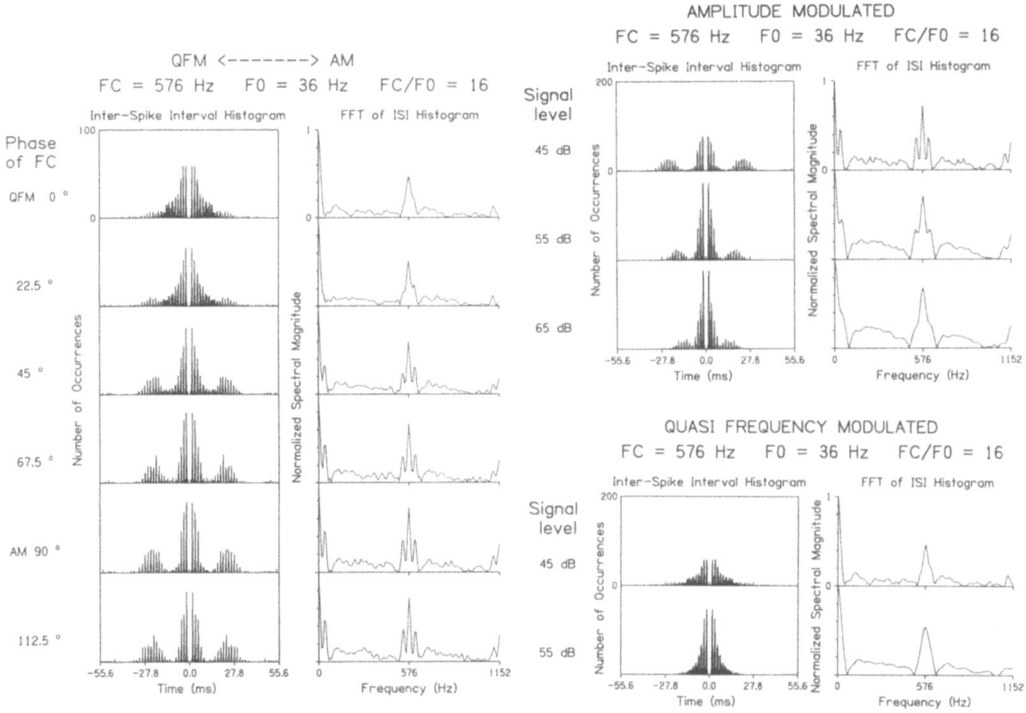

Fig. 2a The data of Fig. 1a expressed as interspike-interval histograms (ISIHs) and the spectra of the ISIHs. The ISIHs are reflected with respect to an interval length of 0 ms. Divisions on the horizontal axis represent integral multiples of the fundamental period of 27.8 ms.
Fig. 2b Responses to an AM stimulus for various stimulus levels.
Fig. 2c Responses to a QFM stimulus for various stimulus levels.

Obviously, the prior knowledge of the waveform necessary to compile PHs is not available to the auditory system. So, other types of information, such as correlations within spike trains or between spike trains of different fibers have to be used by the CNS to extract important features of the stimulus. An often used means of analyzing spike trains is the ISIH (Johnson, 1974; Goldstein and Srulovicz, 1977; Sachs and Young, 1980; Horst et al., 1986a). Fig. 2a shows how this type of analysis works out for the AM/QFM tones. In the ISIHs the modulation is most prominent for the AM stimulus. In the spectrum of the ISIH, the amplitude of the response at F_0 is also maximal for the AM stimulus. This is in agreement with Johnson's (1974) prediction that the magnitudes of individual frequency components in the ISIH are approximately equal to the squares of the synchronization indices in the period histograms. Also for the AM stimulus, individual stimulus components are best resolved. Figs. 2b,c show how the response at F_0 degrades with stimulus level and how poor it is for the QFM stimulus.

The above changes in response came about by a change in the phase of only one component. In the following we will present examples of various changes of the whole phase spectrum. A simple case occurs when all frequency components of a stimulus are shifted by the same phase angle. In this case the temporal envelope of the stimulus waveform is retained but the fine structure of the waveform shifts in time within the envelope. The same behaviour can be observed in the PH. Fig. 3a shows period histograms of responses to multi-component stimuli with a flat amplitude spectrum described before by Horst et al. (1985, 1986abc, 1990). The spectrum was one octave wide centered around the CF (2649 Hz) of the nerve fiber. All components were harmonics of a common fundamental frequency. In this case it was CF/16. That is, the stimulus components ranged from 12 F_0 to 22 F_0. As in the case of the AM/QFM tones the fundamental itself was not present. The period histogram in fig. 3a clearly shows the shift in time within the temporal envelope. Perceptually these types of stimuli are usually not distinguishable (Duifhuis, 1972), since they possess the same temporal envelope in addition to the same amplitude spectrum. In agreement with this, the spectra of the PHs show no essential differences and the same holds for the ISIHs and their spectra (Fig. 3b).

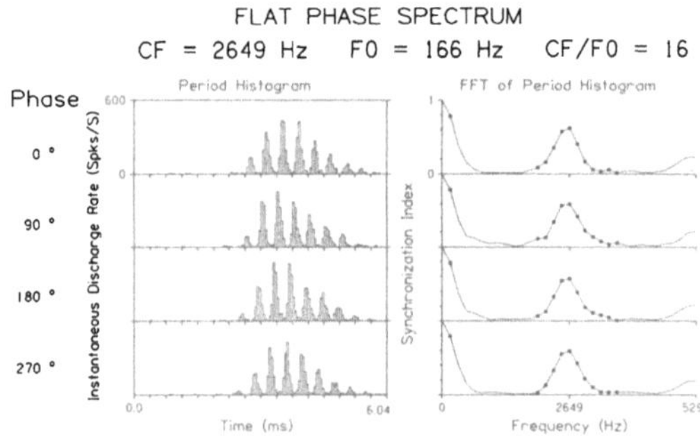

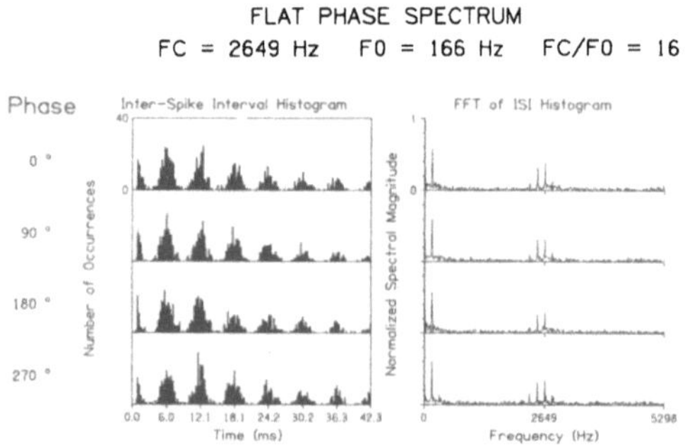

Fig. 3a Period histograms and spectra of the period histograms in response to multi-tone complexes with flat phase spectra.
Fig. 3b The data of Fig. 3a expressed as ISIHs (single sided) and the spectra of the ISIHs.

The majority of possible realisations of phase spectra, however, results in quite different waveform envelopes, although the amplitude spectra are the same. If single-fiber responses were essentially linear (except for half-wave rectification) no changes in response spectra would be observed. Horst et al. (1985, 1986c, 1990) have shown, however, that different temporal envelopes may result in quite different spectra of PHs, and we will show here that it has drastic consequences for the coding of the fundamental frequency.

Fig. 4a shows responses for the same stimulus type. FC was 1444 Hz and F_0=FC/16 was 90.3 Hz. The three different choices for the phase spectrum are flat phase spectrum (top), randomly chosen phase spectrum (middle), resulting in a more even temporal envelope of the stimulus waveform, and alternating phase spectrum (Horst et al., 1986c, 1990; Patterson, 1987), which results in a modulation of the temporal envelope with twice F_0. The changes in the temporal envelope of the PH are considerable, and in agreement with this the synchronization at F_0 decreases. Fig. 4a shows a stepwise decrease from almost 1 to almost 0, when we compare responses to the flat phase spectrum, the randomly chosen phase spectrum and the alternating phase spectrum. This is just another demonstration that the PH does not generate a measure of the fundamental frequency as suggested by Greenberg (1986) but rather of the frequency of the temporal envelope.

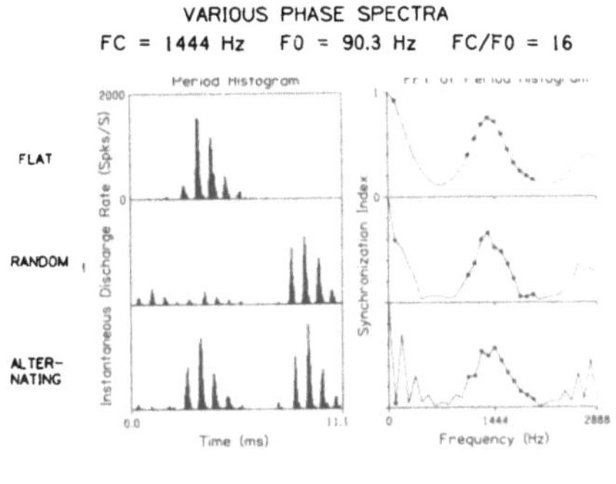

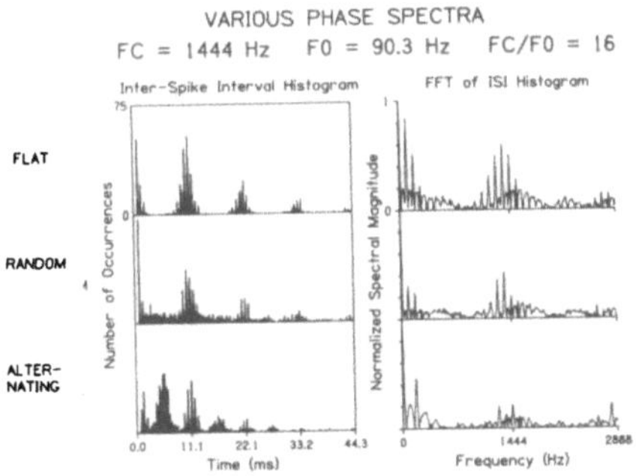

Fig. 4a Period histograms and spectra of the period histograms in response to multi-tone complexes with various phase spectra.

Fig. 4b The data of Fig. 4a expressed as ISIHs (single sided) and the spectra of the ISIHs.

The consequences of the changes in the phase spectrum for the ISIHs (Fig. 4b) are even stronger. First, the modulation of the ISIH decreases as a consequence of the flattening of the envelope of the PH. In addition to that, the spike rate is higher in cases of flatter waveform envelopes. So the number of short intervals increases at the cost of intervals of the order of the fundamental period. This also reduces the modulation of the ISIH. The most conspicuous spectral counterpart is a reduction of the strength of the F_0 component. Besides, the amplitudes of the responses to the stimulus components also decrease considerably. This means that a mechanism to determine F_0 and its strength indirectly would also encounter more difficulty in those cases where the temporal envelope of the stimulus waveform is suboptimal.

Some of the data above might suggest that sharpness of peaks in the ISIH spectrum for individual stimulus components is necessary for sharpness of the response component at F_0. However, good synchronization at F_0 may occur when synchronization to the stimulus components is poor. In the example in Fig. 5a the synchronization to the stimulus components was poor as a consequence of their high frequencies (FC was 4585 Hz). Still, this nerve fiber could easily produce synchronization to the waveform envelope (top panel). Scrambling of the phases resulted again in a considerable decrease of synchronization at the fundamental frequency. The ISIH (Fig. 5b, bottom) did not have appreciable information on F_0 and no peak could be detected in the spectrum of the ISIH. The response to the stimulus with the flat phase spectrum yielded a distinct peak in the spectrum of the ISIH.

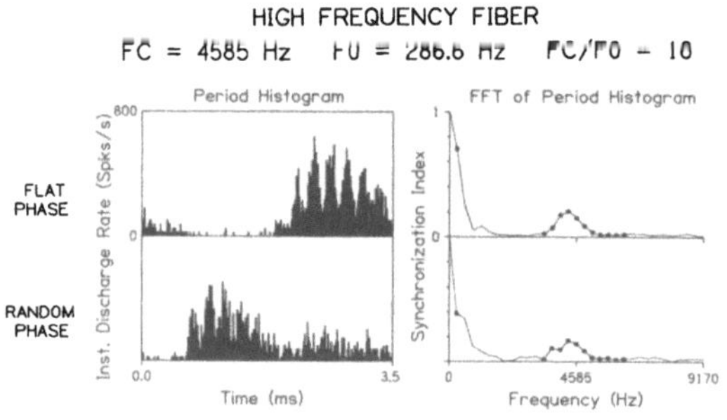

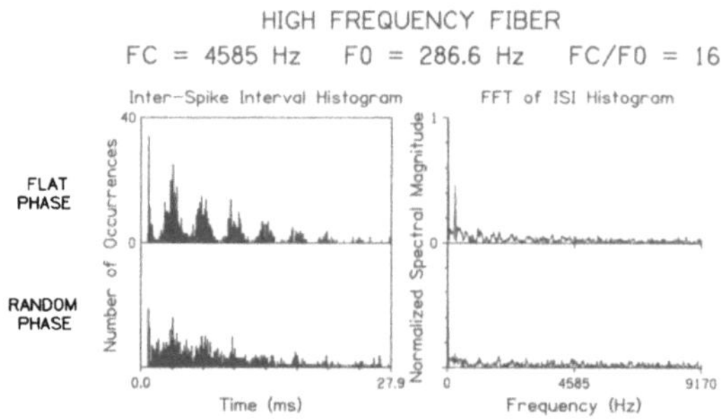

Fig. 5a Period histograms and spectra of the period histograms in response to high-frequency multi-tone complexes with flat and random phase spectrum.
Fig. 5b The data of Fig. 5a expressed as ISIHs (single sided) and the spectra of the ISIHs.

3. Discussion

The above data give another confirmation that single fiber responses can show a strong response synchronized to the frequency of the temporal envelope of the stimulus waveform. Often this frequency is the same as the fundamental frequency of the stimulus. This, however, does not permit the general statement that the cochlea produces synchronization to the fundamental frequency (Greenberg, 1986). The inability to synchronize to F_0 for various phase spectra of the stimulus (e.g. the QFM case) cannot easily be reconciled with "an efficient FM demodulation process in the inner ear" (Khanna and Teich, 1989). The ability at higher levels of the auditory system, e.g. the cochlear nucleus, to synchronize to the fundamental frequency of speech sounds claimed by Kim and Leonard (1988) should be checked with various phase spectra of the stimuli.

The strength of the response in the period histograms to the fundamental frequency generally decreased with stimulus level. This was shown for AM stimuli, in agreement with Javel's (1980) period histograms for AM stimuli. In ISIHs this was even more the case. For other phase relations the response to F_0 was generally smaller, so that in many cases the response to F_0 was often weak or absent. Similar observations could be made for multi-component stimuli. The best response to F_0 occurred for flat phase spectra at fairly low to intermediate stimulus levels. Increase of the stimulus level generally gave some decrease of the amplitude of the response at F_0 (Horst et al. 1986a, 1990) in agreement with Delgutte's (1980) and Delgutte and Kiang's (1984) period histograms in response to artificial vowels. Deviations of the phase spectrum from the flat case resulted in a dramatic decrease of the amplitude of response to F_0 in the spectra of the PHs, and an even greater decrease in the spectra of the ISIHs. In addition to that, resolution and strength of individual components around FC decreased, so that indirect information about F_0 also degraded.

These data may be important for modelling of the extraction of various features of speech from physiological responses (e.g. Assmann and Summerfield, 1989, 1990; Palmer, 1990). In everyday situations the phase spectra of speech may be seriously affected, e.g. by room acoustics, and still be of sufficient quality. Therefore, it seems important to use stimuli with various phase spectra to test models of speech processing in the auditory system and to incorporate adequate stimulus level dependence in such models.

Houtsma and Smurzynski (1990) have shown that just noticeable differences (jnds) of fundamental frequency for stimuli containing only high harmonics may increase by a factor of less than two when the phase spectrum is changed from flat to a "Schröder-phase" spectrum (producing maximally flat temporal envelope). The present data would rather suggest an increase of the jnd by an order of magnitude. This in turn suggests that for frequency discrimination and possibly pitch perception more efficient use is made of temporal information than only first order intervals from spike trains.

References

Assmann, P.F. and Summerfield, Q. (1989). Modelling the perception of concurrent vowels: Vowels with the same fundamental frequency, *J. Acoust. Soc. Am.*, 85, 327-338.

Assmann, P.F. and Summerfield, Q. (1990). Modelling the perception of concurrent vowels: Vowels with different fundamental frequencies, *J. Acoust. Soc. Am.*, 88, 680-697.

Delgutte, B. (1980). Representation of speech-like sounds in the discharge patterns of auditory-nerve fibers, *J. Acoust. Soc. Am.*, 68, 843-857.

Delgutte, B. and Kiang, N.Y.S. (1984). Speech coding in the auditory nerve: I. Vowel-like sounds, *J. Acoust. Soc. Am.*, 75, 866-878.

Duifhuis, H. (1972). *Perceptual analysis of sound*, Doctoral Dissertation, Eindhoven University of Technology.

Goldstein, J.L and Srulovicz, P. (1977). Auditory nerve spike intervals as an adequate basis for aural frequency measurements, in: *Psychophysics and Physiology of Hearing*, edited by E.F. Evans and J.P. Wilson, Academic Press, London, 337-346.

Greenberg, S.R. (1986). Possible role of low and medium spontaneous rate nerve fibers in the encoding of waveform periodicity, in: *Auditory Frequency Selectivity*, (B.C.J. Moore and R.D. Patterson, eds.), Plenum, New York, 241-252.

Hoekstra, A. (1979). *Frequency discrimination and frequency analysis in hearing*, Doctoral dissertation, University of Groningen.

Horst, J.W., Javel, E., and Farley, G.R. (1985). Extraction and enhancement of spectral structure by the cochlea, *J. Acoust. Soc. Am.*, 78, 1898-1901.

Horst, J.W., Javel, E., and Farley, G.R. (1986a). Coding of spectral fine structure in the auditory nerve. I. Fourier analysis of period and interspike interval histograms, *J. Acoust. Soc. Am.*, 79, 398-416.

Horst, J.W., Javel, E., and Farley, G.R. (1986b). New effects of cochlear nonlinearity in temporal patterns of auditory nerve fiber responses to harmonic complexes, in: *Peripheral*

Auditory Mechanisms, edited by J.B. Allen, J.L. Hall, A. Hubbard, S.T. Neely, and A. Tubis (Springer-Verlag, Berlin, Heidelberg, New York), 298-305.

Horst, J.W., Javel, E., and Farley, G.R. (1986c). Effects of phase and amplitude spectrum in the nonlinear processing of complex stimuli in single fibers of the auditory nerve, in: *Auditory frequency selectivity*, edited by B.C.J. Moore and R.D. Patterson, Plenum Publishing Corporation, New York and London, 229-239.

Horst, J.W., Javel, E., and Farley, G.R. (1990). Coding of spectral fine structure in the auditory nerve. II. Level-dependent nonlinear responses, *J. Acoust. Soc. Am.*, 88, 2656-2681.

Houtsma, A.J.M. and Smurzynski, J. (1990). Pitch identification and discrimination for complex tones with many harmonics, *J. Acoust. Soc. Am.*, 87, 304-310.

Javel, E. (1980). Coding of AM tones in the chinchilla auditory nerve: Implications for the pitch of complex tones, *J. Acoust. Soc. Am.*, 68, 133-146.

Johnson, D.H. (1974). *The response of single auditory-nerve fibers in the cat to single tones: Synchrony and average discharge rate*. Doctoral Dissertation, Massachusetts Institute of Technology, Cambridge, MA.

Khanna, S.M. and Teich, M.C. (1989). Spectral characteristics of the responses of primary auditory-nerve fibers to frequency-modulated signals, *Hear. Res.*, 39, 159-176.

Kim, D.O. and Leonard, G. (1988). Pitch-period following response of cat cochlear nucleus neurons to speech sounds, in: *Basic issues in Hearing*, (H. Duifhuis, J.W. Horst and H.P. Wit, eds.), Academic Press, London, 252-260.

Moore, B.C.J. and Glasberg, B.R. (1988). Effects of the relative phase of the components on the pitch discrimination of complex tones by subjects with unilateral cochlear impairments, in: *Basic Issues in Hearing*, edited by H. Duifhuis, J.W. Horst, and H.P. Wit, Academic Press, London, 421-428.

Palmer, A.R. (1990). The representation of the spectra and fundamental frequencies of steady-state single- and double-vowel sounds in the temporal discharge patterns of guinea pig cochlear-nerve fibers, *J. Acoust. Soc. Am.*, 88, 1412-1426.

Patterson, R.D. (1987). A pulse ribbon model of monaural phase perception, *J. Acoust. Soc. Am.*, 82, 1560-1586.

Ritsma, R.J. and Hoekstra, A. (1974). Frequency selectivity and the tonal residue, in: *Facts and Models in Hearing*, (E. Zwicker and E. Terhardt, eds.), Springer, Berlin, 156-163.

Sachs, M.B. and Young, E.D. (1980). Effects of nonlinearities on speech encoding in the auditory nerve, *J. Acoust. Soc. Am.*, 68, 858-875.

Coding of the Pitch of Harmonic and Inharmonic Complex Tones in the Interspike Intervals of Auditory-Nerve Fibers.

Bertrand Delgutte and Peter Cariani

Research Laboratory of Electronics
Massachusetts Institute of Technology
Cambridge, Massachusetts

Eaton-Peabody Laboratory
Massachusetts Eye and Ear Infirmary
and Department of Otolaryngology
Harvard Medical School
Boston, Massachusetts

1. INTRODUCTION

An issue in the auditory processing of speech that has received much attention is how the gross spectral pattern associated with the formant frequencies is coded at the early stages of the auditory nervous system (Sachs and Young, 1979; Delgutte and Kiang, 1984; Delgutte, 1987; Sachs, this volume). This paper addresses another important problem in auditory processing: the coding of the fine spectral structure associated with voice pitch. The pitch of voice conveys important linguistic information, provides cues to the speaker's identity, and helps segregate the speaker's voice from other sources of sound. Because, over short times, voiced speech can be considered to be a complex periodic tone, voice pitch is a special case of the pitch of complex tones, which has long been an topic of interest for psychoacousticians (for reviews, see De Boer, 1976; Evans, 1978). This paper examines how the pitch of complex tones, particularly speech-like sounds, is represented in the activity of auditory-nerve fibers.

Information about the pitch of complex tones might be available either in the profiles of average discharge rates of auditory-nerve fibers as a function of their point of innervation along the cochlea, or in the fine temporal patterns of discharge. According to "rate-place" models, discharge rate should be higher when a fiber characteristic frequency (CF) coincides with a harmonic of the fundamental frequency of a complex tone than when the CF falls between two harmonics. The available data from auditory-nerve fibers (Sachs and Young, 1979) do not support these models: Profiles of average rates against CF for vowel stimuli do not show obvious peaks at harmonics of the fundamental, even at low stimulus levels where fiber discharge rates are not saturated. Although these results do not rule out the possibility that small, but significant rate-place cues to the fundamental frequency might be available, the present paper focuses on how the pitch of complex tones is encoded in the interspike intervals of auditory-nerve fibers. Most auditory-nerve fibers show prominent interspike intervals at the fundamental period in response to complex periodic tones (eg. Evans, 1978; Delgutte, 1980; Javel, 1980; Delgutte and Kiang, 1984; Miller and Sachs, 1984; Horst et al., 1986, this volume; Palmer and Winter, 1991). While this result is not surprising for harmonic complex tones, in which all stimulus components are integer multiples of the fundamental, a stronger test of temporal models of pitch is provided by the inharmonic tones that have been studied psychophysically (e.g. Schouten et al., 1962). Although these stimuli have no fundamental period, they can produce strong, reproducible pitch sensations. It has been reported that auditory-nerve fibers can show interspike intervals corresponding to the pitch of inharmonic tones (Javel, 1980; Evans, 1983; Greenberg, 1986), but such data are available only for small numbers of stimuli and auditory-nerve fibers. This paper presents systematic data on the responses of auditory-nerve fibers to both harmonic and inharmonic complex tones covering a broad range of pitch frequencies and spectral characteristics.

2. Method

Fig. 1 shows the waveforms and magnitude spectra of four stimuli that are representative of the types of sounds used in our experiments. Single-formant (SF) vowels are simple harmonic stimuli that provide a good approximation to the low-frequency region of the spectra of voiced speech sounds, the region most important for pitch perception (Plomp, 1967; Ritsma, 1967). Their spectrum shows a prominent peak at the formant frequency F_1, and their waveform a periodicity at the fundamental frequency F_0, which is perceived as voice pitch. In these experiments we used SF stimuli whose fundamental frequency varied in the range of the human voice (100-450 Hz).

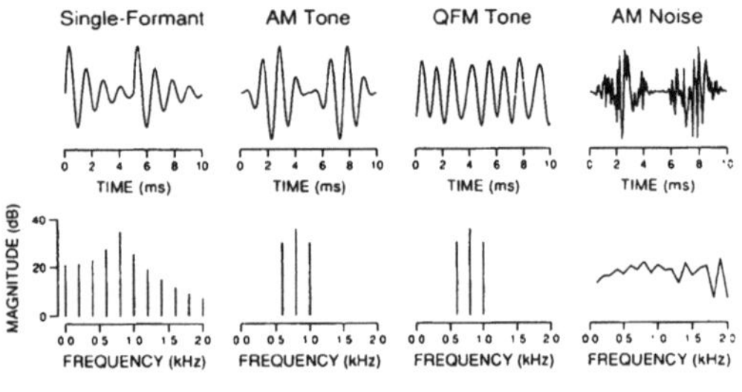

Fig. 1 Waveforms (top) and magnitude spectra (bottom) of 4 acoustic stimuli that produce a pitch at 200 Hz. The single-formant stimulus has a formant frequency of 800 Hz and a fundamental frequency of 200 Hz. The AM and QFM tones both have a carrier frequency of 800 Hz and a modulation frequency of 200 Hz, and are 100% modulated. The AM white noise has a modulation frequency of 200 Hz.

Sinusoidally amplitude-modulated (AM) tones are three-component tones centered at the carrier frequency F_c. When F_c is an integer multiple of the modulation frequency F_m, this stimulus is periodic, and produces a strong pitch at F_m (Ritsma, 1962)[1]. When F_c is not a multiple of F_m, the stimulus becomes inharmonic, but still produces a pitch at frequency that differs systematically from F_m, a phenomenon known as "pitch shift" (Schouten et al., 1962). Quasi frequency-modulated (QFM) tones are three component tones that have the same magnitude spectra as AM tones with the same F_m and F_c, but differ in their phase spectra and time waveforms. In general, the two stimuli produce the same pitches, although pitch strengths may differ somewhat (Ritsma and Engel, 1964; Wightman, 1973a; Moore, 1977). Unlike AM and QFM tones, sinusoidally amplitude-modulated white noise has a flat long-term spectrum. For low (< 500 Hz) modulation frequencies, this stimulus produces a weak pitch at the modulation frequency (Burns and Viemeister, 1976), which therefore differs from the pitch of an inharmonic AM tone with the same F_m. Thus, comparison of neural responses to AM tones, QFM tones, and AM noise can help identify features of these responses that are associated with pitch. In our experiments, we used all three types of stimuli

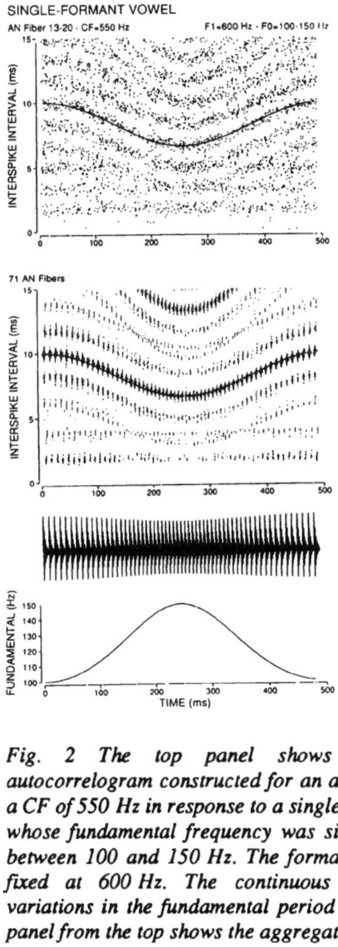

Fig. 2 The top panel shows the short-time autocorrelogram constructed for an auditory fiber with a CF of 550 Hz in response to a single-formant stimulus whose fundamental frequency was sinusoidally varied between 100 and 150 Hz. The formant frequency was fixed at 600 Hz. The continuous line shows the variations in the fundamental period $1/F_0$. The second panel from the top shows the aggregate short-time autocorrelogram for 71 auditory-nerve fibers from the same cat. The two bottom panels show the stimulus waveform and the variations in F_0.

with modulation frequencies in the range of 100-450 Hz.

In order to study a wide range of stimulus conditions within the limited times that single fibers are contacted, we designed stimuli in which variables associated with pitch are slowly varied. For example, the bottom panel of Fig. 2 shows the waveform of an SF stimulus whose fundamental frequency varies sinusoidally between 100 and 150 Hz over the 480-ms duration of the stimulus. The r.m.s. amplitude was kept constant for each "period", so that the peak amplitude varied somewhat with F_0. We also generated AM and QFM tones in which either F_m or F_c was sinusoidally varied, and AM noise with variable F_m.

All stimuli were generated by a 16-bit digital-to-analog converter using a sampling rate of 100 kHz, and were played repeatedly without interruption during the collection of neural responses. Stimulus level was always 60 dB SPL, except for the AM noise, whose spectrum level was approximately 23 dB re. 20 μPa/$\sqrt{\text{Hz}}$ for frequencies below 10 kHz. Techniques for recording from auditory-nerve fibers in Dial-anaesthetized cats were standard for our laboratory (Kiang et al., 1965; Liberman, 1978). Our results are based on recordings from about 200 auditory-nerve fibers in 2 cats.

3. Results

The temporal patterns of discharge of auditory-nerve fibers in response to both harmonic and inharmonic complex tones were analyzed in the form of short-time autocorrelograms (Licklider, 1951; Evans, 1983; Greenberg, 1986). Autocorrelograms were used rather than the more traditional period histograms because inharmonic stimuli lack a well-defined period. The short-time autocorrelogram technique is like examining the first-order interspike interval distribution as a function of time (Chung et al., 1970; Bourk, 1976; Young et al., 1988), except that intervals of all orders are considered. The short-time autocorrelogram is illustrated at the top of Fig. 2 for one auditory-nerve fiber in response to an SF stimulus whose F_0 was varied between 100 and 150 Hz. The CF of the fiber was 500 Hz, close to the 600-Hz formant frequency F_1. Each point at coordinates X and Y indicates that one spike occurred X ms after the onset of the stimulus, and that another spike (not necessarily the preceding one) occurred Y ms before. At the beginning of the stimulus, when F_0 is near 100 Hz, spikes tend to occur at intervals of $1/6F_0$ and its multiples, indicating a response to the 6th harmonic, the one closest to F_1. As F_0 gradually increases to 150 Hz, interspike intervals tend to correspond to the 5th, then to the 4th harmonic, whichever is closest to F_1. This sequence of events is reversed as F_0 is lowered from 150 to 100 Hz. Although the responses do show intervals corresponding to the fundamental period $1/F_0$ (solid line), these are not particularly salient for this fiber. This poor representation of F_0 in the responses of fibers whose CF is close to a formant frequency has been noted previously (Delgutte, 1980; Delgutte and Kiang, 1984).

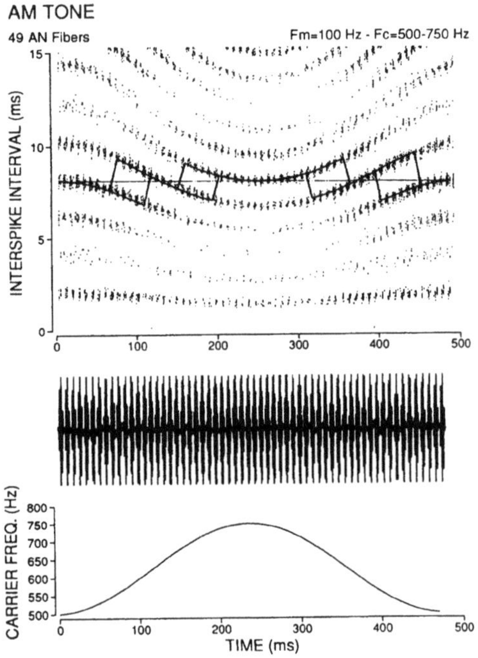

Fig. 3 Aggregate short-time autocorrelogram in response to an AM tone whose carrier frequency F_c was sinusoidally varied between 500 and 750 Hz, while the modulation frequency F_m was fixed at 125 Hz. The thin line shows the modulation period ($1/F_m$). The thick line shows the pitch period that would be perceived by human listeners for a steady-state stimulus having the same F_c and F_m at each point in time (Schouten et al., 1962).

In order to display responses for populations of auditory-nerve fibers, "aggregate autocorrelograms" were constructed by summing the autocorrelograms for many single fibers, and displaying only the bins containing more than a threshold number of spikes. The second panel of Fig. 2 shows such an aggregate autocorrelogram for 71 auditory-nerve fibers from the same cat in response to the same SF stimulus as in the top panel. Most (89%) of the fibers included in this aggregate autocorrelogram had CF's below 2 kHz, although a few had CF's as high as 20 kHz. We chose to record primarily from low CF fibers because low frequencies are known to be the most important for pitch (Ritsma, 1967; Plomp, 1967). The aggregate autocorrelogram shows a prominent dark band coinciding with the fundamental period $1/F_0$. This result suggests that pitch may correspond to the most frequent interspike interval in the array of auditory-nerve fibers.

Fig. 3 shows aggregate short-time autocorrelograms for an inharmonic AM tone whose carrier frequency F_c was sinusoidally varied between 500 and 750 Hz, while the modulation frequency F_m was kept at 125 Hz. The thick solid line indicates the perceived pitch period, derived from the psychophysical data of Schouten et al. (1962). The pitch varies sinusoidally over small ranges of Fc, and shows abrupt jumps when the ratio F_c/F_m is not close to an integer. Between integer values of F_c/F_m, the pitch is ambiguous, an effect shown by regions where two thick lines overlap in time in Fig. 3. Results show a good match between the darkest bands of the aggregate autocorrelogram and the human pitch judgements. In particular, the intervals do not, in general, correspond to the modulation period $1/F_m$ (shown by a thin line), except in the harmonic case.

The top panel of Fig. 4 shows an aggregate autocorrelogram for another AM tone in which F_m rather than F_c was varied. Specifically, F_m varied sinusoidally between 100 and 150 Hz, while F_c was fixed at 600 Hz. Small changes in F_m produce minimal changes in pitch, but if these changes become large enough that the ratio F_c/F_m changes by more than unity, the pitch jumps abruptly. As in Fig. 3, the most frequent intervals in the autocorrelogram follow the perceived pitch, and in particular do not correspond to $1/F_m$ (thin line). The bottom panel of Fig. 4 shows an aggregate short-time autocorrelogram for a QFM tone with the same F_m and F_c as the AM tone shown on top. The aggregate autocorrelograms are broadly similar for the two stimuli, consistent with the psychophysical observation that these stimuli produce the same pitches (Wightman, 1973a), and are in fact hard to distinguish. However, the autocorrelogram for the QFM tone shows a larger number of intervals near 3-5 ms than does the AM-tone autocorrelogram. This observation is consistent with psychophysical reports that, for QFM stimuli, pitches in the vicinity of (but not exactly at) 2 F_m are occasionally perceived (Ritsma and Engel, 1964).

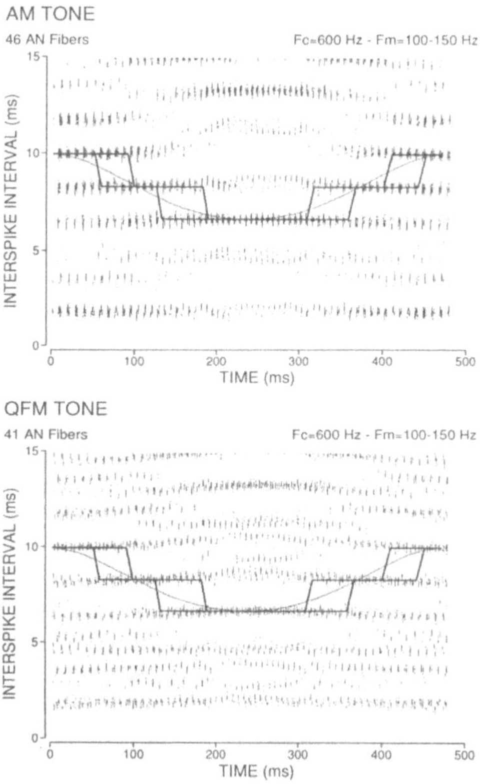

Fig. 4 Aggregate short-time autocorrelograms for AM (top) and QFM (bottom) tones whose modulation frequencies were sinusoidally varied between 100 and 150 Hz, while F_c was fixed at 600 Hz. The thick and thin lines are as in Fig. 3.

Fig. 5 shows aggregate autocorrelograms for an AM tone and AM white noise whose F_m were sinusoidally varied between 200 and 300 Hz. As noted in Fig. 4 for an AM tone with a lower F_m, the most frequent interspike intervals for the AM tone differ systematically from $1/F_m$, as does the perceived pitch. The aggregate autocorrelogram for the AM noise clearly differs from that for the AM tone in that intervals are much less concentrated near specific values. Nevertheless, there is a tendency for intervals to occur more frequently near $1/F_m$ and its multiples. These results are consistent with psychophysical data showing (1) that the pitch of AM noise is much weaker than that of AM tones, and (2) that the former is at the modulation frequency, while the latter in general is not.

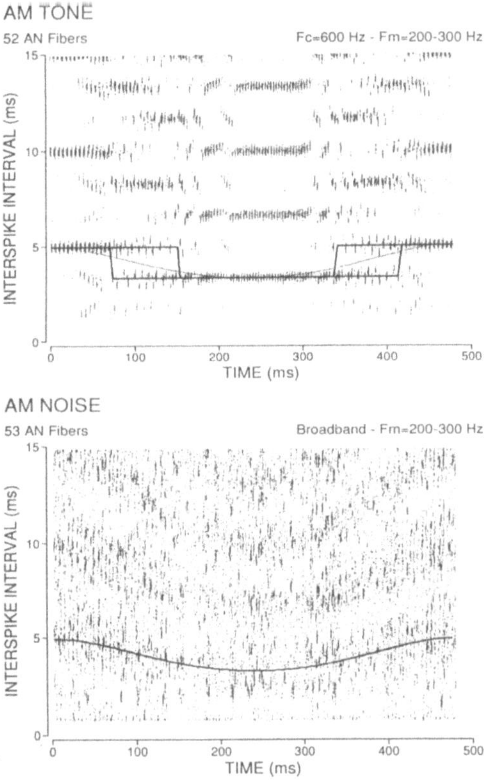

Fig. 5 Aggregate short-time autocorrelograms for AM tone (top) and AM broadband noise (bottom) whose modulation frequencies were sinusoidally varied between 200 and 300 Hz. The thick and thin lines are as in Fig. 3.

4. Conclusion

We have studied the responses of auditory-nerve fibers to a wide range of harmonic and inharmonic complex tones that produce pitches in the range appropriate for human voice and musical sounds. Responses were analyzed in terms of short-time autocorrelograms (Licklider, 1951) that display the distribution of interspike intervals over time. The autocorrelograms were summed for large samples of fibers in order to obtain an approximate picture of the distribution of interspike intervals for the entire array of auditory-nerve fibers. This summation of intervals from the entire auditory-nerve array is the basis for several temporal models of pitch perception (Moore, 1983; Van Noorden, 1982; Meddis and Hewitt, 1991). Qualitatively, the results showed good correspondence between the most frequent interspike intervals in the aggregate autocorrelogram, and the most salient pitches perceived by human listeners. This correspondence was true both for a given stimulus, in that the darkest bands in the aggregate autocorrelogram tended to coincide with the pitch, and when comparing across stimuli, in that stimuli that produce the most salient pitches showed a greater concentration of intervals near the pitch period. Aggregate autocorrelograms for perceptually similar stimuli such as AM and QFM tones with the same F_m and F_c were broadly similar. Clearly, more quantitative measures of relative interspike interval densities need to be developed, and a wider range of stimulus conditions needs to be investigated. Nevertheless, the good match between human pitch judgements and the most salient features of aggregate interspike interval distributions supports the temporal models of pitch perception cited above.

A potential difficulty for these temporal models is the poor pitch discrimination of cochlear-implant patients for sinusoidal stimuli or periodic pulse trains applied through a single electrode (e.g. Eddington et al., 1978). Discharges of auditory-nerve fibers are precisely phase-locked to sinusoidal electric stimuli (Dynes and Delgutte, 1992), so that the majority of stimulated fibers would be expected to show prominent interspike intervals at the fundamental period. If such interval information were available, the temporal models based on interspike intervals from the entire auditory nerve would predict equally good pitch discrimination for electric stimulation and for acoustic stimulation, contrary to psychophysical observations. Despite this difficulty, if the pitch of complex tones is extracted by a form of interval analysis, the challenge for the physiologist is to identify how this analysis is carried out in the central nervous system.

Acknowledgements

We thank K. Jacob and K. Whitley for surgical assistance, and N.Y.S. Kiang and D.K. Eddington for valuable comments. This work was supported by NIH grants DC00019 and DC00006.

Notes

1. A stimulus is said to produce a pitch at frequency *F* when human listeners reliably match the pitch of that stimulus to that of a harmonic complex having a fundamental of frequency *F*.

References

Bourk, T.R. (1976). *Electrical responses of neural units in the anteroventral cochlear nucleus of the cat,* Doctoral Dissertation, MIT, Cambridge, MA.

Burns, E.M. and Viemeister, N.F. (1976). Nonspectral pitch, *J. Acoust. Soc. Am.* 60, 863-869.

Chung, S.H., Lettvin, J.Y., and Raymond, S.A. (1970). Multiple meaning in single visual units, *Brain, Behavior and Evolution*, 3, 72-101.

De Boer, E. (1976). On the "residue" and auditory pitch perception, in: *Handbook of Sensory Physiology*, V/3, edited by W.D. Keidel and W.D. Neff, Springer-Verlag, Berlin, 479-583.

Delgutte, B. (1980). Representation of speech-like sounds in the discharge patterns of auditory-nerve fibers, *J. Acoust. Soc. Am.*, 68, 843-857.

Delgutte, B. (1987). Peripheral auditory processing of speech information: Implications from a physiological study of intensity discrimination, in: *The Psychophysics of Speech Perception*, edited by M.E.H. Schouten, Nijhof, Dordrecht, 333-353.

Delgutte, B., and Kiang, N.Y.S. (1984). Speech coding in the auditory nerve I: Vowel-like sounds, *J. Acoust. Soc. Am.*, 75, 866-878.

Dynes, S.B.C., and Delgutte, B. (1992). Phase locking of auditory-nerve fiber discharges to sinusoidal electric stimulation of the cochlea, *Hearing Res.*, 58, 79-90.

Eddington, D.K., Dobelle, W.H., Brackman, D.E., Mladejovsky, M.G., and Parkin, J.L. (1978). Auditory prostheses research with multiple channel intracochlear stimulation in man, *Ann. Otol. Rhinol. Laryngol.*, 87, Suppl 53.

Evans, E.F. (1978). Place and time coding of frequency in the peripheral auditory system: Some physiological pros and cons, *Audiol.*, 17, 369-420.

Evans, E.F. (1983). Pitch and cochlear nerve fibre temporal discharge patterns, in: *Hearing Physiological Bases and Psychophysics*, edited by R. Klinke and R. Hartmann, Springer-Verlag, Berlin, 140-145.

Greenberg, S. (1986). Possible role of low and medium spontaneous rate cochlear nerve fibers in the encoding of waveform periodicity, in: *Auditory Frequency Selectivity*, edited by B.C.J. Moore and R.D. Patterson, Plenum, New York, 241-248.

Horst, J.W., Javel, E., and Farley, G.R. (1986). Coding of spectral fine structure in the auditory nerve I: Fourier analysis of period and interval histograms, *J. Acoust. Soc. Am.*, 79, 398-416.

Javel, E. (1980). Coding of AM tones in the chinchilla auditory nerve: Implications for the pitch of complex tones, *J. Acoust. Soc. Am.*, 68, 133-146.

Kiang, N.Y.S., Watanabe, T., Thomas, E.C., and Clark, L.F. (1965), *Discharge Patterns of Single Fibers in the Cat's Auditory Nerve*, M.I.T. Press, Cambridge.

Liberman, M.C. (1978). Auditory-nerve responses from cats raised in a low-noise chamber, *J. Acoust. Soc. Am.*, 63, 442-455.

Licklider, J.C.R. (1951). The duplex theory of pitch perception, *Experimentia*, 7, 128-137.

Meddis, R. and Hewitt, M.J. (1991). Virtual pitch and phase sensitivity of a computer model of the auditory periphery. I: Pitch identification, *J. Acoust. Soc. Am.*, 89, 2866-2882.

Miller, M.I. and Sachs, M.B. (1984). Representation of voice pitch in the discharge patterns of auditory-nerve fibers, *Hearing Res.*, 14, 257-279.

Moore B.C.J. (1977). Effects of relative phase of the components on the pitch of three-component complex tones, in: *Psychophysics and Physiology of Hearing*, edited by E.F. Evans and J.P. Wilson, Academic, London, pp 349-358.

Moore, B.C.J. (1983). Introduction to the Psychology of Hearing (Academic, London).

Palmer, A.R. and Winter, I.M. (1991). Cochlear nerve and cochlear nucleus responses to the fundamental frequency of voiced speech sounds and harmonic complex tones, *International Hearing Symposium*, Carcans, France.

Plomp, R. (1967). Pitch of complex tones, *J. Acoust. Soc. Am.*, 41, 1526-1533.

Ritsma, R.J. (1962). Existence region of the tonal residue I, *J. Acoust. Soc. Am.*, 34, 1224-1229.

Ritsma, R.J. (1967). Frequencies dominant in the perception of the pitch of complex sounds, *J. Acoust. Soc. Am.*, 42, 191-198.

Ritsma, R.J. and Engel, F.L. (1964). Pitch of frequency-modulated signals, *J. Acoust. Soc. Am.*, 36, 1637-1644.

Sachs M.B. and Young, E.D. (1979). Encoding of steady-state vowels in the auditory nerve: Representation in terms of discharge rate, *J. Acoust. Soc. Am.*, 56, 1835-1847.

Schouten, J.F., Ritsma, R.J., and Cardozo, B. (1962). Pitch of the residue, *J. Acoust. Soc. Am.*, 34, 1418-1424.

Van Noorden, L. (1982). Two channel pitch perception, in: *Music, Mind and Brain*, edited by M. Clynes, Plenum, New York.
Wightman, F.L. (1973a). Pitch and stimulus fine structure, *J. Acoust. Soc. Am.*, 54, 397-406.
Young, E.D., Robert, J.M., and Shofner, W.P. (1988). Regularity and latency of units in the ventral cochlear nucleus: Implications for unit classification and generation of response properties, *J. Neurophysiol.*, 60, 1-29.

Processing of the Auditory-Nerve Code for Speech by Populations of Cells in the Anteroventral Cochlear Nucleus

Murray B. Sachs,
Carol C. Blackburn,
M.I. Banks*,
Xiaoqin Wang
Department of Biomedical Engineering and Center for Hearing Sciences
The Johns Hopkins University School of Medicine
Baltimore, Maryland, USA 21205

*and Department of Neurophysiology
University of Wisconsin Medical School
Madison Wisconsin 53076.

1. Introduction

The encoding of speech-like sounds in the firing patterns of auditory-nerve fibers (ANFs) has been studied intensively over the past fifteen years or more. The spectra of vowels and consonants can be represented in the auditory nerve both in terms of rate responses and temporal (phase-locked) responses (Delgutte and Kiang, 1984a; Delgutte and Kiang, 1984b; Miller and Sachs, 1983; Palmer et al., 1986; Sachs and Young, 1979; Young and Sachs, 1979). The AN code must be processed by the central nervous system in order to produce the perception of sound and other appropriate behavior. The first step in that processing occurs in the cochlear nucleus. In this paper we consider some recent results relating to the processing of spectral features of vowels in the anteroventral cochlear nucleus (AVCN). An issue that has been the focus of auditory research for at least half a century concerns the mechanism(s) by which the auditory system is able to discriminate between sounds on the basis of spectral features over a broad range of stimulus levels, given the limited dynamic range of ANFs (Palmer and Evans, 1980; Sachs and Abbas, 1974; Sachs et al., 1989). We concentrate this discussion on results that relate directly to this issue.

2. Representation of Vowel Spectrum in the Auditory Nerve

Rate-place profiles are plots of discharge rate to a fixed stimulus vs. best frequency (BF) for a population of neurons. As shown in Fig. 1a, rate-place profiles for high spontaneous rate (SR>19/s; (Liberman, 1978)) ANFs provide a good representation of the spectrum of the vowel /ε/ at low sound levels in the sense that there are peaks in rate at BF places corresponding to the vowel formant frequencies (arrows; Sachs and Young, 1979). At moderate sound levels (about 50 dB SPL), the formant peaks disappear, primarily because of rate saturation (Sachs and Young, 1979); however, as shown in Figs. 1b-c, at these and higher levels rate-place profiles for low- and medium SR ANFs provide a good neural representation of spectrum because of their relatively higher thresholds and wider dynamic ranges (Liberman, 1978; Sachs and Young, 1979; Schalk and Sachs, 1980). As we and others have pointed out, the central nervous system (CNS) could derive a rate-place representation for vowel spectra that is practically invariant across sound levels by "selectively listening" to high-SR ANF inputs at low sound levels and to low-SR inputs at high levels (Delgutte, 1982; Sachs and Blackburn, 1988). By selective listening to one SR group we mean a process by which the output of a population of CNS neurons is determined predominantly by the inputs from that SR group.

Fig. 2 shows examples of phase-locked responses of three ANFs whose BFs are near the

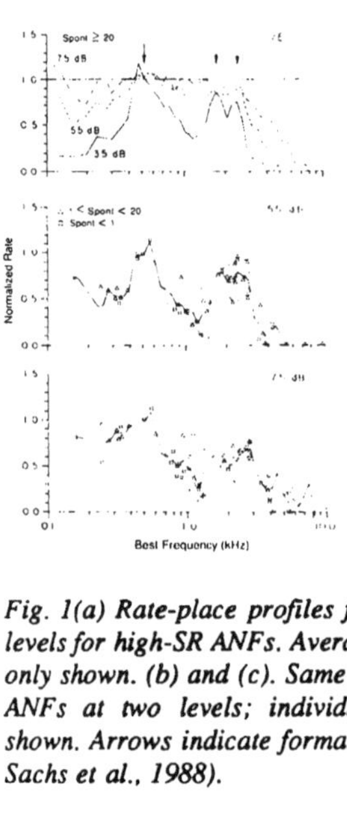

Fig. 1(a) Rate-place profiles for /ε/ at three sound levels for high-SR ANFs. Average of single unit data only shown. (b) and (c). Same for high- and low-SR ANFs at two levels; individual unit data points shown. Arrows indicate formant frequencies. (From Sachs et al., 1988).

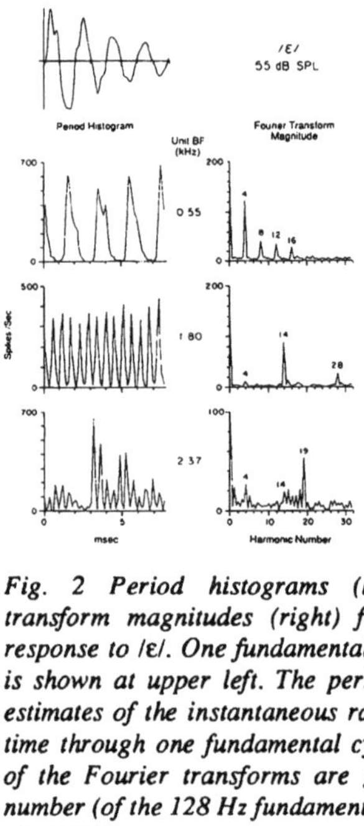

Fig. 2 Period histograms (left) and Fourier transform magnitudes (right) for three ANFs in response to /ε/. One fundamental cycle of the vowel is shown at upper left. The period histograms are estimates of the instantaneous rate as a function of time through one fundamental cycle. The abscissae of the Fourier transforms are given as harmonic number (of the 128 Hz fundamental). (From Sachs et al., 1988).

first three formant frequencies of /ε/. The left side shows period histograms computed from the spike trains; the right side shows the Fourier transforms of the corresponding histograms. All three units are phase-locked to the formant nearest the BF. For example, the middle unit has a BF just above the second formant frequency (1.792 kHz, which is the fourteenth harmonic of the vowel's 128 Hz fundamental frequency). The fourteen peaks in the histogram indicate a strong phase-locked response to the second formant and the Fourier transform shows a peak at the second formant (see Young and Sachs (1979) for detailed discussion of temporal responses). We have shown that a clear representation of the spectrum of speech sounds can be generated by computing the magnitude of the synchronized response at various stimulus frequencies. By magnitude of the synchronized response we mean the magnitude of

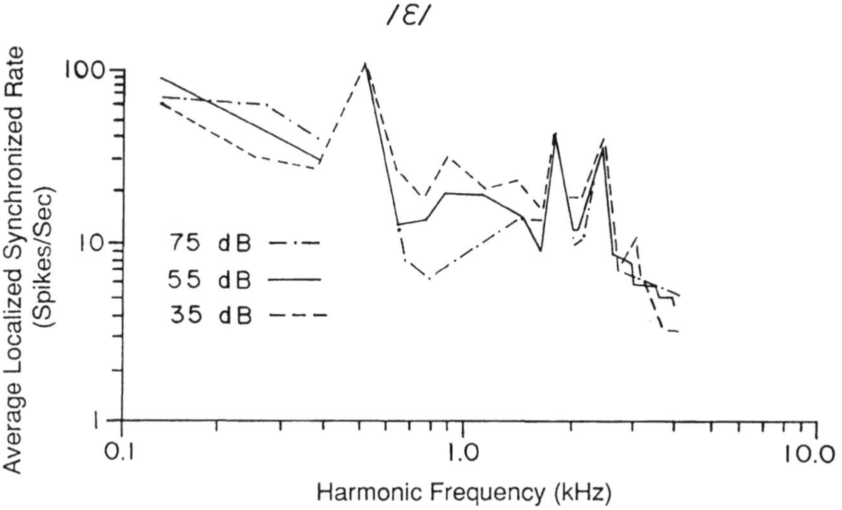

Fig. 3 Average localized synchronized rate (ALSR) for /ε/ at three sound levels. (From Sachs et al., 1988).

the Fourier transform of the period histogram. We take advantage of the fact that synchronized response to each stimulus component is generally largest among fibers tuned to the component (Young and Sachs, 1979). We define the average localized synchronized rate, ALSR (Young and Sachs, 1979) at any frequency as the average value of the amplitude of the Fourier transform component ("synchronized rate", spikes/s) at that frequency. The average is computed over all fibers whose BFs are within 0.25 octaves of the frequency. Fig. 3 shows that the ALSR provides a clear representation of the vowel stimulus over all levels tested; there are clear formant peaks at all levels.

3. Signal Transformations in the Anteroventral Cochlear Nucleus

Thus we have two complementary representations for the spectra of vowels in the AN. Note, however, that both of these representations place certain demands on signal processing in the central nervous system (CNS). In order that a rate-place representation be stable even over a moderate range of stimulus levels, some form of selective listening process must occur. In order that a temporal-place representation be viable the CNS must be able to deal with phase-locked spike trains up to frequencies at least in the range of the third formant (about 3.0 kHz). In this section we consider the processing of both of these representations by two populations of cells in the AVCN: bushy cells and stellate cells.

Two morphologically defined principal cell types, called bushy and stellate cells, have been described in the anteroventral cochlear nucleus (Fig. 4a; Cant & Morest, 1984). These differ from one another in terms of their cellular morphology, patterns of synaptic organization, sources of descending efferent input, and the patterns of their axonal projections

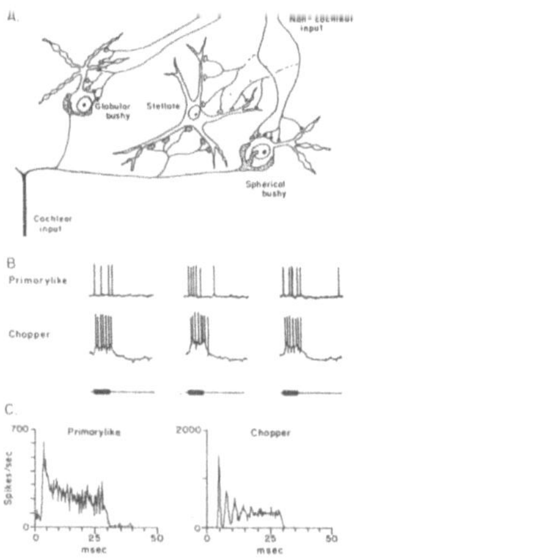

Fig. 4 (a) Schematic illustration of afferent connections and synaptic organization of spherical bushy cells, globular bushy cells, and stellate cells in the anteroventral cochlear nucleus (AVCN; from Cant and Morest, 1984). (b). Examples of spike trains recorded intracellularly from a primarylike and a chopper unit; stimuli were 25 ms BF tone bursts. (Redrawn from Romand, 1978). (c). Post stimulus-time histograms for a primarylike and a chopper unit.

onto more central auditory nuclei. Corresponding differences in the complexity of their physiological responses have also been demonstrated. The bushy cells receive relatively few large synaptic terminals (the end bulbs of Held) from the auditory nerve directly on their somas (Cant and Morest, 1984; Roullier et al., 1986). They have small dendritic trees which receive few synaptic terminals. Bushy cells differ in the number and size of their endbulbs; spherical bushy cells have a few larger endbulbs and globular bushy cells have more, smaller endbulbs (Brawer and Morest, 1975). Intracellular labelling studies have allowed at least a preliminary identification of some response characteristics of bushy cells (Rhode et al., 1983a; Roullier and Ryugo, 1984). As a result of their synaptic input pattern responses of bushy cells appear to be very similar to those of auditory-nerve fibers. Figs. 4b,c illustrate those response properties which are relevant to this discussion and which we take as the physiologically distinguishing features of bushy cells. At the onset of a tone burst, bushy cells give a high rate of discharge followed by a gradual decline to a more or less steady level (Fig. 4c). This tone burst response is called primarylike and is associated with spherical bushy cells (Rhode et al., 1983a; Roullier and Ryugo, 1984). The tone burst response of globular bushy cells is similar to the primarylike pattern except that there is a brief pause ("notch", about one msec) in firing after the initial rapid increase in rate; this pattern is called primarylike with notch (Smith and Rhode, 1987). The responses of the great majority of spherical and globular bushy cells to the vowel stimuli of interest here are thus far indistinguishable and so we will consider them to be one class which we will call *primarylike*. An important distinguishing feature of the primarylike units is the extent to which their firing patterns are irregular. As shown in Fig. 4b, the responses of these units to successively presented, identical stimuli are not the same; even the number of spikes during the stimulus interval varies from presentation to presentation. Furthermore, the intervals between spikes are highly variable.

Stellate cells on the other hand, receive a large number of small bouton inputs on their dendritic trees and, in some cases, on their cell bodies (Fig. 4a; Cant and Morest, 1984). Stellate cells appear to produce *chopper* response patterns to BF tones (Fig. 4c; Rhode et al. 1983a). This pattern is characterized by fluctuations in response rate synchronized to the stimulus onset, which are reflected in the "chopping" pattern in the post-stimulus-time histogram in Fig. 4c. The spike trains of these units are very regular. The number of spikes is quite constant from one stimulus presentation to the next and the interval between spikes shows little variability (Fig. 4b). The chopping pattern in their tone burst responses is related to this regularity of firing. These units have a very precise onset time to the tone bursts and the following rate fluctuations simply reflect the regularity of the spike trains following the onset spike.

The behavior of AVCN chopper units suggests that these cells may be performing a selective listening operation (Blackburn and Sachs, 1990). Fig. 5 compares rate profiles for a population of irregular or transient chopper units (ChT (Blackburn and Sachs, 1989; Bourk, 1976; Young et al., 1988)) with those of high-SR and low- and medium-SR ANF's. The spectrum of the vowel /ɛ/ used as stimulus is shown at the top in Fig. 5. At the lowest sound level tested (25 dB SPL) only a small group of chopper units with BFs near the second and third formants of the vowel were studied. The rate profile for these units (solid line) is similar to that for high-SR ANF's with BFs in the same range (dashed line) and shows a clear peak in the second/third formant regions. At all other stimulus levels studied (35-75 dB SPL) the chopper profile closely resembles that of the low- and medium-SR ANF's. Even at 75 dB SPL, where rate saturation has obliterated formant peaks in the high-SR ANF profile, the chopper rate profile maintains a clear separation between the first and second formants. Thus at medium and high sound levels the chopper representation is at least as good as that provided by the low- and medium-SR ANFs. Although most of the data in Fig. 5 can be explained by a selective connection of low- and medium-SR ANFs with CN choppers, it is clear from cross-correlation analysis of ANF-CN chopper unit pairs (Young and Sachs, 1988) that choppers receive inputs from high-SR units as well. Under the selective listening hypothesis this high-SR input would account for the low stimulus level (25 dB) responses illustrated at the bottom of Fig. 5.

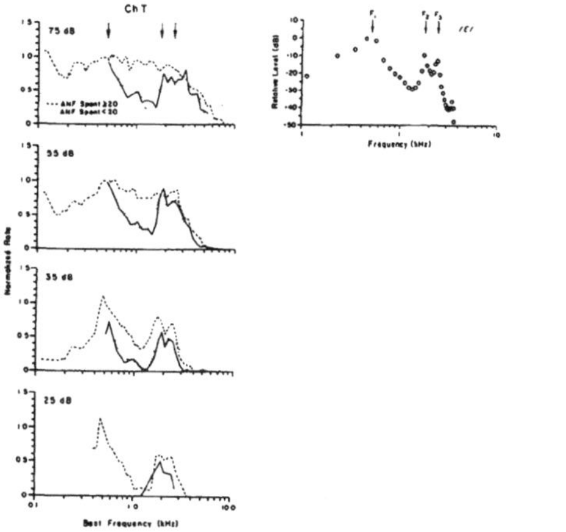

Fig. 5 Normalized average rate plotted vs. BF for high-SR ANFs (dashed lines), low and medium SR ANFs (dotted lines), and ChT units (solid lines). (Redrawn from Blackburn and Sachs, 1991).

An important functional difference between primarylike and chopper units is found in their ability to phase-lock to tones. The ability of choppers to phase-lock is limited to lower frequencies than is that of primarylike units (Blackburn and Sachs, 1989; Bourk, 1976; Rhode and Smith, 1986). The dependence of phase-locking on stimulus frequency in primarylike units is similar to that found for ANFs (Blackburn and Sachs, 1989; Bourk, 1976; Johnson, 1980; Rhode and Smith, 1986). In both cases, phase locking is maximum and roughly constant at frequencies below about 1.0 kHz., falls to half maximum at about 2.5 kHz, and is unmeasurable above about 6.0 kHz. Thus, very little temporal information is lost across the auditory nerve to bushy cells synapse. This efficiency in transmitting temporal information is related both to the large, secure synaptic endings on the bushy cell soma and to specializations of the postsynaptic cell membrane which allow it to follow rapid changes in synaptic potentials (Oertel, 1983).

Phase-locking in choppers, on the other hand, declines at frequencies above 100 Hz and is very much smaller than that of primarylike units at higher frequencies. This loss of phase locking in choppers is consistent with the dendritic configuration of the stellate cells. The effect of large dendritic trees on synaptic inputs far from the soma can be viewed as a low pass filter effect (Koch, 1984; Young et al., 1988b). For example, under assumptions consistent with what is known about stellate cell membrane properties, Young et al. (1988b) have computed the voltage response at the soma to a current source located on a dendritic tree one and a half space constants from the soma. At a frequency of 1.0 kHz, the soma voltage

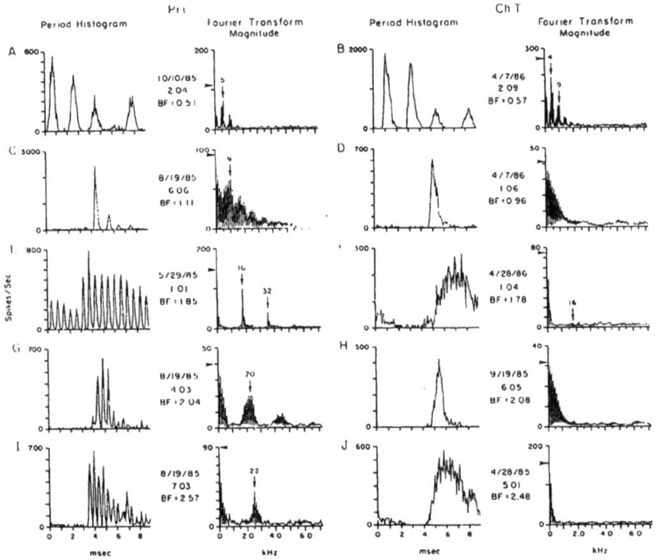

Fig. 6 Period histograms and Fourier transform magnitudes for primarylike and chopper units with /ɛ/ as the stimulus. (Redrawn from Blackburn and Sachs, 1990.)

is attenuated more than 40 dB relative to the voltage generated by a 1.0 kHz current applied directly to the soma.

Fig. 6 compares the temporal representation for /ɛ/ in a number of primarylike units with those in chopper units. They are arranged so that each row has data from units with similar BFs. Period histograms are shown in the left columns and Fourier transform magnitudes are shown in the right columns for each unit type. The responses of primarylike units with BFs near the formant frequencies are strongly phase-locked to the formant frequencies, as would be expected on the basis of their ability to phase-lock to tones in this frequency region. At the stimulus level shown, units with BFs between the formants are phase-locked to stimulus components near their BFs. All of the histograms show envelope modulations locked to the pitch period of the stimulus; the envelope modulation of the units with BFs between the formants is stronger than that at the formants. The period histograms of these primarylike units resemble those of corresponding ANFs in Fig. 2.

Like primarylike units, chopper units with BFs near the first formant are phase-locked to stimulus components near that frequency. However, the period histograms of choppers with BFs above the first formant have envelopes locked to the vowel fundamental but do not show the higher frequency oscillations that would reflect phase-locking to frequencies above the first formant. The period histograms of these units resemble the envelopes of the corresponding period histograms for primarylike units. In particular the envelopes of responses of both primarylike and choppers with BFs between the formants are sharper than those with BFs near one of the formant peaks. The failure of choppers to phase-lock to frequencies above the first formant is expected on the basis of their poor phase-locking to BF tones at these frequencies.

The ALSRs for primarylike and chopper units reflect the differences illustrated in Fig. 6. Fig. 7 shows ALSRs for two types of choppers (ChT and ChS; see Blackburn and Sachs (1989) for definition of chopper types) and for primarylike units. While the ALSR for the primarylike units resembles that for the ANFs, in that there are clear peaks at the second and third formant frequencies, there are no such peaks in the chopper ALSRs. The trough in the ChT ALSR just below the second formant frequency can be attributed to the corresponding trough in the rate-place profile shown above in Fig. 5 (Blackburn and Sachs, 1990).

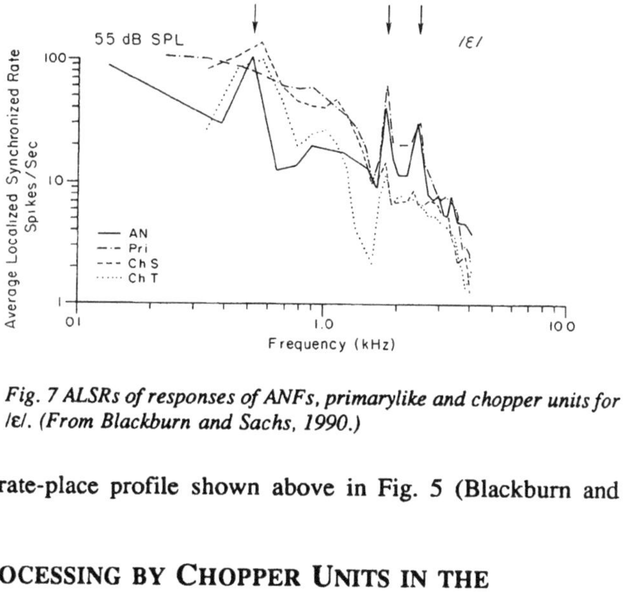

Fig. 7 ALSRs of responses of ANFs, primarylike and chopper units for /ɛ/. (From Blackburn and Sachs, 1990.)

4. Model for Signal Processing by Chopper Units in the Anteroventral Cochlear Nucleus

We have illustrated two important signal processing properties of AVCN chopper units: they maintain a robust rate-place representation of vowel spectra over a range of stimulus levels that encompasses the range of operation of the high- and low-SR ANFs in a manner consistent with the selective listening hypothesis, and they do not maintain a temporal representation of spectra at frequencies above the first formant frequencies. In this section we discuss these properties in terms of a model for the stellate cell, from which chopper responses are recorded (Rhode et al., 1983; Roullier and Ryugo, 1984; Smith and Rhode, 1989).

One way in which selective listening could be accomplished involves inhibitory inputs to stellate cells. In the model suggested by Winslow et al. (1987), stellate cells receive on-BF inputs from high-SR ANFs distally on their dendritic trees, inhibitory inputs more proximally from either off-BF high-SR or on-BF low-SR ANFs via an inhibitory interneuron, and excitatory inputs from low-SR ANFs near the soma. At low sound levels the only active inputs are the excitatory high-SR ANFs. At high levels, the inhibitory inputs are activated (either by spread of excitation to off-BF ANFs or to high-threshold low-SR on-BF units) and the high-SR inputs are effectively isolated from the spike generating mechanisms of the soma. The responses are thus dominated by the low-SR excitatory inputs near the soma at high sound levels. Such a model is similar to the one suggested for retinal ganglion cell motion processing by Koch and Poggio (1986).

Motivated by this conceptual model, Banks and Sachs (1991) constructed a simulation model of a chopper unit. The model cell (Fig. 8a) is a hypothetical "exemplar cell" that was constructed on the basis of descriptions of CN chopper cells that had been filled with HRP (Rhode et al., 1983; Roullier and Ryugo, 1984). The basic electrical parameters chosen are within the range of the standard values (Rall, 1977; Rall, 1989), adjusted to fit intracellular records and data. These parameters yield time constants and input resistances that are close to those recently estimated for stellate cells on the basis of responses to current injection (White et al., 1990). The dendritic tree of the hypothetical exemplar cell can be collapsed into a single equivalent cylinder (Rall, 1977; Rall, 1989); the cylinder is separated into 10 compartments of equal electrotonic length ($\Delta Z = 0.1$).

The model used for the dendritic compartments is similar to the one developed by Rall (1977). As illustrated in Fig. 8b, Banks models isopotential sections of the dendritic cylinder as electrical circuits with four branches: a resting branch with battery $E_r = 62$ mv and resting conductance $g_r = 0.25 \times 10^{-8}$ S; a capacitive branch with $C_i = 0.75 \times 10^{-4}$ F; an excitatory input branch with battery $E_e = 0$ mv and conductance $g_e(t)$; and an inhibitory input branch with battery $E_j = E_{Cl} = -68$ mv (Wu and Oertel, 1986) and conductance $g_j(t)$. The compartments are connected to one another by axial conductances $g_{ij} = 2.48 \times 10^{-7}$S. The soma is modeled as an electrical circuit with a leakage branch, a capacitive branch, excitatory and inhibitory input branches (identical to the dendritic input branches), and two branches with voltage and time dependent Na^+ and K^+ conductances comprising the spike generator. The axonal segment is modeled as a single compartment with circuit branches nearly identical to the somatic compartment but with no input branches. The spike generating mechanism used is a slight modification of the model proposed by Hodgkin and Huxley (1952). It consists of a fast, inactivating sodium conductance $g_{Na}(V,t)$, a slower, delayed rectifier potassium conductance $g_r(V,t)$, and a linear leakage conductance g_l.

Excitatory and inhibitory inputs to each compartment are similar to shot noise (Papoulis, 1965) with alpha-wave conductance impulse responses; the underlying input processes used by Banks are nonstationary Poisson processes modified by a deadtime $t_d = 1.2$ ms (Young and Barta, 1986). We have recently modified the model so that the input process can be the sequence of spike times recorded experimentally from an ANF. The amplitudes and time

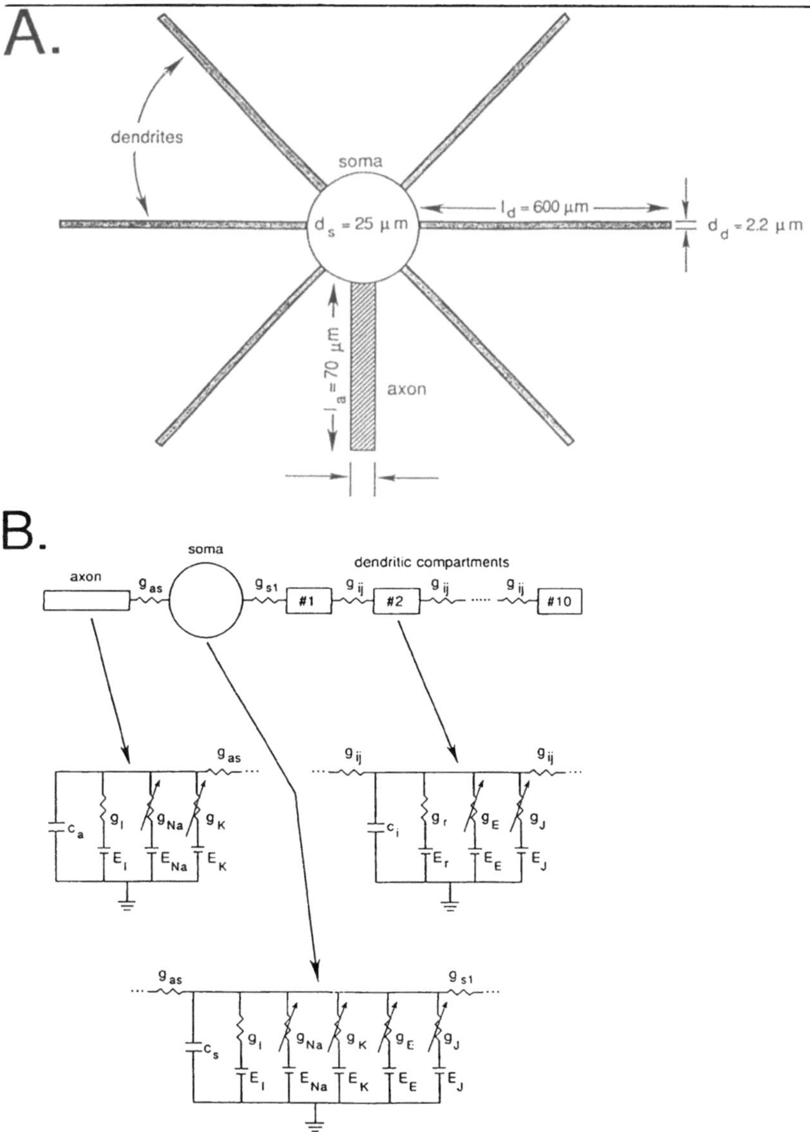

Fig. 8 (a) Schematic diagram of the "exemplar" cell showing six dendrites, axonal segment and soma and the anatomical parameters relevant to the model. (b). Top: Compartmental model with axon compartment connected by axial conductance g_{as} to the soma, the soma connected by axial conductance g_{s1} to compartment #1 and so on. Bottom: The corresponding electrical circuit representations for the axon compartment, the soma and the ith dendritic compartment. (From Banks and Sachs, 1991).

course of the alpha waves are set to give EPSPs and IPSPs at the soma comparable to those reported *in vitro* (Oertel, 1983; Oertel et al., 1988; Wu and Oertel, 1984; Wu and Oertel, 1986). Fig. 9a shows the PST histogram of the model output, which has an easily discernible chopping pattern. The peaks disappear after about 20 ms because of accumulated jitter in the output spike times.

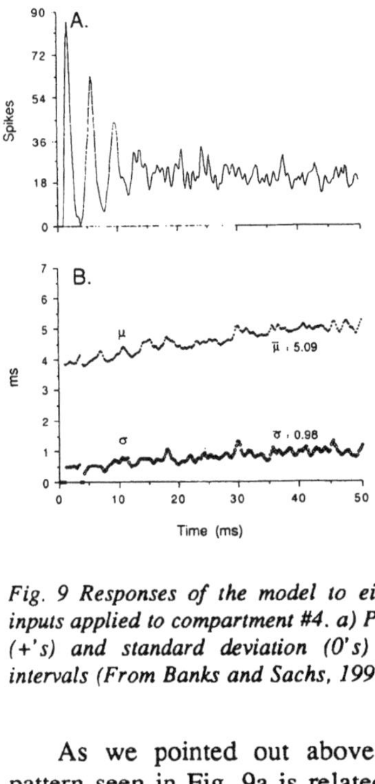

Fig. 9 Responses of the model to eight excitatory inputs applied to compartment #4. a) PSTH. b) Mean (+'s) and standard deviation (0's) of interspike intervals (From Banks and Sachs, 1991).

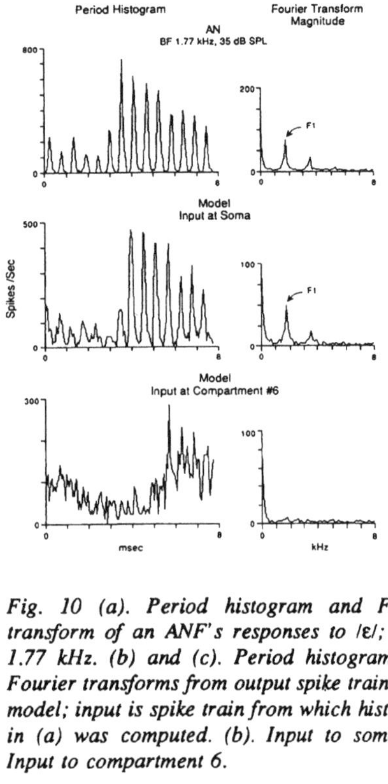

Fig. 10 (a). Period histogram and Fourier transform of an ANF's responses to /ε/; BF = 1.77 kHz. (b) and (c). Period histograms and Fourier transforms from output spike train of the model; input is spike train from which histogram in (a) was computed. (b). Input to soma. (c). Input to compartment 6.

As we pointed out above, the chopping pattern seen in Fig. 9a is related to the regular firing pattern of the chopper units. As shown in Fig. 9b there is little variability in the mean interspike interval throughout the stimulus duration (ratio of standard deviation to mean interval, (μ/σ) is 0.19). This very regular firing pattern is in contrast to that seen in ANFs where μ/σ is typically 0.7 or greater (Young et al., 1988a). This transformation from irregular to regular firing patterns is easily interpreted in terms of this model. The statistical properties of the model output change in a predictable manner when the number or location of excitatory inputs is varied. A large number of distally located inputs result in an output process that is extremely regular, while fewer, proximally located inputs elicit a much less regular response. Inputs farther from the soma are subject to greater low-pass filtering by the dendritic tree so that the somatic membrane potential, which is the input to the spike generator, resulting from distal inputs has a smoother waveform than that resulting from proximal inputs. Hence the output spike train is more regular for distal inputs. The effect of convergence reflects the increased regularity of the conductance input signal (Banks and Sachs, 1991; Goldberg and Brownell, 1973; Molnar and Pfeiffer, 1968).

The effects of dendritic low-pass filtering can also produce the reduction in phase-locking in choppers observed in Fig. 6 (Young et al., 1988b). Fig. 10a shows the period histogram for the responses to the vowel /ε/ of an auditory-nerve fiber with BF near the second formant frequency. The unit is phase-locked to the second formant and its histogram shows strong envelope modulation at the fundamental frequency. Figs. 10b and c show period histograms computed from the output of the model; the input is the spike train from which the histogram in Fig. 10A was computed. In Fig. 10b the input spike train is applied directly to the soma in the model and the output in this case is similar to the input in that it is phase-locked to the second formant and shows envelope modulation at the fundamental. On the other hand, if the input is moved distally on the dendritic tree to compartment four, as in Fig. 10c, phase-locking to the second formant is lost because of dendritic filtering and the only phase-locking is to the fundamental frequency as is the case for the chopper units shown in Fig. 6.

We have not explored the behavior of this model in detail with respect to the selective listening hypothesis. However, we have obtained some model results related to the effects of proximal inhibitory input on excitatory responses that resemble some recent experimental results on the effects of adding off-BF inputs to BF tones (Banks and Sachs, 1991; Blackburn and Sachs, 1991).

Acknowledgements

This work was supported by research and training grants from the National Institute of Deafness and other Communications Disorders.

Summary

Vowel spectra are encoded in the auditory-nerve in terms of rate-place and temporal-place representations. Populations of primarylike units in AVCN preserve the temporal place code, whereas chopper units do not. Auditory-nerve rate-place representation is viable only if the CNS listens selectively to low-SR units at high sound levels. Populations of chopper units could be performing such a process in that their rate-place representation closely resembles that of low-SR ANFs at high sound levels. Properties of chopper units are well summarized in terms of a simple model of dendritic processing.

References

Banks, M.I. and Sachs, M.B. (1991). Regularity analysis in a compartmental model of chopper units in the anteroventral cochlear nucleus, *J. Neurophysiol.*, 65, 606-629.

Blackburn, C.C. and Sachs, M.B. (1989). Classification of unit types in the anteroventral cochlear nucleus: post-stimulus time histograms and regularity analysis, *J. Neurophysiol.*, 62, 1303-1329.

Blackburn, C.C. and Sachs, M.B. (1990) The representations of the steady-state vowel /eh/ in the discharge patterns of cat anteroventral cochlear nucleus neurons, *J. Neurophysiol.*, 63, 1191-1212.

Blackburn, C.C. and Sachs, M.B. (1991). Effects of off-BF tones on the responses of chopper units in the ventral cochlear nucleus. I: Regularity and temporal adaptation patterns, *J. Neurophysiol.*, in press.

Bourk, T.R. (1976). *Electrical Responses of Neural Units in the Anteroventral Cochlear Nucleus of the Cat*, Ph.D. Thesis, Massachusetts Institute of Technology.

Cant, N.B. and Morest, D.K. (1984). The structural basis for stimulus coding in the cochlear Nucleus of the cat, in: *Hearing Science Recent Advances*, edited by C.I Berlin, San Diego: College Hill Press, 371-422.

Delgutte, B. (1982). Some correlates of phonetic distinctions at the level of the auditory nerve, in: *The representation of speech in the peripheral auditory system*, edited by Carlson, R. and Granstrom, B. Amsterdam: Elsevier Biomedical Press, 131-149.

Delgutte, B. and Kiang, N.Y.S. (1984a). Speech coding in the auditory nerve: IV. Sounds with consonant-like dynamic characteristics, *J. Acoust. Soc. Am.*, 75, 897-907.

Delgutte, B. and Kiang, N.Y.S. (1984b). Speech coding in the auditory nerve: I. Vowel-like sounds, *J. Acoust. Soc. Am.*, 75, 866-878.

Goldberg, J.M. and Brownell, W.E. (1973). Discharge characteristics of neurons in anteroventral and dorsal cochlear nuclei of cat, *Brain Res.*, 64, 35-54.

Hodgkin, A.L. and Huxley, A.F.A (1952). Quantitative description of membrane current and its application to conduction and excitation in nerve, *J. Physiol. (Lond.)*, 117, 500-544.

Johnson, D.H. (1980). The relationship between spike rate and synchrony in responses of auditory-nerve fibers to single tones, *J. Acoust. Soc. Am.*, 68, 1115-1122.

Koch, C. and Poggio, T. (1986). Computations in the vertebrate retina: motion discrimination, gain enhancement and differentiation, *Trends Neurosci.*, 9, 204-211.

Liberman, M.C. (1978). Auditory-nerve responses from cats raised in a low-noise chamber, *J. Acoust. Soc. Am.*, 63, 442-455.

Miller, M.I. and Sachs, M.B. (1983). Representation of stop consonants in the discharge patterns of auditory-nerve fibers, *J. Acoust. Soc. Am.*, 74, 502-517.

Molnar, C.E. and Pfeiffer, R.R. (1968). Interpretation of spontaneous spike discharge patterns in neurons of the cochlear nucleus, *Proc. IEEE*, 56, 993-1004.

Oertel, D. (1983). Synaptic responses and electrical properties of cells in brain slices of the mouse anteroventral cochlear nucleus. *J. Neuroscience*, 3, 2043-2053.

Oertel, D., Wu, S.H., and Hirsch, J.A. (1988). Electrical characteristics of cells and neuronal circuitry in the cochlear nuclei studied with intracellular recording from brain slices, in: *Auditory Function.*, edited by Edelman, G.M., Gall, W.E., and Cowan, W.M. New York: John Wiley and Sons.

Palmer, A.R. and Evans, E.F. (1980). Cochlear fiber rate intensity functions: no evidence for basilar membrane nonlinearities, *Hear. Res.*, 2, 319-326.

Palmer, A.R., Winter, I.M., and Darwin, C.J. (1986). The representation of steady-state vowel sounds in the temporal discharge patterns of the guinea pig cochlear nerve and primary-like cochlear nucleus neurons, *J. Acoust. Soc. Am.*, 79, 100-113.

Papoulis, A. (1965). *Probability, Random Variables and Stochastic Processes,* New York: McGraw Hill.

Rall, W. (1977). Core conductor theory and cable properties of neurons, in: *Handbook of Physiology - The Nervous System.,* edited by Kandel, E. and Geiger, S. Washington, D.C.: Am. Physiol. Soc., 39-97.

Rall, W. (1989). Cable theory for dendritic neurons, in: *Methods in Neuronal Modeling.,* edited by Koch, E. and Segev, I. Cambridge, Massachusetts: MIT Press, 9-62.

Rhode, W.S., Oertel, D., and Smith, P.H. (1983). Physiological response properties of cells labeled intracellularly with horseradish peroxidase in cat ventral cochlear nucleus, *J. Comp. Neurol,* 213, 448-463.

Rhode, W.S. and Smith, P.H. (1986). Encoding timing and intensity in the ventral cochlear nucleus of the cat, *J. Neurophysiol.,* 56, 261-286.

Romand, R. (1978). Survey of intracellular recording in the cochlear nucleus of the cat, *Brain Res.,* 148, 43-65.

Roullier, E.M. and Ryugo, D.K. (1984). Intracellular marking of physiologically characterized cells in the ventral cochlear nucleus of the cat, *J. Comp. Neurol.,* 255, 167-186.

Sachs, M.B. and Abbas, P.J. (1974). Rate versus level functions for auditory nerve fibers in cats: tone-burst stimuli, *J. Acoust. Soc. Am.,* 81, 680-691.

Sachs, M.B. and Blackburn, C.C. (1988). Rate-place and temporal-place representations of vowels in the auditory-nerve and anteroventral cochlear nucleus, *J. Phonetics,* 16, 37-43.

Sachs, M.B., Winslow, R.L., and Sokolowski, B.A.H. (1989). A computational model for rate-level functions from cat auditory-nerve fibers, *Hear. Res.,* 41.

Sachs, M.B. and Young, E.D. (1979). Encoding of steady-state vowels in the auditory nerve: Representation in terms of discharge rate, *J. Acoust. Soc. Am.,* 66, 470-479.

Schalk, T.B. and Sachs, M.B. (1980). Nonlinearities in auditory-nerve fiber responses to bandlimited noise, *J. Acoust. Soc. Am.,* 67, 903-913.

Smith, P.H. and Rhode, W.S. (1989). Structural and functional properties distinguish two types of multipolar cells in the ventral cochlear nucleus, *J. Comp. Neurol.,* 282, 595-616.

White, J.A., Young, E.D., and Manis, P.B. (1990). Application of new electrotonic modeling methods: Results from Type I cells in guinea pig ventral cochlear nucleus, *Soc. Neuro. Abs.,* 16, 870.

Winslow, R.L., Barta, P.E., and Sachs, M.B. (1987). Rate coding in the auditory nerve, in: *Auditory Processing of Complex Sounds.,* edited by Yost, W.A. and Watson, C.S. Hillsdale, N.J.: Lawrence Erlbaum Assoc., 212-224.

Wu, S.H. and Oertel, D. (1984). Intracellular injection with horseradish peroxidase of physiologically characterized stellate and bushy cells in slices of mouse anteroventral cochlear nucleus, *J. Neuroscience,* 4, 1577-1588.

Wu, S.H. and Oertel, D. (1986). Inhibitory circuitry in the ventral cochlear nucleus is probably mediated by glycine, *J. Neuroscience,* 6, 2691-2706.

Young, E.D. and Barta, P.E. (1986). Rate responses of auditory-nerve fibers to tones in noise near masked threshold, *J. Acoust. Soc. Am.,* 79, 426-442.

Young, E.D., Robert, J.M., and Shofner, W.P. (1988a). Regularity and latency of units in the ventral cochlear nucleus: implications for unit classification and generation of response properties, *J. Neurophysiol.,* 60, 1-29.

Young, E.D. and Sachs, M.B. (1979). Representation of steady-state vowels in the temporal aspects of the discharge patterns of populations of auditory-nerve fibers, *J. Acoust. Soc. Am.*, 66, 1381-1403.

Young, E.D. and Sachs, M.B. (1988). Interactions of auditory nerve fibers and cochlear nucleus cells studied with cross-correlation, *Soc. Neuro. Abs.*, 14, 646.

Nonlinearities in the Peripheral Encoding of Spectral Notches

P.A.J. Oomens,
A.J. Breed,
E. de Boer
Laboratory of Auditory Physics, D2-211
Academical Medical Centre
Meibergdreef 9
1105 AZ, Amsterdam
The Netherlands

M.E.H. Schouten
Research Institute for Language and Speech
University of Utrecht
Trans 10, 3512 JK Utrecht
The Netherlands

1. Introduction

The transformation from sound pressure at the tympanic membrane to discharge patterns in the auditory nerve involves nonlinear properties of the transduction system, especially if both strong and weak frequency components are simultaneously present. Sinex and Geisler (1984) suggested that one function of peripheral suppression may be to enhance the neural representation of spectral features such as formants. Earlier, the same suggestion had been made by Houtgast (1974), after a psychoacoustical study with vowel-like sounds. Spectral enhancement of formants relative to the 'valleys' in between was supposed to assist spectral analysis at more central levels.

This study investigates whether spectral contrasts in strongly stylized stimuli are encoded in a nonlinear way. The spectra of these stimuli were derived from those of nasal consonants. Nasal consonants are characterized by the presence of a strong antiformant, due to resonances of the nasal cavity. The net effect of interacting resonances and antiresonances is a band of low amplitude in the steady-state spectrum. The antiformants of [m] (around 800- 1000 Hz), [n] (around 1500-2000 Hz), as well as [ng] (above 3000 Hz) are likely to function as an acoustic cue for place of articulation. Considering nasal-vowel transitions, Kurowski and Blumstein (1987) have shown that there is a major spectral change in lower frequency regions for labial nasals, and for high frequencies in alveolar nasals. Thus, the presence of a spectral zero may be expected to be an important cue in the perception of nasals.

In our stimuli this spectral zero was simulated by band-filtering pseudo-random noise symmetrically around the characteristic frequencies (CF) of the nerve fibres. Firstly, we investigated how these spectral 'notches' are encoded in each nerve fibre. Secondly, we wanted to assess in a quantitative way how enhanced frequency components at the lower edge of the notch interfere with the encoding of the notch. The enhanced edges can be interpreted as abstract versions of a formant-like structure.

2. METHODS

Single auditory-nerve fibre recordings were made with glass microelectrodes from five Mongolian gerbils (Meriones unguiculatus, 12-18 months old). The auditory nerve of the right ear was exposed by a ventral approach (Sokolich, 1977; Chamberlain, 1977). Animals were anaesthetized by a combination of Nembutal® and Thalamonal®.

All stimuli were based upon pseudo-random noise centred around the CF (the spectrum extended from 0.1 CF to 3.0 CF). Four sets of stimuli were constructed.

The first set contained only one element: flat-spectrum noise. The second set contained four elements: noise with the same spectrum except for a spectral notch which was 0.05 CF, 0.1 CF, 0.15 CF, or 0.2 CF wide and was at least 50 dB below the overall spectral level. Each notch was symmetrically placed around CF. The spectral edges of the notches had a slope of more than 100 dB per octave. The third set contained four stimuli with the same spectrum as the first set except for a spectral peak of 0.01 CF width and 10 dB height above the overall spectral level at 0.975 CF, 0.950 CF, 0.925 CF, or 0.900 CF. The fourth set contained four stimuli that had both a notch and a peak as in the second and in the third set; the peak was immediately adjacent to the notch.

The stimuli were presented at three levels of intensity: 20, 40, and 60 dB SPL/third-octave. The lowest level at which a stimulus was presented had to be at least 10 dB higher than the threshold for pure tones at CF. In the recording sessions the centre frequency of the notch was scaled to the CF of the fibre under study.

All stimuli were made to contain only odd-order frequency components so that the waveform in one period was an antisymmetrical function of time. The responses to repeated presentations of the stimuli were accumulated in histograms with a length of 4096 bins. For each histogram 6144 spikes were collected. The second half of the histogram was subtracted from the first half to remove even-order nonlinearities. From these combined histograms autocorrelation functions (512 bins to each side) were computed, which were windowed with a raised cosine taper and Fourier transformed to obtain power spectra. Each power spectrum was normalized by dividing it by the spectrum of the response to the flat-spectrum control stimulus. This normalization made it possible to compare the responses of different fibres irrespective of the shape of their tuning curves.

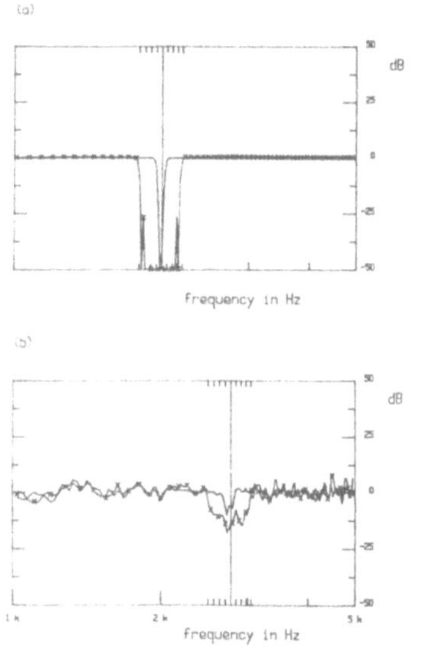

***Fig. 1** (a) Spectra of two notched stimuli. Relative notch is 50 dB.*
(b) Corresponding response spectra from a fibre with a CF of 2712 Hz.

3. RESULTS

In Fig. 1 the spectra of two stimuli and their responses are compared. In Fig. 1a the spectra of the stimuli are presented. The notches are 0.05 CF and 0.2 CF. We can observe small disturbances at the sides of the spectral edge, just within the notch. The disturbances have no consequences for the analyses that we performed on the spectra. Fig. 1b shows an example of response spectra to these stimuli from a fibre with a CF of 2712 Hz. The difference between components inside and outside the notch is much smaller in the responses than it is in the stimuli. The 50 dB contrast is reduced to some 10-15 dB in the nerve fibres.

Fig. 2a shows the "contrast reduction" in dB (vertical axis) between the stimuli and the nerve fibre responses for the four "dipwidths", and for each presentation level (different symbols). It is clear that presentation level has no influence on contrast reduction, which is generally between 35 and 45 dB.

Fig. 2b contains the results of the third stimulus set, in which a spectral peak was introduced at specified distances from CF; the figure shows that such a peak had no effect on the response (a difference of 0 dB).

In Fig. 2c, we see the effect of combining a spectral notch with a spectral peak. Contrast reduction is still considerable for a nerve fibre at CF, but it is somewhat smaller than in Fig. 2a, where only a notch was present. This means that the spectral peak caused a reduction of the response at CF, in the centre of the notch; this is probably a form of suppression. Fig. 3 gives a clearer picture of this suppressive effect: it displays the differences (averaged over presentation levels) between the response to stimuli with only a notch and stimuli with both a notch and a peak. In most cases, the suppressive effect of the peak is of the order of 5 dB. The effect is almost independent of notch width.

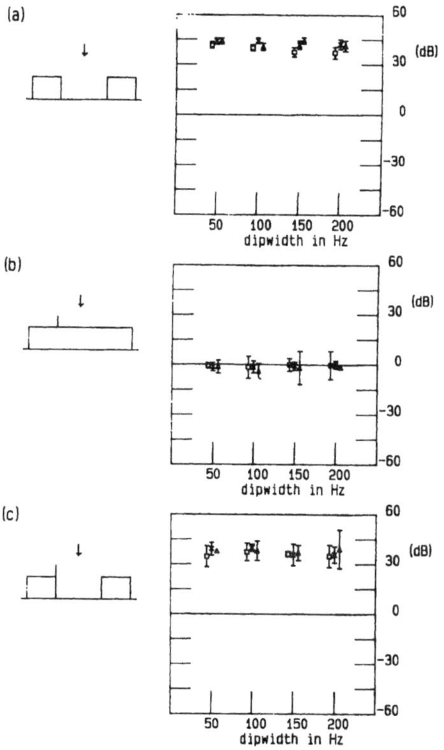

Fig. 2 Contrast reduction in dB from stimulus to response when one or two components are added to a pseudo-random noise stimulus. (a) A notch of 50 dB produces a response at CF that is 35-45 dB less deep - a contrast reduction of 5-15 dB. (b) A spectral peak at 50, 100, 150, or 200 Hz below CF has no effect on the response at CF. (c) The combination of a notch and a peak leads to a smaller contrast reduction (i.e. a greater contrast) than a notch by itself. Squares indicate stimulation at 20 dB(SPL), crosses at 40 dB(SPL), and triangles at 60 dB(SPL).

4. Discussion

We have observed a net reduction of the contrast between components within and outside spectral notches to as little as 10-15 dB at the level of a single fibre. However, a simulation study with a poisson noise generator indicated that this is to be expected if the generation of spikes in the nerve fibres is a poisson process. This does not mean that the signal-to-noise ratio in the firing of the nerve fibre is 10-15 dB because in our experiments as well as in our simulations we accumulated the spikes over near to a hundred presentations. One may ask whether the timing information is of any interest because of the very poor signal-to-noise ratio in the nerve fibre itself. If, however, it is assumed that the timing information of a few hundred fibres is summed somewhere in the brain, it can be speculated that a signal-to-noise ratio that is not too different from what is presented here could be achieved.

One point that has not been mentioned so far is the generation of even-order distortion products by the rectification that occurs in the hair cells of the inner ear. Inevitably, even-order distortion products are present in the response of the auditory nerve to broad-band noise. In this study they have been eliminated, as explained in the methods section.

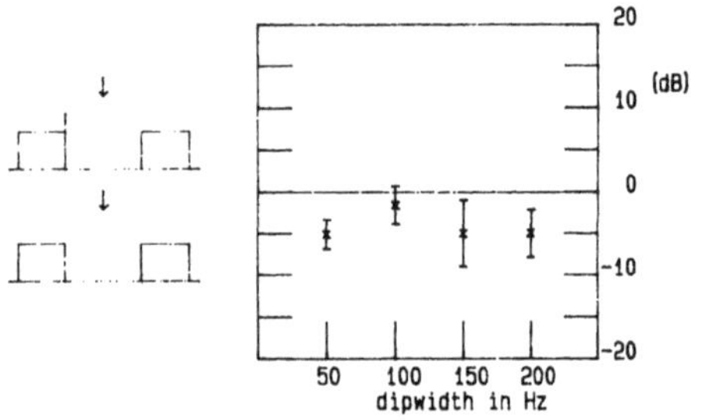

Fig. 3 Spectral quotients between [+peak+notch] and [+notch]. The values of this plot summarize the specific effect of edge enhancement upon centre components within the notches.

We have been able to show that a formant-like peak at the lower edge of a notched noise suppresses components that occur in the notch next to it. This effect improves auditory contrasts between frequency components inside and outside the notch. The suppressive effect of formant-like features may be a first step to overcome effects of noisy signal transmission in the auditory periphery.

Acknowledgements

We would like to thank Luc-Johan Kanis for being a resisting opponent in numerous discussions and M.B. Sachs and O. Ghitza for their valuable comments after the presentation.

References

Chamberlain, S.C. (1977). Neuroanatomical aspects of the gerbil inner ear: light microscopic observations, *J. Comp. Neur.*, 171, 193-204.

Houtgast, T. (1974). *Lateral Suppression in Hearing* (Free University, Amsterdam).

Kurowski, K. and Blumstein, S.E. (1987). Acoustic properties for place of articulation in nasal consonants, *J. Acoust. Soc. Am.*, 81, 1917-1927.

Oomens, P.A.J. (1991). *Peripheral encoding of nasal-like stimuli. Physiological and psychophysical investigations*, Laboratory of Auditory Physics, Amsterdam

Sinex D.G. and Geisler, C.D. (1984). Comparison of the responses of auditory nerve-fibers to consonant-vowel syllables with predictions from linear models, *J. Acoust. Soc. Am.*, 76, 116-121.

Sokolich, W. (1977). Some electrophysiological evidence for a polarity-opposition mechanism of interaction between inner and outer hair cells in the cochlea, *Special Report* (ISR-S-15), Institute for Sensory Research, Syracuse University, NY, USA.

Auditory Models as Preprocessors for Speech Recognition

Roy D. Patterson,
John Holdsworth, and
Michael Allerhand
MRC Applied Psychology Unit
15 Chaucer Road
Cambridge CB2 2EF UK

1. Introduction

Over the past decade, hearing scientists have developed a number of time-domain models of the processing performed by the cochlea in an effort to develop a reasonably accurate multi-channel representation of the pattern of neural activity flowing from the cochlea up the auditory nerve to the cochlear nucleus. When these models are applied to speech sounds, the neural activity patterns of vowel sounds reveal an elaborate formant structure that is absent in the more traditional representation of speech -- the spectrogram. This has led to the suggestion that the performance of speech recognition systems could be improved if their traditional spectrographic preprocessors were replaced by a comprehensive auditory preprocessor. In the first part of this paper we review several of these auditory models and argue that some form of periodicity-sensitive temporal integration should be included in the auditory preprocessing.

Speech scientists are typically receptive to the concept of auditory models as preprocessors for speech sounds until they realise that the data rate at the output of these auditory models is on the order of 1-10 megabyte per second (Mbps). Speech scientists concerned with developing recognition systems that might become practical some time this decade are working with input data rates on the order of 1-10 Kbps! The data rates and the reasons for the discrepancy between the auditory and speech rates are presented in the second part of the paper. In the third and final part of the paper, we describe a method for reducing the data rate of the auditory representation of speech. The result is a Stabilised Auditory Spectrogram (SAS) that has the same data rate as the traditional spectrogram and which can be compared directly with it in terms of the recognition performance that it supports.

2. Cochlear Models and Auditory Images

A variety of computational models of cochlear processing have been developed to provide representations of the complex neural activity patterns that arise in the auditory nerve in response to broadband sounds like speech and music (Lyon, 1982, 1984; Lyon and Dyer, 1986; Seneff, 1988; Shamma, 1988; Deng, Geisler and Greenberg, 1988; Ghitza, 1988; Assmann and Summerfield, 1990; Patterson and Holdsworth, 1991; Patterson and Hirahara, 1989; Meddis and Hewitt, 1991a). In each case, the cochlea simulation is composed of an auditory filterbank which simulates the motion of the basilar partition, and some form of compressive adaptation which simulates neural transduction.

2.1 Spectral Analysis: The Auditory Filterbank

The auditory filterbanks of these models all reflect our knowledge of cochlear filtering inasmuch as the bandwidths of filters increase quasi-logarithmically with the centre frequency of the filter, and the filters are distributed across frequency in proportion to filter bandwidth. The filterbanks have many channels when the modellers are primarily concerned with the accuracy of the simulation (Lyon, 92; Shamma, 128; Assman and Summerfield, 256; Deng, Geisler and Greenberg, 1400!), and many fewer channels when the models are intended for use as speech preprocessors (Seneff, 40; Ghitza, 43; Patterson and Hirahara, 32).

The output of an 87 channel auditory filterbank in response to four cycles of the vowel /æ/ from the word 'hat' is presented in Fig. 1. Each line in the Fig. shows the output of an individual auditory filter. In the low-frequency channels, where the auditory filter is relatively narrow, the output is essentially sinusoidal in shape, indicating that the filter has isolated a harmonic of the fundamental frequency. In this vowel, the fundamental is close to 125 Hz and the lowest harmonic in the figure is the second harmonic (250 Hz), which is seen to rise and fall twice per cycle of the wave. The first formant of the vowel falls in the region of the fourth and fifth harmonics which are those that have the greatest amplitude in the lower half of the figure. The fact that these harmonics are largely resolved shows that the vocal resonance that created this formant is broader than the auditory filters that analysed it. The width of the auditory filter increases with centre frequency and the filters that analyse the higher formants are wider than the vocal resonances that create them. As a result, the upper formants appear as sets of impulse responses, with the longest occurring in the centre of the formant and the shortest occurring between formants. The repetition rate of the pattern corresponds to the pitch of the vowel. The surface defined by the full set of lines in Fig. 1 represents basilar membrane motion (BMM) as a function of time in response to the vowel. It was generated by the gammatone auditory filterbank advocated by Patterson, Holdsworth, Nimmo-Smith and Rice (1988) and Patterson and Holdsworth (1991). These landscape displays of the microstructure of speech sounds are what led to recent attempts to use these models as speech preprocessors.

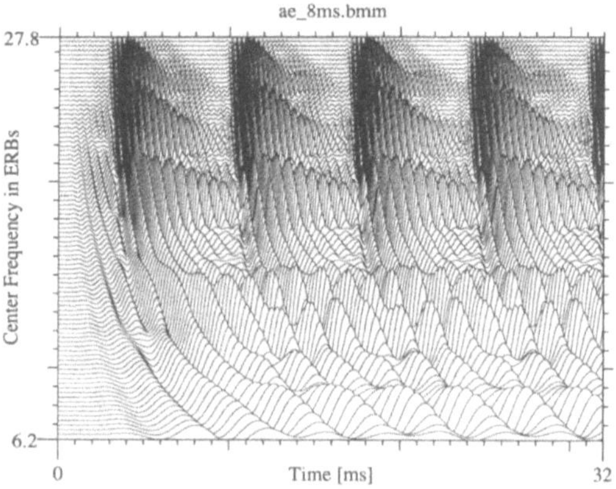

Fig. 1 Simulation of the basilar membrane motion produced in response to four cycles of the vowel /æ/, produced by a gammatone auditory filterbank. Each line shows the output of one auditory filter. The triangular concentrations of activity are the upper formants of the vowel; the repetition rate of the pattern is the voice pitch.

The shape of the BMM surface is largely determined by the bandwidth of the auditory filters and whether the filters are asymmetric, and it is primarily these parameters that distinguish auditory models functionally. With regard to bandwidth, there are two groups; those who use generally broader filters (in line with the bark scale of Zwicker, 1961), and those who use generally narrower filters (in line with the ERB scale of Glasberg and Moore, 1990). With regard to asymmetry, there are those who use highly asymmetric filters as indicated by passive basilar membrane models, and those who use mildly asymmetric filters as indicated by more recent measures of human auditory masking (see Patterson and Moore, 1986, for a review). From the point of view of a hearing scientist, these are important issues; a filterbank with relatively broad, highly asymmetric filters produces basilar membrane motion in which the formants are much less well defined than those shown in Fig. 1 (which was generated with narrow, symmetric filters). However, from the point of view of the speech scientist, these are not yet crucial issues inasmuch as broad and narrow filters yield roughly similar levels of recognition performance. For example, Robinson, Holdsworth, Patterson and Fallside (1990) contrasted a bank of 20 relatively broad filters with a bank of 36 relatively narrow filters. The recogniser size was scaled up to ensure that it had the power to handle the extra channels in the larger filterbank. Nevertheless the recognition performance of the high resolution system was identical to that of the low resolution system. To the hearing scientist, at least, this suggests that recognition systems may not yet be sufficiently sophisticated to make full use of auditory resolution. In any event, the differences between the models will not be pursued in this paper since they have not yet been shown to be critical.

2.2 Feature Enhancement: Compressive, Adaptive, Neural Transduction

The neural activity pattern in the auditory nerve is not simply a digitised version of basilar membrane motion. The strip of hair cells along the basilar membrane applies compression, rectification, adaptation, and suppression to the basilar membrane motion before passing the activity to the auditory nerve. The compression is necessitated by the large dynamic range of the basilar membrane which has to be reduced for neural transmission. Traditional speech preprocessors also include compression. By its nature, however, compression reduces contrasts within and across channels and makes features less discriminable. The suppression and adaptation processes sharpen features that appear in the compressed basilar membrane motion and so restore contrast for the larger features at the expense of smaller features. Virtually all models of auditory processing intended for use as speech preprocessors include auditory models of neural transduction. Together, the auditory filterbank and the model of neural transduction form a time-domain cochlea simulation.

The output of the cochlea simulation is intended to represent the pattern of neural activity that flows from the cochlea up the auditory nerve to the cochlear nucleus. A neural activity pattern (NAP) for the 32-ms sample of the vowel sound /æ/ is shown in Fig. 2. As is typical, there is one neural transduction unit for each channel of the auditory filterbank in this model (Patterson and Holdsworth, 1991), and thus one channel of NAP activity for each auditory filter channel. The important information concerning the precise timing of the glottal pulses and the position of the formants has been sharpened, and the neural activity away from the vowel pattern has been suppressed. Each of the small rounded pulses that form the fine structure of the NAP results from sharpening of the positive half of one cycle of a wave from one auditory filter. The base of each NAP pulse is less than half the time between pulses, indicating that the adaptation and suppression mechanisms operate at the level of the fine structure of the NAP and sharpen the individual pulses as well as the overall pattern. The process is referred to as two-dimensional adaptive thresholding since it operates in the frequency domain as well as in the time-domain. The importance of this sharpening for speech recognition will be discussed in terms of spectrograms when they are introduced in Section 3.

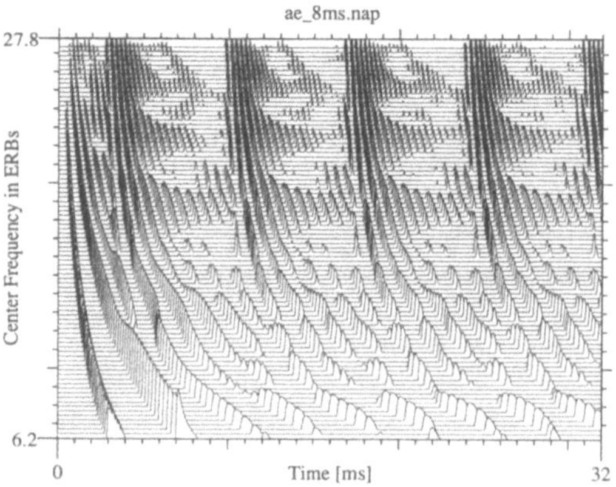

Fig. 2 Simulation of the multi-channel, neural activity pattern arriving at the cochlear nucleus in response to four cycles of the vowel /æ/, produced by applying two-dimensional adaptation to the basilar membrane motion shown in Fig. 1 The adaptation mechanism enhances the formant information and it sharpens the individual pulses of the fine structure of the pattern.

This model is typical in the sense that it provides a functional representation of the operation performed by the hair cells along the basilar membrane. The output pattern is not intended to represent the neural firing pattern that arises in single fibres of the auditory nerve. Rather, the individual rounded pulses in the fine structure of each channel of the NAP are intended to represent all of the activity that collects on the dendrites of a tonotopic unit in the cochlear nucleus. That is, it is the sum of all of the activity from all of the primary fibres connected to all of the inner hair cells associated with that part of the basilar membrane represented by one auditory filter. A physiological model which represented all of the individual primary fibres and simulated their firing pattern as well as the recombination of these firing patterns at the level of the cochlear nucleus would clearly be vastly more complex.

The model of Ghitza (1988) is a little different in that it has four primitive level-crossing detectors for each filter and the temporal intervals from each detector are analysed separately. The resulting interval distributions are, however, similar to those that would be produced by one more sophisticated transduction unit.

2.3 Auditory Image Construction: Periodicity-Sensitive Temporal Integration

The centre section of the vowel /æ/ in the word 'hat' is a highly regular sound, as can be seen in the neural activity pattern presented in Fig. 2. At the start of the period, when the glottal pulse occurs there is a burst of activity in most channels of the auditory filterbank. In the high-frequency channels associated with the third and fourth formants, the activity dies away by about the middle of the period; in the channels associated with the second and first formants the level of activity decreases after the glottal burst, but it does not decay away entirely before the next glottal pulse. From the point of view of auditory modelling, these rapid changes in the level of neural activity in the auditory nerve present a problem because they are not heard as changes in the loudness of the sound. Indeed, periodic sounds produce the most stable auditory images that we hear. If the pitch of the vowel falls, the pattern in Fig. 2 will expand and we will hear a change in the sound to a lower pitch. If the vowel begins to change and the formants move, we will also hear this change. But we do not hear the rapid fluctuations in auditory nerve activity as changes in loudness when the sound is periodic.

The fact that we hear a static image for a periodic sound indicates that some form of temporal integration (TI) has occurred prior to our initial sensation. In most models of auditory processing, a leaky integrator in the form of a lowpass filter is used to perform TI and smooth the output of the cochlea. The problem with this approach is that one needs to integrate over 5-10 cycles to get a stable output from an oscillating input, and since we hear stable images for pitches as low as 50 Hz (20-ms period), the integration time of the lowpass filter would have to be on the order of 100-200 ms. This integration time is far too long. It would smear out many small temporal changes that we hear, for example, the temporal jitter of glottal pulses that helps make a voice distinctive.

Patterson and Holdsworth (1991) have proposed a solution to the TI problem in the form of triggered, quantised, temporal integration. Briefly, the mechanism is as follows: A bank of delay lines is used to form a buffer store for the neural activity pattern flowing from the cochlea. As the neural activity proceeds down the delay lines it decays with a half life of about 20 ms so that the activity is largely attenuated by 80 ms. Each channel is assigned a TI unit which begins by monitoring the activity in the neural activity pattern as it flows past looking for large pulses. The trigger is assumed to be on the order of 5 ms into the NAP buffer away from the point where the pattern is flowing from the cochlea into the buffer. When a large pulse occurs in a given channel, it is detected by the TI unit, which then transfers the entire record in that channel of the NAP buffer to the corresponding channel of a static image buffer, where it is added, point for point, with whatever is already in that channel of the image buffer. The multi-channel result of this quantised TI process is the auditory image.

For quasi-periodic sounds, the trigger mechanism rapidly adapts to the period of the sound and initiates TI roughly once per period of the sound. In this way, it matches the TI period to the period of the sound and, much like a stroboscope, it produces a static display of the repeating temporal pattern of the NAP from the moving record flowing through the NAP buffer. What is more, it converts the NAP of a dynamic sound like a syllable with a dipthong into a flowing image in which the motion of the formants occurs at the rate that we hear the vowel change, and the grid of the pattern expands or contracts in time with the decrease or increase in pitch.

The auditory image of the vowel /æ/ is shown in Fig. 3. The pattern is similar to that which appears in the NAP because the sound is periodic. Thus, fine-structure pulses in one NAP record tend to fall at points in the image where pulses from earlier NAP records fell previously. Similarly fine-structure gaps tend to fall where gaps fell previously. Note, however, that there are important differences: The NAP is a moving record like a multi-channel chart recording flowing from a cochlea positioned at the right-hand edge of Fig. 2, and the rate of flow is very high. If the image in Fig. 3 had been reproduced to occupy about

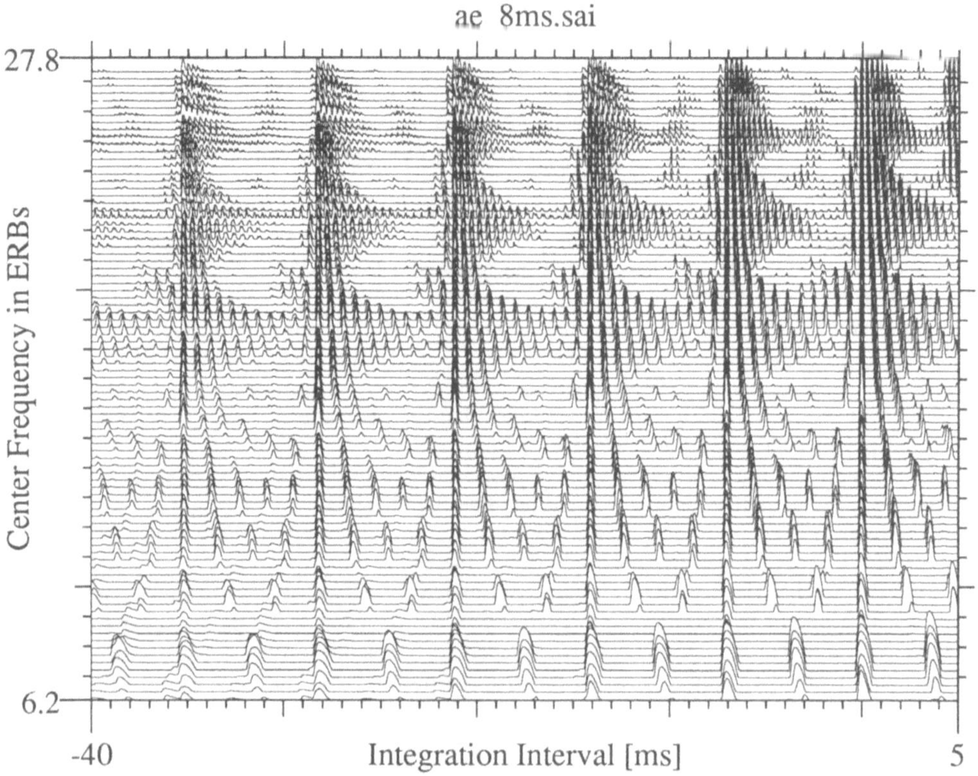

Fig. 3 An auditory image of the vowel /æ/ produced by periodicity-sensitive temporal integration of an 80-ms sample of the neural activity pattern shown in Fig. 2. The real-time display of the NAP flows very rapidly and is blurred; the auditory image is static and aligned.

half of an A4 page, the corresponding multi-channel chart recording for the vowel would flow down the NAP buffer at a rate of about 2.5 metres per second! In contrast, the auditory image is static so long as the sound is periodic, and it would seem likely that it would be much easier to extract the pattern associated with this vowel from the static image than it would to extract the same information from the fast flowing neural activity buffer.

The abscissa of the auditory image is 'temporal integration interval', that is, the time between a point in the NAP and the peak of a succeeding trigger pulse. In general terms, activity on a vertical line in the auditory image shows that there is a correlation in the sound at that temporal interval. The mechanism does not compute a correlation directly; rather, it combines events separated by a particular time interval. It superimposes NAP records that have been aligned on the larger peaks, and to the extent that these large peaks are periodic, the events combine to produce above average activity at the appropriate integration interval.

Once in the auditory image, information about past events does not move. Thus, it is at this point in the auditory image model that the fine-grain temporal information is converted to a position code and the need to preserve phase-locking in a temporal code is removed once and for all. Since the triggering and TI are done on a channel by channel basis, and since the peak of a large NAP pulse is always centred on the trigger point in the auditory image, the mechanism induces phase alignment; that is, global phase changes across channels of the neural activity pattern are removed. This form of phase alignment predicts phase sensitivity in the auditory system within reasonable limits (see Patterson, 1987b, for a review).

At every point in the auditory image, the level of activity decays continuously and exponentially with a half life of about 10 ms. As a result, transients die away quickly and the image of a periodic sound grows rapidly over the first four cycles. Thereafter, it asymptotes to a relatively fixed level as the summation and decay processes come into balance. The trigger point is assumed to be 5 ms into the NAP buffer, and the trigger point is plotted 5 ms into the auditory image buffer, in order to ensure that the activity produced by events that generate trigger pulses is represented in the auditory image and represented near the trigger point.

2.4 Alternative Periodicity-Sensitive TI Mechanisms

The auditory image model of Patterson and Holdsworth (1991) is unique in its emphasis on the temporal integration problem and the importance of periodicity-sensitive TI for the production of a good representation of our auditory images. It is not unique, however, in its production of what might be regarded as auditory images, and the recognition of the importance of having such a representation. The first identifiable auditory image appears to have been produced by Lyon (1984, Fig. 2) who implemented a version of Licklider's (1951) Duplex Theory of pitch perception. A running autocorrelation is performed on the output of each channel of Lyon's (1982) cochlea simulation and the result is plotted as a grey scale display with autocorrelation lag on the abscissa and channel centre frequency on the ordinate. Although the motivation for implementing the autocorrelation mechanism was pitch extraction, Lyon points out that the 'autocorrelogram' contains information about the position of the formants as well as the pitch. Another prototype auditory image appears in Patterson (1987a), where the output of a spiral pitch extractor was used to create a 'cylindrical timbre display' that was, in essence, a stabilised auditory image. More recently, Assmann and Summerfield (1990) and Meddis and Hewitt (1991b) have implemented modified versions of Licklider's duplex model of pitch, using a hair cell simulation developed by Meddis (1986). They have used autocorrelograms to study the perception of concurrent vowels and the images these models produce can also be regarded as auditory images.

All of these models employ a form of periodicity-sensitive TI and the resulting representations have an integration-interval dimension that provides a basis for a phase-aligned, temporal display of timbre information to reinforce the timbre information available in the frequency dimension. The main difference between the auditory image of Patterson and Holdsworth (1991) and the other forms of auditory image is that the former preserves more of the asymmetry observed in the NAP while the latter produces largely symmetric images.

To this point, however, no systematic advantage for preserving asymmetry has been demonstrated in speech recognition.

2.5 Speech Sounds in the Auditory Image

Real-time 'auditory cartoons' of sounds can be produced by calculating the auditory image every 30-40 ms and then rapidly replaying a sequence of these cartoon frames in synchrony with the sound. And again, it appears to be Lyon (1984) who first recognised the value of this representation. The auditory cartoons of vowel sounds can largely be predicted from the /æ/ shown in Fig. 3. A stationary vowel appears as a more or less populated grid of activity in which the spacing of the verticals of the grid represents the pitch of the sound and the position of the activity on the verticals specifies the formants. In the auditory image model, when the pitch of the vowel decreases, the grid expands towards the left and down; in the autocorrelogram, the grid expands to the right and down. In both cases the formants remain stationary to the extent that the vowel does. Vowel changes are observed as motion chiefly in the first and second formants, and the motion is largely independent of pitch changes. The fine structure of the vowel is well defined when the vowel is sustained and in this case the grid pattern extends across the entire auditory image. When the pitch changes relatively rapidly or the formants move rapidly, the image becomes blurry in the region of longer integration intervals, and the level of activity decreases in this region because the sound no longer contains correlations at relatively long integration intervals.

Plosive consonants appear as transients in the auditory image; that is, they appear as a vertical set of impulse responses aligned on the trigger point in the auditory image model or the zero-lag line of the autocorrelogram. The plosives are distinguished by the distribution of activity along the trigger point vertical and by the aspiration and temporal gaps that surround the plosive burst in time. Liquid and nasal sounds appear as rather poorly formed vowel sounds with a restricted frequency range. The noise of fricative sounds and aspiration appears as a random pattern of pulses in the portion of the image away from the trigger point. The pulses in high frequency channels are still narrow and the pulses in low-frequency channels are still broad, but their size and position in time is random. In the region of the trigger point, the activity is never entirely random, even for white noise, because the wave has passed through a bank of relatively narrow auditory filters which apply a continuity constraint that appears as short-term correlations in the noise. Thus, in the auditory image model, whenever there is activity of any sort there is at least a ghost of the general impulse response of the system along the trigger point vertical. In the case of fricatives, the 'impulse response' is broader and less well defined than in the case of plosive bursts. It also lasts longer in the case of fricatives and so they are readily discriminable.

When an auditory cartoon of speech is presented synchronously with the sound, it produces a very compelling form of 'visible speech' in which voiced sounds and plosives appear as auditory figures, distinct from any background noise. This suggests that the auditory image might provide a better representation than the spectrogram for speech recognition systems. A description of the basic principles for extracting Fig. components from individual channels of the auditory image and assembling auditory figures from the Fig. components is presented in the last section of Patterson et al (1991). With regard to speech, it would appear possible to set up three phonology mechanisms to monitor the auditory image and extract patterns of activity that indicate the presence of a) periodic sounds indicative of vowels, liquids, and nasals, b) transients indicative of plosives, and c) bursts of noise indicative of fricatives or aspiration. For example, the vowel mechanism would attempt to locate grids in the individual frames of the auditory cartoon and determine where the concentrations of activity appear on the grid verticals. These statistics would be summarised and passed forward to a phonology assembly mechanism along with the streams from the other two phonology extractors. By performing pattern recognition directly on the auditory image and by including phonology constraints in the pattern recognition process, we would hope to reduce the data rate dramatically while at the same time preserving a good representation of the phonology.

Finally, it should be noted that, in the course of producing stabilised speech images, both quantised TI and autocorrelation perform a kind of triggered computer averaging. In so doing they enhance periodic components of the sound at the expense of aperiodic components of the sound; that is, they improve the signal-to-noise ratio of periodic components of the sound. A similar process occurs in the construction of the interval histograms of the EIH model (Ghitza, 1988), and it is this property which is assumed to provide the basis for the improved performance in noise demonstrated in that paper.

3. The Data-Rate Problem

Although logically feasible, extraction of phonology from the auditory image is not yet available. Consequently, a practical method of reducing the data rate of the auditory image has been developed. It is presented in Section 4 of the paper. Before proceeding, we turn to a detailed discussion of the discrepancy between the data rate leaving the typical auditory model and that entering the typical recognition system.

3.1 The Appropriate Data Rate for the Cochlea Simulation

Hearing scientists have traditionally been more concerned with the fidelity of the auditory representation they produce than the speed with which they produce the output. To ensure that an auditory model is capable of representing all of the discriminations that humans hear, one must digitise the incoming wave with 16-bit accuracy and a sample rate no less than 32 kHz. The filterbank must have no less than 100 channels, and so the total data rate is around 3.2 million 2-byte words per second. For speech signals, it is reasonable to reduce the sampling rate to, say 16 kHz, and to reduce the number of channels to around 64 without losing a great deal of fidelity. Beyond this, however, further reductions are likely to lead to the loss of phonetic distinctions. Thus, for the hearing scientist, the data rate at the output of the auditory filterbank is on the order of 2 million bytes per second (Mbps)!

In contrast, existing real-time recognition systems typically use some form of LPC or FFT preprocessor which segments the wave into frames about 20 ms in duration and converts the time waveform into a vector of values that specify the level of activity in a set of different frequency channels. When a sequence of such frames is presented in a grey scale format, it is referred to as a spectrogram. Existing commercial recognisers use 10-20 channels in the analysis and existing research systems use 20-50 channels. Thus, a fairly high fidelity

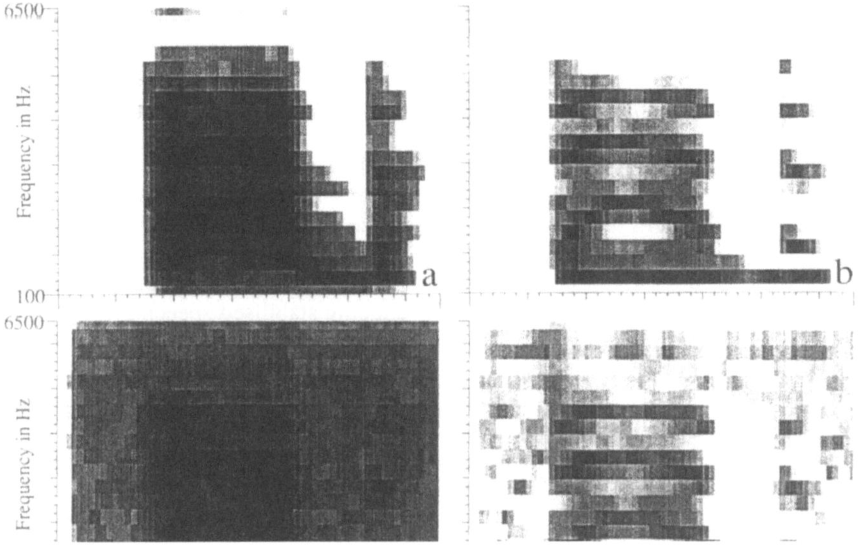

Fig. 4 Spectrograms of the syllable 'bab' occurring on its own (a) and in the presence of a soft background noise (c), and cochleograms of 'bab' on its own (c) and in noise (d). The contrast around the speech features is better in the cochleograms.

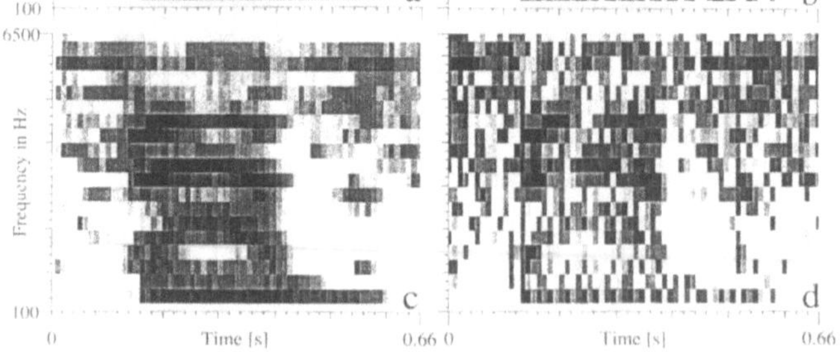

Fig. 5 Stabilised auditory spectrograms of 'bab' occurring on its own (upper panels) and in the presence of a soft noise (lower panels). The integration limits used to convert the auditory image to a spectrogram were chosen to enhance voiced speech sounds (a) and (c) or unvoiced speech sounds (b) and (d).

commercial system, or a moderate fidelity research system, with a 10 ms frame width and 20 channels in the spectrogram would have a data rate of 2 Kbps — three orders of magnitude lower than the data rate at the output of a competent auditory filterbank!

One can get some impression of the discrepancy between a Mbps data rate and a Kbps data rate by comparing the spectrogram of the syllable 'bab' shown in Fig. 4a with the segment of the /æ/ shown in Fig. 1. The vowel in bab is similar to /æ/. In Fig. 4a, the vowel appears as the horizontal bands in the centre of the spectrogram, and four of the fine vertical strips represent a 40-ms sample of the vowel. In Fig. 1, a 32-ms segment of the vowel occupies the entire width of the Fig. and the segment is represented by 640 points per channel. Thus, the representation that recognition systems take as input is very coarse in comparison to that at the output of an auditory model; indeed, it is coarse in comparison to the spectrograms traditionally published by phoneticians and other speech researchers where the temporal resolution is on the order of 1-3 ms. The lack of detail in the recogniser input is another reason why some research groups have decided to look to auditory models for a better input representation.

There is no question that the data rate of a competent auditory filterbank is on the order of 2 Mbps, and there is no question that this data rate is excessive for the information content of the original sound. The question is 'Why does the auditory system expand the data rate?' 'How long does it maintain the high-data-rate representation?' And 'How does it eventually reduce the data rate?' The time domain models presented in this paper appear to assume that the data rate is expanded in order to encode the initial spectral analysis adequately. The high data rate is maintained through the compressive/adaptive transduction process because it is more realistic in terms of auditory simulation, and it supports better feature enhancement. An example of the feature enhancement is presented in Fig. 4. The spectrogram in Fig. 4a is the rectified, compressed output of the gammatone filterbank. The spectrogram in Fig. 4b is the output when auditory suppression and adaptation are included in the processing. The fundamental and the formants are more pronounced in Fig. 4b. Furthermore, the feature enhancement operates well in noise. The spectrograms in Figures 4c and 4d show the compressed filterbank output and the cochlea simulation output, respectively, when the 'bab' is presented in a moderate level of noise that begins before and continues after the speech sound. The contrast around the speech features is better when suppression and adaptation are included in the processing, and this is one of the main attractions of auditory preprocessing for speech sounds. Thus, it is generally assumed by hearing scientists that the minimum data rate required to represent the neural activity patterns of broadband sounds *in the format in which they occur* in the auditory nerve is around 1 Mbps, and that auditory preprocessors for speech should operate at this rate throughout the spectral analysis and feature enhancement stages at least.

With the advance of computing power, and in particular with the advance of special purpose DSP chips, data rates that seemed prohibitive at the start of the last decade should be available by the end of the current decade and so we need not be unduly concerned by this rate. It is perfectly reasonable to assume that a special purpose cochlear processing chip like that designed by Lyon and Mead (1988) will be in commercial production before the end of the decade. The problem comes when we argue that this Mbps data rate should be preserved in yet further stages of auditory processing, and when we suggest that recognition systems should take these high-data-rate representations as input.

3.2 The Appropriate Data Rate for Temporal Integration

The simple temporal averaging that was originally proposed as a model of auditory TI smooths the NAP activity as it proceeds and, as a result, the data rate at the output of that TI process could be reduced in accordance with the degree of temporal averaging. Unfortunately, the same is not true for periodicity-sensitive TI. The individual channels of the auditory image and the correlogram have the same resolution as the channels of the NAP from which they are generated. If the auditory image is summarised as an auditory cartoon in which the time between frames of the cartoon is 40 ms and the width of the auditory image is 40 ms, then the inclusion of this form of TI in the system causes neither an expansion nor a contraction of the data rate. This rate is probably satisfactory for speech, although the auditory window is not really sufficiently wide for speakers with a very low voice pitch, and the frame rate is rather slow for the plosives of speech. The decay rate of the auditory image is on the order of 10 ms and so a burst that occurs just after a frame has been calculated will have decayed to about 1/8th its size by the time the next frame is calculated. In any event, it is clear that the auditory image construction process does not reduce the data rate even though it involves integration, because the preferred range of integration intervals (up to 80 ms) is greater than the preferred inter-frame interval of the auditory cartoon (preferably about 10 ms).

With regard to computational load, triggered, quantised TI is relatively inexpensive; at worst, for 100 channels, an 80 ms segment of the NAP is added to the corresponding channel of the auditory image every 10 ms. In contrast, the computational load of autocorrelation is relatively high; the calculation requires the addition of an extra dimension in which delayed copies of the wave are stored -- one copy for each of the possible delays. If the delay resolution has to be as small as 1 ms to account for temporal pitches up to 0.5 kHz, and if the capacity of the delay line has to be 80 ms to account for the perception of very low pitches, and if the basic operation requires multiplication and scaling (Meddis & Hewitt, 1991a), the computation becomes prohibitive -- especially for a real-time system. Following Licklider's original suggestion, Lyon (1984) notes that addition can be substituted for multiplication when dealing with unipolar functions. This reduces the problem somewhat, but it does not eliminate the major problem, which is that a full length correlation calculation has to be performed for every lag, every time a frame of the cartoon is required.

With regard to data reduction, the stabilised figures produced by periodicity-sensitive TI would appear to provide a particularly good basis for phonological pattern recognition, and it seems reasonable to assume that it is constrained recognition systems operating at this level in the auditory system that finally curtail the data rate expansion and reduce it by orders of magnitude in preparation for syllable and/or word recognition. And by analogy, this is probably the correct place to reduce the data rate in a speech recognition machine. However, low-level phonological recognition systems of this sort have yet to be developed, and so we turn to an interim solution for reducing the data rate of the auditory image and preserving some of the advantages that accrue from periodicity-sensitive TI -- a solution that can be used with existing speech recognition systems.

4. Stabilised Auditory Spectrograms

The auditory image has two obvious advantages as a representation of voiced speech sounds. Firstly, in the region away from the trigger point or zero-lag point, periodicity-synchronous TI enhances the signal-to-noise ratio of periodic sounds at the expense of aperiodic sounds. Thus we might expect a recognition system operating on this representation to be more resistant to background noise (Ghitza, 1988; Patterson & Hirahara, 1989). Secondly, periodicity-synchronous TI leads to a more stable estimate of the strength of periodic sounds. In traditional preprocessors there is a *fixed* temporal integration window with an integration time of between 5 and 40 ms. If the integration time is, for example, 8 ms, then for the average male voice with a pitch of 125 Hz, there will be one glottal pulse per spectrogram frame on average. As the speaker's voice rises the frame rate of the system and the period of the voice will go out of synchrony, and frames will sometimes contain two or even three pulses. Worse still, when the voice pitch decreases below 125 Hz, there will be a reasonable number of cases where there is no glottal pulse in the frame whatsoever. Thus as the voice pitch varies over an octave about its average, the level in the output frame can go from nothing at all to about four times that associated with a single glottal pulse. In this way, the traditional spectral analysis introduces variability into the spectrogram that is not a characteristic of the speech signal itself but rather a characteristic of the beating that arises between the fixed frame rate and the variable glottal rate. In a periodicity-sensitive system, this problem does not arise because there is always a period available to match the period of the voice.

The data rate of the auditory image can be reduced dramatically while preserving some of the advantages of periodicity-sensitive TI if we simply add the activity in each channel across Integration-Interval and provide the vector of resultant values as a frame of a spectrogram. If we match the number of channels and the frame rate to that of the traditional spectrogram, then the output data rate will be reduced to that of the traditional spectrogram. Furthermore, the data will be in a format that current recognition systems are accustomed to use -- a not insignificant consideration. We refer to the result as a 'Stabilised Auditory Spectrogram' or SAS, and examples for 'bab' in silence and in noise are presented in Figures 5a and 5c. In the absence of noise, the SAS for the vowel (Fig. 5a) is comparable to the spectrogram computed from the cochlea simulation (Fig. 4b). In the presence of noise (Figures 5c and 4d), we find greater contrast for the vowel sound in the SAS; that is, the formants are darker and the noise in the region of the vowel is more attenuated in the SAS (Fig. 5c).

4.1 The SAS Preprocessor with an HMM Recogniser

The first recognition tests based on an SAS were performed by Patterson and Hirahara (1989) and Hirahara (1990), using a recognition system based on Hidden Markov Modelling (Waibel, Hanazawa, Hinton, Shikino, and Lang,1988). The recogniser takes spectrographic input and it was carefully tuned to operate in conjunction with a bark-scaled DFT analyser and compressor. The resolution of the spectrogram was 16 frequency channels by 10 ms frames -- a data rate of 1.6 Kbps. In order to produce comparable stabilised spectrograms, the auditory image model was run with 32 normal-width filters spanning the same frequency region and then adjacent pairs of channels were averaged to produce a 16 channel output. Frames of the auditory image were calculated at 10 ms intervals and summed across the Interval dimension to produce the vector of frequency values for that frame. Both the DFT and the SAS recognition system were then trained on a large corpus of syllables extracted from continuous speech, in which the initial consonant was /b/, /d/, or /g/. The syllables were either presented in no background noise or in a relatively loud background noise like that of a noisy computer room where one would be inclined to raise the voice. The original database was randomly divided into two sets, one which was used both for training and testing, and one which was just used for testing. The system was trained and tested using clean speech, and trained and tested using noisy speech. There were also cross-over performance tests in which a system trained with clean speech was tested with noisy speech and vice-versa, to assess the ability of the system to generalise.

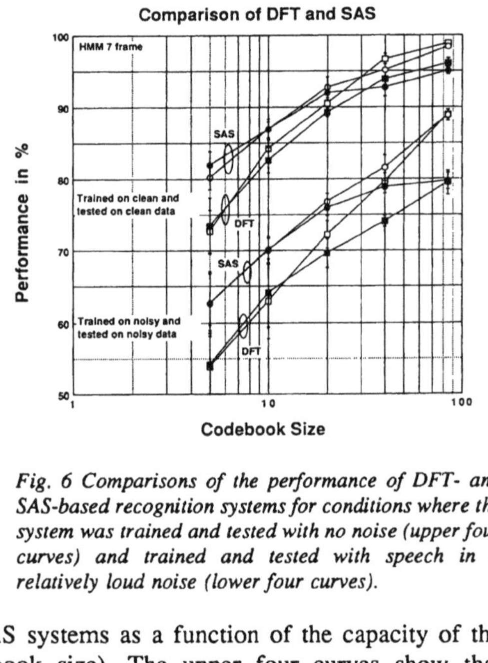

Fig. 6 Comparisons of the performance of DFT- and SAS-based recognition systems for conditions where the system was trained and tested with no noise (upper four curves) and trained and tested with speech in a relatively loud noise (lower four curves).

The results for the uncrossed conditions are presented in Fig. 6, which shows the performance of the DFT and SAS systems as a function of the capacity of the memory of the recognition system (codebook size). The upper four curves show that performance for the two systems is comparable when the codebook size is large, but as the system is stressed by reducing the codebook size, the performance of the traditional DFT system falls off faster than that of the SAS system. The lower four curves show a similar pattern; however, the added stress of the noise background causes the performance of the DFT system to fall off even sooner and separate even farther from that of the SAS system. The cross-over conditions produce a similar pattern of results and their overall level of performance falls, as expected, between that shown by the two sets of curves in Fig. 6. Hirahara (1990) extended the research with tests at intervening signal-to-noise ratios and tests with a larger phoneme set and found similar results.

These results confirm Ghitza's (1988) finding that an auditory preprocessor can lead to a more noise-resistant recognition system to the extent that the bottom four curves in Fig. 6 diverge more than the top four. They extend his results inasmuch as they show that an auditory preprocessor can improve the performance of the smaller, faster recognisers -- a result that was confirmed by Hirahara (1990) for a wide range of noise levels. This suggests that an auditory model with periodicity-sensitive TI extracts a better representation of voiced speech and one that is more noise resistant.

4.2 Separate SAS Processing for Voiced and Unvoiced Speech Sounds

In the course of examining stabilised auditory spectrograms and comparing them with traditional spectrograms, we noted that the differences were not as great as we might have expected. We also observed that the transients in speech were not well represented in the SAS, particularly when they followed a vowel. Note, for example, that the final burst in bab is only poorly represented in the SAS's of Figs. 5a and 5c. Both effects follow directly from the fact that we integrated across the entire width of the auditory image from the trigger point leftwards in these initial studies. All sounds, including noise, cause activity in the region of the trigger point, and so integrating from the trigger point means that noise activity is recombined with activity from voiced sounds. This suggests that we might be able to produce better representations of voiced and unvoiced speech by integrating separately across different regions of the auditory image and producing two parallel spectrograms, one with enhanced periodic information and one with enhanced transient information. The motivation for this approach was provided by Wu, Schwartz, and Escudier (1989) who refer to periodic and transient activity as 'tonic' and 'phasic' information. They pointed out that tonic information tends to be narrowly defined in frequency and extend over time, whereas phasic information tends to extend across frequency and be localised in time, and they recommended separate processors for the two kinds of information.

The auditory image was extended to the right of the trigger point to include a range of negative Integration Intervals as shown in Fig. 3. Conceptually, this is equivalent to moving the trigger point into the NAP buffer by a small amount, say 5 ms, and including this part of the NAP record in the transfer to the auditory image. The importance of this modification is that it enables the image to show the events that occur immediately after the large NAP pulses that trigger TI. When the stimulus is an isolated acoustic event like a plosive, the activity is confined to the trigger-point region and it dies away quickly; when the stimulus is extended in time the activity extends across the image and persists for the duration of the sound. With this extended auditory image, two auditory spectrograms can be generated using two different sets of integration limits. For the tonic information the auditory image is integrated from about 3.5 *cycles* of the centre frequency of the channel over to the lefthand edge of the window. For the phasic information the integration limits are from -3.5 *cycles* to +1.5 *cycles*, that is, a column about the trigger point vertical that is broader at the base than at the apex, and which is asymmetric in the same direction as the impulse response of the filterbank.

Auditory spectrograms that emphasise the phasic information in 'bab' are shown in Figs. 5b and 5d. In the absence of background noise, the bursts of the b's are well marked (Fig. 5b). In noise the burst position is not so clear (Fig. 5d), although there is a consistent increase in activity across channels at the intants of the bursts. The SAS's in Figures 5b and 5d were generated with narrow integration limits about the trigger point vertical; the decay time of the auditory image was 8 ms. The SAS's in Figures 5a and 5c were generated by summing from 4-24 ms in the auditory image; the decay time was increased to 30 ms to increase the stability of tonic information.

The SAS's in Figs. 5b and 5d show activity throughout the region of the vowel because all activity entering the auditory image must have a contribution on the trigger point vertical, namely, the NAP pulse that caused triggering. Thus, this version of the SAS is an 'activity' spectrogram, and it is similar to a traditional spectrogram with a short time constant. It would be reasonably easy, following the example of Wu et al., to implement a processor that monitored this version of the SAS looking for coordinated onsets across a range of frequency channels, and which only produced output in the event of coordinated activity across channels. This would remove most of the activity in the activity spectrogram aside from the bursts and so convert it into the desired phasic auditory spectrogram.

The tonic and phasic auditory spectrograms have the same format and because of the nature of speech, activity in one tends to be minimal when activity in the other is maximal. Thus it seems likely that we could combine the tonic and phasic auditory spectrograms by simple addition and produce a single auditory spectrogram that would contain vowel information that had been processed to enhance its tonic character and consonant burst information that had been processed to enhance its transient nature. Efforts to produce and test this representation are proceeding.

Acknowledgements

The authors would like to thank Ken Robinson for assistance with figures in the paper, and James McQueen and Brit van Ooyen for providing the speech materials. The work presented in this paper was supported by the MRC and grants from Esprit BRA (3207) and MOD PE (2239). The HMM recognition work was performed while the first author was a visiting researcher at ATR Auditory and Visual Perception Research Laboratories in Kyoto, Japan.

References

Assmann, P.F. and Summerfield, Q. (1990). Modelling the perception of concurrent vowels: Vowels with different fundamental frequencies, *J. Acoust. Soc. Am.*, 88, 680-697.

Deng, L., Geisler, C.D., and Greenberg, S. (1988). A composite model of the auditory periphery for the processing of speech, *J. of Phonetics*, 16, 93-108.

Ghitza, O. (1988). Temporal non-place information in the auditory-nerve firing patterns as a front-end for speech recognition in a noisy environment, *J. of Phonetics*, 16, 109-123.

Glasberg, B.R. and Moore, B.C.J. (1990). Derivation of auditory filter shapes from notched-noise data, *Hearing Research*, 47, 103-138.

Hirahara, T. (1990). *HMM speech recognition using DFT and auditory spectrograms* (Part 2), ATR Technical Report TR-A-0075.

Licklider, J.C.R. (1951). A duplex theory of pitch perception, reprinted in: E.D. Schubert (ed), *Psychological Acoustics*, Stroudsburg, P.A., Dowden, Hutchinson and Ross, Inc (1979).

Lyon, R.F. (1982). A computational model of filtering, detection, and compression in the cochlea, *Proc. IEEE Int. Conf. Acoust., Speech, Signal Process.*, Paris, France, May 1982.

Lyon, R.F. (1984). Computational models of neural auditory processing, *Proc. IEEE Int. Conf. Acoust., Speech, Signal Processing*. San Diego, CA, March 1984.

Lyon, R.F. and Dyer, L. (1986). Experiments with a computational model of the cochlea, in: *Proc. IEEE Int. Conf. Acoust., Speech, Signal Processing*. Tokyo, Japan, April 1986.

Lyon, R.F. and Mead, C.A. (1988). *Cochlear hydrodynamics demystified*, Caltech Comput. Sci. Tech. Rep. Caltech-CS-TR-884, Pasadena, CA, February 1988.

Meddis, R. and Hewitt, M.J. (1991a). Virtual pitch and phase sensitivity of a computer model of the auditory periphery: I pitch identification, *J. Acoust. Soc. Am., submitted.*

Meddis, R. and Hewitt, M.J. (1991b). Modelling the perception of concurrent vowels with different fundamental frequencies, *J. Acoust. Soc. Am.*, submitted.

Meddis, R. (1986). Simulation of mechanical to neural transduction in the auditory receptor, *J. Acoust. Soc. Am.*, 79, 702-711.

Patterson, R.D. (1987a). A pulse ribbon model of peripheral auditory processing, in: *Auditory Processing of Complex Sounds* (W.A. Yost and C.S. Watson (eds)), pp 167-179. New Jersey, Erlbaum.

Patterson, R.D. (1987b). A pulse ribbon model of monaural phase perception, *J. Acoust. Soc. Am.*, 82, 1560-1586.

Patterson, R.D. and Hirahara, T. (1989). *HMM speech recognition using DFT and auditory spectrograms*, ATR Technical Report TR-A-0063.

Patterson, R.D. and Holdsworth, J. (1991). A functional model of neural activity patterns and auditory images, in: *Advances in Speech, Hearing and Language Processing* (W.A. Ainsworth, ed.), Vol 3, JAI Press, London, in press.

Patterson, R.D., Holdsworth, J., Nimmo-Smith, I., and Rice, P. (1988). SVOS Final Report: The Auditory Filterbank, *APU report*, 2341.

Patterson, R.D. and Moore, B.C.J. (1986). Auditory filters and excitation patterns as representations of frequency resolution, in: *Frequency Selectivity in Hearing* (B.C.J. Moore, ed.), London: Academic Press Ltd., 123-177

Patterson, R.D., Robinson, K., Holdsworth, J., McKeown, D., Zhang, C., and Allerhand, M. (1991). Complex sounds and auditory images, *9th International Symposium on Hearing: Auditory physiology and perception*, June 9-14, Carcans, France

Robinson, T.J., Holdsworth, J., Patterson, R.D., and Fallside, F. (1990). A comparison of preprocessors for the Cambridge recurrent error propagation network speech recognition system, *Int. Conference on Spoken Language Processing*, Nov 18-22, Kobe, Japan.

Seneff, S. (1988). A joint synchrony/mean-rate model of auditory speech processing, *J. Phon.*, 16, 77-91.

Shamma, S. (1988). The acoustic features of speech sounds in a model of auditory processing: vowels and voiceless fricatives, *J. Phon.*, 16, 77-91.

Slaney, M. and Lyon, R.F. (1990). A perceptual pitch detector, *Proc. ICASSP 90 - 1990 International Conference on Acoustics, Speech, and Signal Processing*. Albuquerque, New Mexico, April 3-6 1990.

Zwicker, E. (1961). Subdivision of the audible frequency range into critical bands (frequenzgruppen), *J. Acoust. Soc. Am.*, 33, 248.

Temporal Resolution and Modulation Analysis in Models of the Auditory System

Armin Kohlrausch,[1]
Dirk Püschel, and
Henning Alphei
Drittes Physikalisches Institut
Universität Göttingen
Bürgerstraße 42-44
D-3400 Göttingen
Germany

[1]now at:
Institute for Perception Research
P.O. Box 513
NL-5600 MB Eindhoven
The Netherlands

1. INTRODUCTION

One of the important properties of the human auditory system is its ability to follow rapid fluctuations in acoustic signals as they occur for instance in speech. The study of temporal resolution is therefore of major interest not only for the basic understanding of the hearing system and appropriate models, but also for applications such as speech preprocessing. One apparent problem with respect to temporal properties of our hearing system is the wide range of durations over which temporal effects are observed (e.g. de Boer, 1985). On the one hand, the hearing system is able to detect short gaps in an otherwise continuous signal, which can be as short as 2 ms. On the other hand, the system is able to integrate signal intensity in detection tasks over at least 200 ms. From a comparison of these time periods it becomes obvious that the temporal behavior of the auditory system cannot be simply described by a series of integrating stages with different time constants linearly operating on the acoustic signals: in such a simulation, the longest time constant would smear out fast temporal variations and the high resolution seen in e.g. gap-detection experiments cannot be adequately simulated.

An attempt to overcome this obvious problem is to apply a nonlinear transformation prior to the integration (e.g., Penner, 1978). In the first part of this paper, we will use such an approach to model forward masking curves. In a forward-masking condition, the threshold of a short signal, presented after the temporal offset of a masker, is determined for various temporal positions of the test signal. With increasing temporal distance, the signal threshold decreases, and the absolute threshold is typically reached after 200 ms. The involved mechanical and neural processes are, at least quantitatively, not well understood. Duifhuis (1973) described forward masking curves as reflecting two different processes. While the beginning of the decay curve should reflect short-term transient masking, the later part should reflect a neural process with a time constant "of about 75 ms", probably due to neural adaptation.

In the second part of this paper, we apply the model for nonsimultaneous masking to the problem of how temporal properties of the acoustic signal can be used for the segregation of simultaneously perceived sounds. Measurements are described in which a segregation threshold is determined for pairs of superimposed harmonic complex tones differing in, e.g., fundamental frequency or in amplitude modulation. The model calculations make use of the above nonlinear transformation. However, in order to allow a more sophisticated pattern analysis, the preprocessed signals are not only integrated, but also analyzed for envelope periodicities with time windows of 200 ms. In this way, an internal acoustic image (or modulation spectrum) is derived for each auditory channel which is stable over a period of 100 to 200 ms.

2. Basic Properties of Forward Masking

We would like to start the description of forward masking with two figures showing results of our own measurements in a forward masking paradigm. We performed these measurements in order to obtain forward masking curves with a higher temporal resolution than typically found in the literature. The masker was a fixed 300-ms section of a flat-spectrum noise (frozen noise) with an upper cut-off frequency of 5 kHz and with a rectangular temporal envelope. It was presented at a level of 80 dB SPL (spectrum level 43 dB) in a 3 Interval Forced Choice (3 IFC) paradigm. The target was a 2-kHz pulse with a Hanning envelope of 5 ms total duration. By this choice of masker and target, we tried to minimize disturbing effects of cueing and confusion, which seem to reflect very central properties effective in some forward masking conditions (Moore and Glasberg, 1982). Each data point is the outcome of a single adaptive track consisting of about 40 3-IFC trials.

In Fig. 1, the results of three subjects are plotted. The temporal position of the target is indicated on the abscissa for the target's end. As the masker cutoff was at 300 ms, all target positions with END ≤ 300 ms correspond to simultaneous masking, those with END ≥ 305 ms are nonsimultaneous and positions in between indicate the transition between these two conditions. The ordinate indicates signal level at threshold on a relative scale, where 0 dB corresponds to 97 dB SPL. On this relative level scale, the absolute threshold of the target for the three listeners lies between -75 and -80 dB (17 to 22 dB SPL). The transition between simultaneous and nonsimultaneous masking is replotted for two subjects on a larger time scale in Fig. 2.

If we first consider simultaneous masking thresholds, we see a strong modulation in the thresholds for different temporal positions. These variations reflect the direct, phase-sensitive interaction between the frozen-noise waveform and the target, and are typical of frozen-noise measurements (Gilkey et al., 1985). When the signal is partly moved out of the masker, the thresholds start to drop abruptly. At END=305 ms, where the presented signal just has no overlap with the masker, the thresholds are already 20 dB below the simultaneous values. Looking at Fig. 2, it is obvious that for further delays between masker and target, the threshold function decreases more slowly and nearly linearly on this scale. Although it is not obvious from these figures, the initial drop in the threshold is largest for high masker levels (more precisely, for a large difference between simultaneous and absolute thresholds of the target) and for short maskers.

Another interesting observation is the very smooth, monotonic decay in the forward masking curve. The smoothness reflects the earlier finding of e.g. Yost et al. (1982) that in forward masking no phase-sensitive interaction between masker waveform and target can be observed. Thus, forward masking curves are the same for different frozen noise maskers of the same level and duration, even if the simultaneous thresholds are very different.

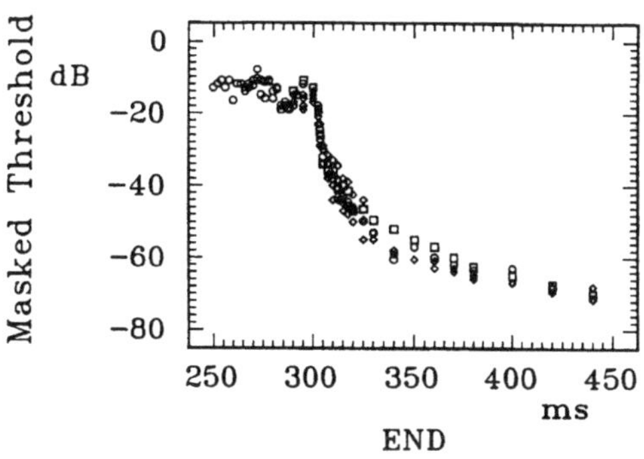

Fig. 1 Forward masked thresholds of a 5-ms 2-kHz target in the presence of a broadband frozen-noise masker. The masker had a level of 80 dB SPL and a duration of 300 ms. The abscissa indicates the temporal position of the signal offset (masker offset occurs at 300 ms), the ordinate gives signal level at threshold on a relative scale (0 dB corresponds to 97 dB SPL). Results for three listeners.

The best possible comparison with literature data is with the results of Carlyon (1988), because he used the same target frequency and duration and a very similar masker duration. He determined simultaneous and nonsimultaneous thresholds at 6 temporal positions corresponding to values of END between 300 ms and 345 ms. Taking into account that his masker had a 10 dB lower level, the values for his most sensitive subject correspond to our data within about 5 dB. Two more effects, already described by other authors, should be recalled here. In contrast with simultaneous thresholds, nonsimultaneous thresholds depend nonlinearly on masker level and masker duration. For shorter maskers, the decay of the target threshold (measured for instance in dB/ms) is steeper. For a masker of only 20 ms duration, the target reaches its absolute threshold 50 ms after the masker's offset. In addition, the steepness of the forward masking curves increases with the masker level.

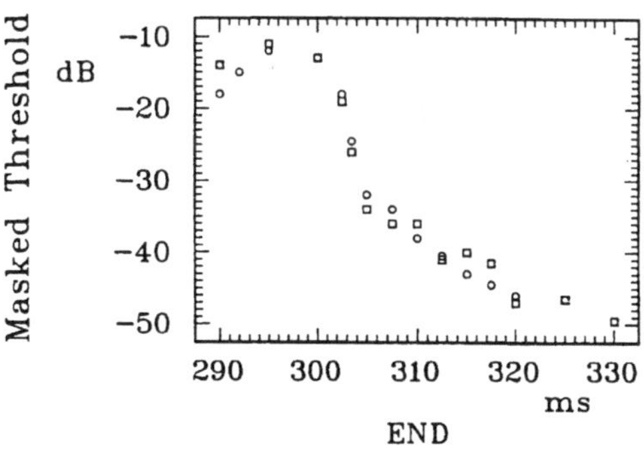

Fig. 2 Results for two listeners from Fig. 1 on an enlarged time scale.

3. Modelling Forward Masking

In this section we will describe attempts to model the experimental data. Some common properties and specifications of all models are outlined first. Later in this section the predictions of various model variants are discussed. In the simulations, we used exactly the same target and sample of frozen noise as in the measurements. We assumed that the signal is detected within a single auditory channel, i.e. all models are single-band models. The input signals were filtered with a linear basilar-membrane model (Strube, 1985) and only the channel tuned to the signal frequency was further examined. This signal was half-wave rectified and lowpass filtered at 1 kHz. This stage simulates the transformation in the inner hair cell and is a common part of many auditory models. In this stage, an absolute threshold for the target was introduced by setting a minimum output value. This value was chosen to match the sensation levels used in the experiments. The output of this stage forms the input x for the various models discussed below.

The next problem was to define a detection threshold for the short target. We first considered the transformation characteristic of the models for stationary conditions. One of the specifications of the models was that, for stationary input, they should have a compressing characteristic, which is nearly logarithmic. This should, on the one hand, reflect the relation between signal amplitude and perceived loudness. On the other hand, a change of the output value by a specific amount, say 1 model unit, should correspond to the just noticeable difference of the input level, which for simplicity we assumed to be about 1 dB at all levels. To allow a comparison of different models, a uniform way of defining "1 model unit" had to be derived. For all models, we calculated the range of output values for stationary input signals covering a range of 100 dB. The range of derived output values was then linearly mapped to the range of 0 to 100 dB_{mod} (for model units). For a perfect logarithmic transformation, a change of 1 dB_{mod} for a stationary signal would correspond to a 1-dB change at the input for all input levels. The threshold definition for shorter signals was now that any change at the output of the model of at least 1 dB_{mod} was detectable. The output time function of the models was always calculated for noise alone and noise plus target. Since all models had compressing

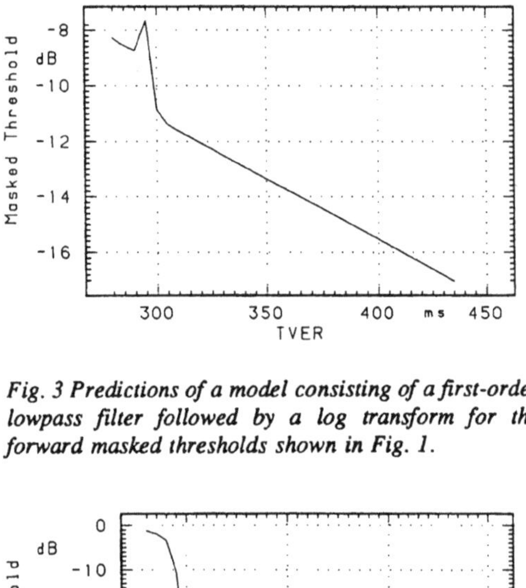

Fig. 3 Predictions of a model consisting of a first-order lowpass filter followed by a log transform for the forward masked thresholds shown in Fig. 1.

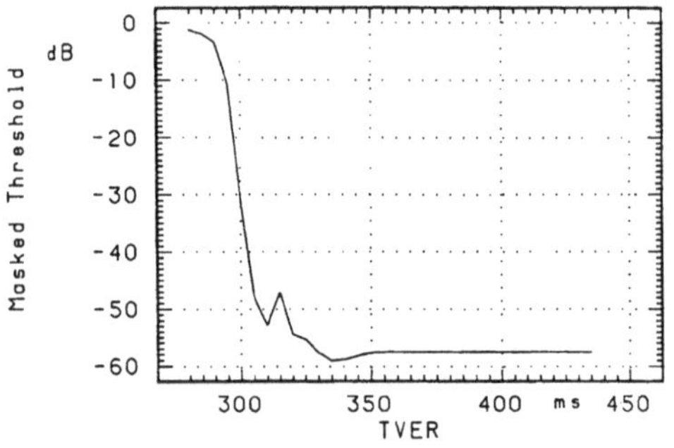

Fig. 4 Predictions of a model consisting of a log transform followed by a first-order lowpass filter for a time constant of 60 ms.

nonlinearities, the signal level leading to a 1-dB_{mod} change at the model output had to be calculated iteratively.

The first model consisted of a simple lowpass filter (time constant 200 ms) with a subsequent logarithmic transformation. Such a model comes very close to energy detection models as proposed and used by e.g. Pfafflin and Matthews (1962). The result of the threshold calculation is shown in Fig. 3. The time axis represents the beginning of the target; for a comparison with the experimental results, the theoretical curves have to be moved 5 ms to the right. The ordinate gives the signal level on the same relative scale as used for the experimental data in Figs. 1 and 2. The prediction for the simultaneous masking thresholds is about 5 to 10 dB too high. Much worse is the prediction for the nonsimultaneous data which leads to a linear decay of much too shallow a slope. By choosing a shorter time constant, the slope could be increased, but it would still be linear.

In the next version, the positions of logarithmic transformation and integrator were exchanged. This arrangement comes close to that of Penner and Shiffrin (1980). The simulated results in Fig. 4 for a lowpass time constant of 60 ms decay much too rapidly and reach the absolute threshold after about 30 ms. A change of the time constant to 200 ms does not affect this slope. Its main effect is a positive shift of all values by about 30 dB.

The last class of investigated models tries to incorporate the adaptive properties of the auditory periphery. Adaptation means a change in the transformation characteristic (or gain) according to the input level. Such an automatic gain control (AGC) can be achieved with a feedback loop and we will concentrate in the following on the most promising version derived in our investigation.

A series of simple feedback elements is shown in Fig. 5. The signal flow is from left to right. Within each single element, the lowpass-filtered output is fed back to form the denominator of the dividing element (the gain control for the input to this element). For stationary signals, each element calculates the square root of the input. Input variations that are rapid compared to the time constant of the lowpass filter are transformed linearly, because the gain in the feedback loop will not follow these fast variations. Thus, each element combines a static compressing nonlinearity with a higher sensitivity for fast temporal variations. In addition, each individual element reacts differently to increments and decrements in the input amplitude. For positive steps, the output shows an overshoot in the beginning with a later adaptation to a stationary value similar to auditory nerve fibers. This high overshoot will "charge" the lowpass filter capacitor rapidly. Therefore, adaptation towards the higher value occurs faster than would be expected from the time constant of the lowpass filter. Because the amount of overshoot increases with increasing input step size, the adaptation time will become even shorter for larger positive changes in input level. In contrast, for a decrease in the input level the capacitor of the lowpass filter only discharges at the rate determined by the filter's time constant. This follows from the fact that the values at all stages of the feedback element are positive and hence the maximal undershoot at the output is limited. Therefore, the readaptation after a negative level step at the input will take more time than adaptation to a higher level. This dichotomy of the time constants for positive and negative changes - as well as the nonlinear dependence of adaptation times on the level change - reflects typical findings in the dynamic responses of single fibers in the eighth nerve (e.g. Westerman and Smith, 1984).

How can we now incorporate such feedback elements into a model for nonsimultaneous masking? The first step is to use several of these elements in series with different time constants for the individual feedback loops. By combining five elements, the stationary transformation is nearly identical to the logarithmic transformation. The time constants of the five feedback stages were spaced at equal increments between 5 and 500 ms. In order to simulate the integrating properties of the ear, the series of five elements was followed by a simple lowpass filter with a time constant of 200 ms (τ_y in Fig. 5). The results of a threshold simulation with this model are shown in Fig. 6. The nonsimultaneous as well as the simultaneous thresholds are now in the same range as the measured data.

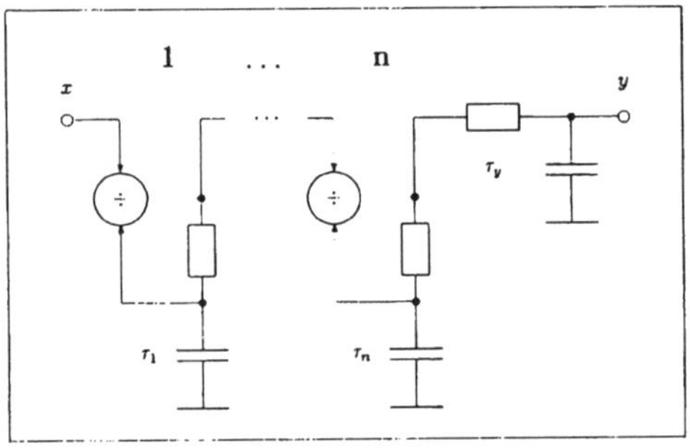

Fig. 5 Final model, consisting of n feedback loops with individual time constants τ_i in series and a final integrator with a time constant of 200 ms.

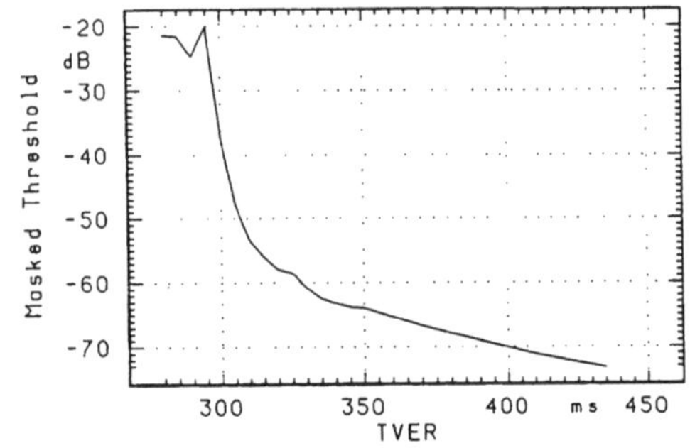

Fig. 6 Predictions of the final model for 5 feedback elements and a linear spacing of the τ_i between 5 and 500 ms.

4. Principal Properties and Further Applications of the Model

We would like to discuss some basic properties of this model and mention its use in auditory preprocessing. In this model, forward masking is not a consequence of a slowly decreasing internal excitation caused by the masker, but follows from the time varying values of the feedback loops. Given a very long masker, all feedback loops have reached a constant value which produces a high compression of the masker. A signal occurring simultaneously with the masker will go through the same compression, and if it changes the input by about 1 dB, it will also change the output by about 1 dB_{mod}. However, after cessation of the masker, the feedback factors return only slowly towards zero, and a target presented just after masker offset will be strongly attenuated. In order to produce a sufficient change at the output of the final lowpass filter, the signal level at the input must be high enough to overcome this internal gain. With increasing distance from the masker offset, the feedback loops return to a low value and the input level of the signal can continuously be decreased in order to produce the same change at the output. Thus the forward masking curve reflects the readaptation of the feedback loops, which depends on the individual time constants $\tau_1 \ldots \tau_n$.

How does masker duration influence the nonsimultaneous masking thresholds? If we use a shorter masker, the capacitors of the "slow" stages are not completely charged at the masker's offset and are therefore less involved in the readaptation process. In this case, forward masking is more dominated by the stages with a shorter time constant and the return to the absolute threshold for the signal will occur within a shorter period, hence with a steeper slope. In a similar way, we can explain the dependence of forward masking on masker level. The higher the level, the higher the gain compression and the larger the dB range of readaptation. Because the duration of readaptation after a long masker does not depend on masker level, the steepness of the forward masking curves, plotted as signal level in dB, increases with masker level (Püschel, 1988).

The model is formulated in terms of a simple filter and can therefore be used for arbitrary input signals. Its overall properties are that of an AGC filter with different effective time constants for positive and negative level changes in the acoustic signal. Such a filter generally enhances the temporal contrast and is similar to an envelope highpass filter. Because it preserves temporal features and reduces the influence of overall level, it is a good candidate for an auditory preprocessing filter followed by feature detectors. As such it has been successfully applied to automatic speech recognition using a neural-network and a dynamic-time-warping approach (Paping, 1991).

The filter as shown in Fig. 5 is of course only a first approach. Because we were interested in signal detection within and after a noise masker, the final stage was modelled by a simple integrator. This integrator simulates the integration of test-signal intensity. While this model works well with noise maskers, it leads to incorrect predictions for complex-tone maskers, where the masked thresholds are significantly lower than the model calculations. One idea to improve the model is to consider in the final stage not only the temporal average of the adapted waveform, but also temporal details like amplitude modulations. For a periodic masker like a harmonic complex, it is more likely that the target is detected due to a change in the regularity of the complex than due to a change in the total energy.

This idea of a modulation analysis following peripheral processing is supported by physiological observations. Schreiner and Langner (1988) found that neurons in different stages of the afferent auditory pathway have a decreasing ability to follow rapid amplitude fluctuations of the sound stimulus. The information about modulation frequencies seems to be coded in space and yields a slowly varying representation with a time constant of about 200 ms. Such a spatial representation of modulation frequencies can be modelled if the final low pass filter in Fig. 5 is replaced by a running short-time fourier transformation with a time window of 200 ms.

Such a representation at a certain instant of time is shown for a speech sound in Fig. 7. The x-axis gives the modulation frequency between 0 and 1000 Hz within each frequency channel. The y-axis represents the center frequency of the individual frequency channels expressed as basilar-membrane segment number. Segment number 0 corresponds to a center frequency of 7 kHz and segment 80 to 100 Hz. The z-axis shows the level of modulation frequencies in model units (MUs). These MUs are scaled in the same way as for the forward masking models: a stationary level change of 1 dB at the input changes the DC component in the modulation spectrum by 1 MU.

In Fig. 7 there are several peaks along the modulation axis. These are the modulation components corresponding to the difference frequencies in the analyzed frequency channel. In all channels we get a peak at the (present or absent) fundamental frequency of the complex sound together with higher harmonics of this fundamental. The maxima along the center-frequency axis (y-axis) represent the energy maxima or formants of the speech sound. It should be mentioned that this representation is roughly the fourier transform of the "stabilized auditory image" (Patterson et al., 1992; and this volume) calculated along the time axis in every frequency channel. We may characterize their approach as the autocorrelation function of the hair cell output signal and ours as the power spectrum of the same signal. Besides this relation there are of course major differences in the overall processing.

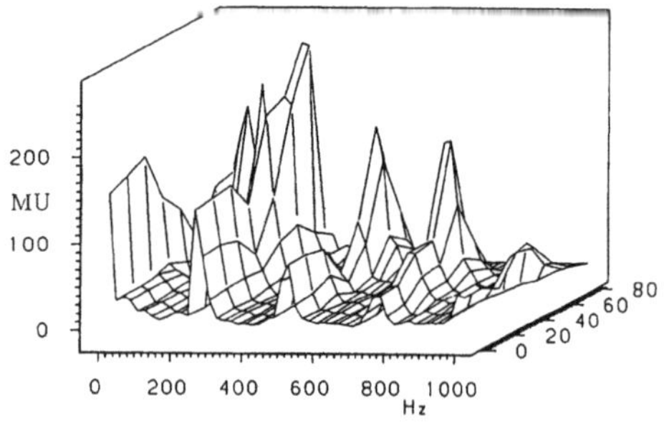

Fig. 7 Modulation spectrum of a vowel sound in model units (MUs, z-axis). The x-axis represents modulation frequency and the y-axis represents basilar-membrane segment number from 0 to 80, corresponding to center frequencies from 7 kHz to 100 Hz.

In the last part of this contribution we will apply this model to the problem of perceptual segregation of simultaneously perceived sounds.

5. Measuring Segregation Thresholds of Simultaneous Complex Sounds

Without any effort we are able in everyday listening conditions to segregate the surrounding sounds into individual sound objects. Possible signal cues in this process are interaural parameters related to the positions of the various objects or differences in temporal properties. The latter may consist of onset differences between competing sounds or of differences in modulation frequencies for speakers with different fundamental frequencies.

Previous attempts to investigate segregation abilities of human listeners have either used a qualitative approach (e.g. Rasch, 1978) or used a paradigm of vowel identification (e.g. Darwin, 1984). In contrast, we tried to establish a quantitative measure for the segregation threshold of a test sound in the presence of a second, interfering sound (Alphei, 1990). The principal approach was as follows. Within a measurement, two different signals were used, labelled as "test" and "interfering" sounds. These two sounds were superimposed in a test interval. The level of the "test" signal was varied within the measurement according to the subject's responses. The task of the subject was to decide after each presentation of the test interval whether the "test" sound could be heard out of or recognized in the mixture. Since such a recognition task can only be performed if the subject has an acoustic reference as to how the "test" signal sounds, a presentation of the "test" sound alone preceded each test interval containing both sounds. This "reference" sound was presented at a fixed level. The level of the "interfering" sound was also fixed.

The measurement was performed in a paradigm resembling a Békésy tracking procedure. As long as the subjects indicated that they heard the "test" sound, its level was decreased, otherwise it was increased. The segregation threshold was calculated as the median of 10 turnaround points of the "test"-sound level. The underlying assumption is that the threshold value will be higher if the test sound is more difficult to segregate. It should be noted that this segregation threshold is not identical with the masked threshold, i.e. the level at which the test sound becomes just audible. The masked threshold was typically 20 dB lower and depended much less on the experimental parameters (see below) than the segregation threshold.

As "interfering" sound we used a harmonic complex tone with a fundamental of 100 Hz, containing only the even harmonics 2,4,6, ... ,30. The "test" sound had a narrower spectrum consisting of the odd harmonics 3,5,7, ... ,19 of a fundamental frequency in the range 100 to 110 Hz. In both complexes, all components had equal amplitudes and zero starting phases. The duration of the sounds was 200 ms, including 10-ms raised-cosine ramps. The (fixed) levels of the "interfering" and the "reference" sounds were 66 dB and 64 dB, respectively. With these parameters the "test" sound is completely embedded - in frequency as well as in time - in the "interfering" sound.

In the first experiment, the segregation threshold was measured for different values of the fundamental frequency of the "test" sound. The individual results of three listeners are shown in Fig. 8. Each data point shows median and interquartile ranges of 5 to 6 measurements. At a threshold value of 0 dB the "test" sound has the same level as the "reference" sound (64 dB). The highest segregation thresholds are measured for 100 Hz fundamental, i.e. if both sounds have the same fundamental. With increasing difference in fundamental frequency the thresholds decrease by about 10 dB for all listeners, indicating that segregation of the "test" sound is easier. A full improvement is reached for a shift of about 5 Hz. This dependence of segregation ability on differences in fundamental frequency is comparable to literature data (e.g. Gardner et al., 1989).

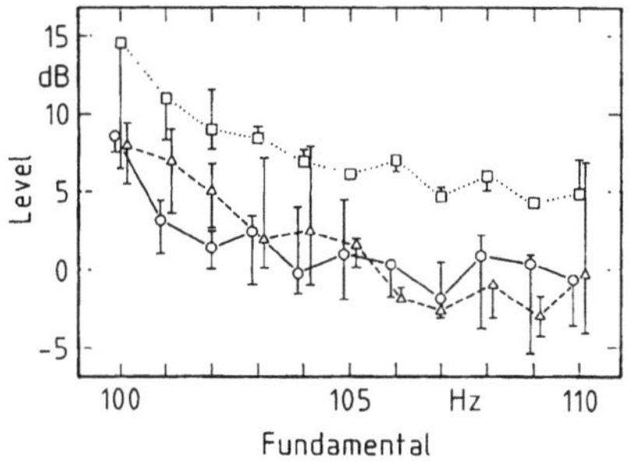

Fig. 8 Segregation thresholds (relative to the "reference"-sound level of 64 dB) for three subjects as a function of the fundamental frequency of the "test" sound. The fundamental frequency of the "interfering" sound was 100 Hz.

In the next experiment, the influence of frequency modulation on the segregation threshold was investigated. The fundamental frequency of the "test" and the "interfering" sound was sinusoidally varied around 100 Hz with a fixed frequency extent of 6 Hz and modulation frequencies of 5, 10, 20 or 30 Hz. The frequency extent of the higher harmonics was correspondingly higher. This modulation was either in phase for the two sounds or in antiphase.

The results for two subjects are shown in Fig. 9. For in-phase modulation (circles), the modulation frequency has hardly any influence on the threshold and the values correspond to the static thresholds for identical fundamental frequency. Thus the parallel variation in fundamental frequency of "test" and "interfering" sound does not help to segregate the "test" sound.

For modulation in antiphase (squares), there is a strong improvement at the lowest modulation frequency. The difference relative to the in-phase modulation of 10 to 12 dB corresponds to the improvement seen in the static case with a 5-Hz difference in fundamental frequency. The improvement in segregation becomes smaller for higher modulation frequencies, but the antiphasic condition always leads to an improvement of 2 to 5 dB.

In the final experiment, "test" and "interfering" sounds were 100% amplitude modulated with modulation frequencies of between 5 and 20 Hz. The results for in-phase and antiphase modulation in Fig. 10 are very similar to the results for frequency modulation. At 5 Hz, a low

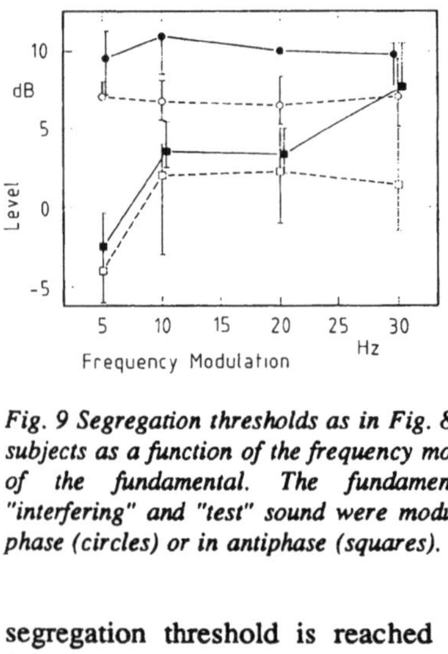

Fig. 9 Segregation thresholds as in Fig. 8 for two subjects as a function of the frequency modulation of the fundamental. The fundamentals of "interfering" and "test" sound were modulated in phase (circles) or in antiphase (squares).

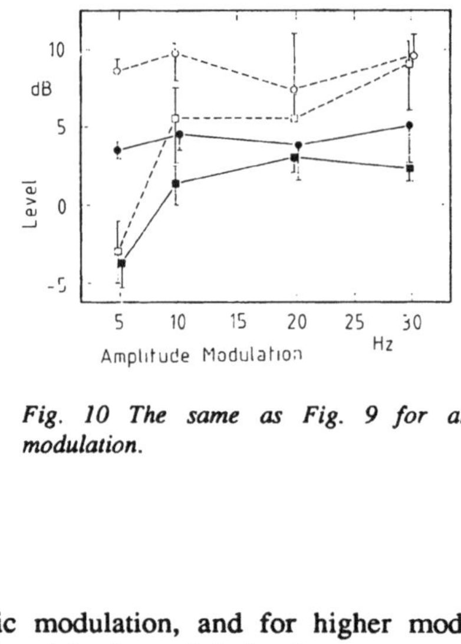

Fig. 10 The same as Fig. 9 for amplitude modulation.

segregation threshold is reached for antiphasic modulation, and for higher modulation frequencies the difference between in-phase and antiphasic modulation becomes very small.

These findings support the interpretation that the sound is statically analyzed with a window length of about 200 ms as was used to compute the modulation spectrum in Fig. 7. Since spectral resolution in such a representation corresponds to the inverse of the window length, two periodic signals will separate if their fundamentals differ by more than 5 Hz. If the fundamentals vary significantly during the analysis period - as is the case for modulation frequencies above 5 Hz - the resolved modulation frequencies are smeared out more and more and the two patterns representing "test" and "interfering" sounds will overlap increasingly. This interpretation corresponds to the findings reviewed and measured by Darwin (this volume) that tone onset allows separation as soon as the onset time differences are of the same order as the proposed window length.

6. Modelling the Internal Representation of Sound

Up to now, we have argued qualitatively that a representation of complex tones in terms of modulation spectra explains the observed dependence of the segregation threshold on different temporal parameters. In this section, we will show some simulations, in which quantitative predictions about the similarity between the "reference" alone and the superposition of "test" and "interfering" sound are derived, using a pattern matching algorithm.

We assume that the listener can store the modulation spectra of the "reference" and of the "interfering" sound in short-time memory. This assumption seems reasonable for the "reference", because it is presented in isolation before each test interval. The corresponding pattern for the "interfering" sound can, of course, be derived in those test intervals, where the "test" sound has a very low level. If a new sound is perceived, e.g. the superposition of the "interfering" sound and the "test" sound, the observer tries to match both stored patterns to the actual modulation representation.

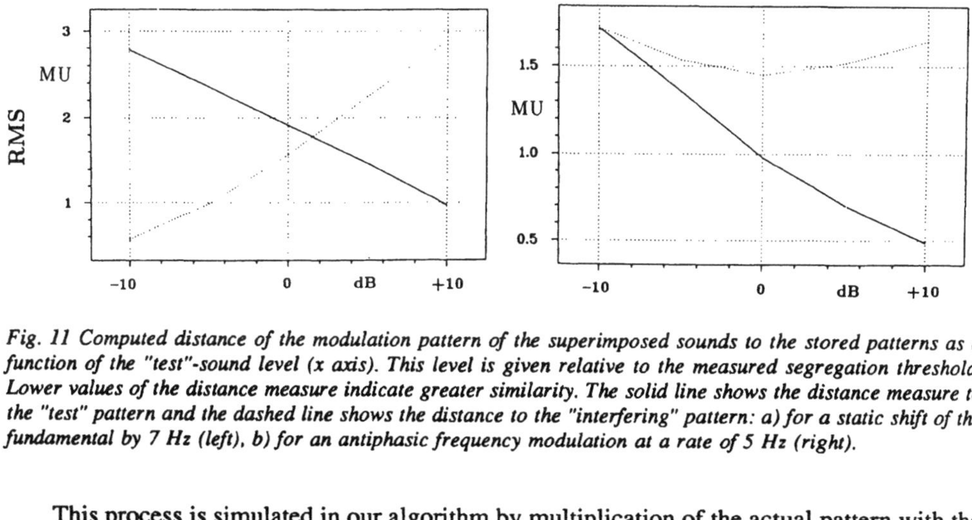

Fig. 11 Computed distance of the modulation pattern of the superimposed sounds to the stored patterns as a function of the "test"-sound level (x axis). This level is given relative to the measured segregation threshold. Lower values of the distance measure indicate greater similarity. The solid line shows the distance measure to the "test" pattern and the dashed line shows the distance to the "interfering" pattern: a) for a static shift of the fundamental by 7 Hz (left), b) for an antiphasic frequency modulation at a rate of 5 Hz (right).

This process is simulated in our algorithm by multiplication of the actual pattern with the stored ones - a process of matched filtering. From this product the square root is taken and the difference with the stored pattern is computed. The rms-value of this difference provides a measure of similarity or distance measure to the stored pattern. In order to model a certain experiment we performed this procedure for several combinations of "interfering" and "test" sounds, in which the level of the "test" sound was varied in a range of +/- 10 dB around the measured segregation threshold. For each level of the "test" sound the modulation spectrum of the test interval had to be computed again, due to the highly nonlinear preprocessing prior to the calculation of the power spectrum. All these computations were done only for one frequency channel at 1 kHz, assuming that other channels give a similar output. This is of course a simplification and certainly not true in low-frequency channels. A more sophisticated algorithm could contain a weighting scheme between the various basilar-membrane frequency channels.

Fig. 11a shows the results of the simulation for a static frequency shift of 7 Hz. The distance of the input pattern to the two stored patterns is shown as a function of the "test"-sound level, where the value 0 dB corresponds to the measured segregation threshold. The continuous line gives the distance to the "reference" and the dotted line the distance to the "interfering" sound. Smaller values of the distance measure correspond to greater similarity. With increasing level of the "test" sound, the modulation spectrum of the sum becomes more similar to the "reference" (solid line) and less similar to the "interfering" sound (dashed line). The two measures of similarity cross near the measured segregation threshold. This result should not be interpreted as a switching between detection of one or the other pattern, but rather as finding a region of levels where both patterns can equally well be "heard out" of the superposition. The corresponding calculation for 5-Hz antiphasic modulation in Fig. 11b shows a similar result. As already observed in the measurements for this low modulation frequency, the antiphasic modulation is treated similarly to a static difference in fundamental frequency.

A different picture results from the analysis of two sounds with identical static fundamental frequency (Fig. 12a) or an in-phase frequency modulation (Fig. 12b). Again the similarity to the stored pattern for the "test" sound increases with increasing "test"-sound level (solid line). The dotted curve for the "interfering" sound, however, shows a nonmonotonic behavior. The right branch of the curve is explained by a greater similarity of the combined pattern to the "test" sound and, therefore, a decreasing similarity to the "interfering" sound

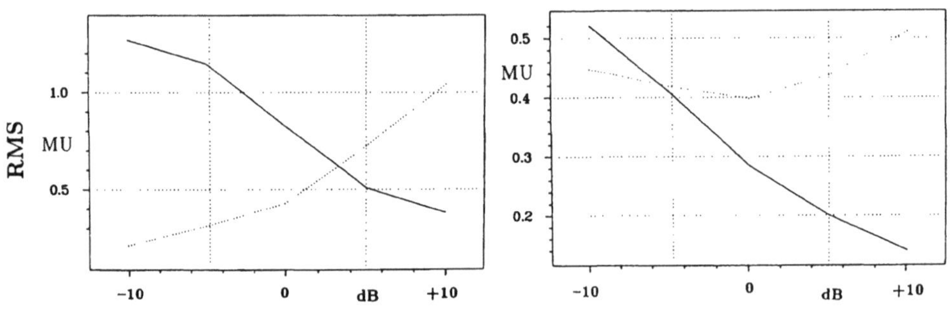

Fig. 12 Similar to Fig. 11 for identical fundamental frequencies of "test" and "interfering" sound (left) and for an in-phase frequency modulation at a rate of 5 Hz (right).

(cf. above arguments for Fig. 11). For decreasing level (left branch of the curve) both sounds are fused into a new complex which differs from the"interfering" as well as from the "test" sound. If the even harmonics of 100 Hz, which form the "interfering" sound, and the odd harmonics of 100 Hz, which form the "test" sound, have the same amplitude, they together perfectly add to a complex with 100 Hz fundamental. This fusion will be perfect at a level of -10 dB in the simulation, because the level axis in Fig. 12 is referred to the measured segregation threshold - which has a value of about 10 dB The resulting new sound has a very distinct pitch corresponding to 100 Hz, while the two individual sounds are usually perceived by the subjects as having a pitch corresponding to 200 Hz. If we could follow the curves further to lower "test"-sound levels, the distance measure for the "interfering" pattern would decrease. In summary, for the case of identical fundamental frequencies or an in-phase modulation, the segregation threshold seems to be reached at a level where the pattern representing the 100-Hz sound disappears.

7. CONCLUSIONS

The present experiments show that amplitude and frequency modulations improve segregation substantially only at low modulation rates (up to 5 Hz). This rate corresponds to the well-known integration time constant of the hearing system of about 200 ms (Zwislocki, 1960). An internal representation of sound is proposed, in which the sounds separate along the modulation frequency axis. In order to make the specific pattern of modulation frequencies less dependent on overall level, a preprocessing algorithm with a (static) level-compressing characteristic, originally designed to model forward masking, is included in the calculations. To perform quantitative comparisons we used a simple pattern matching algorithm. The model calculations show changes of the measure of similarity in the level region of the measured segregation threshold. How critically these results depend on the details of the calculations remains an open question. So far the experimental results can be described as the result of a pattern matching process acting on the modulation spectrum, which has been computed with a window length of about 200 ms.

Acknowledgements

Comments on an earlier draft by M. v.d. Heijden, A.J.M. Houtsma and N. Versfeld are gratefully acknowledged. This work was supported by grants from the Deutsche Forschungsgemeinschaft (Ko 1033/3, Pu 80/1-2).

References

Alphei, H. (1990). *Über die monaurale Trennbarkeit von Tonkomplexen*, Ph.D. thesis, University of Göttingen.

Boer, E. de (1985). Auditory time constants: a paradox?, in: *Time resolution in auditory systems*, edited by A. Michelsen, Springer, 141-158.

Carlyon, R.P. (1988). The development and decline of forward masking, *Hear. Res.*, 32, 65-80.

Darwin, C.J. (1984). Perceiving vowels in the presence of another sound: constraints on formant perception, *J. Acoust. Soc. Am.*, 76, 1636-1647

Duifhuis, H. (1973). Consequences of peripheral frequency selectivity for nonsimultaneous masking, *J. Acoust. Soc. Am.*, 54, 1471-1488.

Gardner, R.B., Gaskill, S.A., and Darwin, C.J. (1989). Perceptual grouping of formants with static and dynamic differences in fundamental frequency, *J. Acoust. Soc. Am.*, 85, 1329-1337.

Gilkey, R.H., Robinson, D.E., and Hanna, T.E. (1985). Effects of masker waveform and signal-to-masker phase relation on diotic and dichotic masking by reproducible noise, *J. Acoust. Soc. Am.*, 78, 1207-1219.

Moore, B.C.J. and Glasberg, B.R. (1982). Contralateral and ipsilateral cueing in forward masking, *J. Acoust. Soc. Am.*, 71, 942-945.

Paping, M. (1991). *Anwendung psychoakustischer und neurobiologischer Modelle in der automatischen Spracherkennung*, Unpublished Master thesis, University of Göttingen.

Patterson, R.D., Robinson, K., Holdsworth, J., McKeown, D., Zhang, C., and Allerhand, M. (1992). Complex sounds and auditory images, in: *Auditory Physiology and Perception*, edited by Y. Cazals, L. Demany, and K. Horner, Pergamon, 429-443.

Penner, M.J. (1978). A power law transformation resulting in a class of short-term integrators that produce time-intensity trades for noise bursts, *J. Acoust. Soc. Am.*, 63, 195-200.

Penner, M.J. and Shiffrin, R.M. (1980). Nonlinearities in the coding of intensity within the context of a temporal summation model, *J. Acoust. Soc. Am.*, 67, 617-627.

Pfafflin, S.M. and Mathews, M.V. (1962). Energy-detection model for monaural auditory detection, *J. Acoust. Soc. Am.*, 34, 1842-1853.

Püschel, D. (1988). *Prinzipien der zeitlichen Analyse beim Hören*, Ph.D. thesis, University of Göttingen.

Rasch, R. (1987). The perception of simultaneous notes such as in polyphonic music, *Acustica*, 40, 21-33.

Schreiner, C.E. and Langner, G. (1988). Coding of temporal patterns in the auditory nervous system, in: *Auditory Function*, edited by G.M. Edelman, W.E. Gall, and W.M. Cowan, John Wiley & Sons, 337-361.

Strube, H.W. (1985). A computationally efficient basilar-membrane model, *Acustica*, 58, 207-214.

Westerman, L.A. and Smith, R.L. (1984). Rapid and short-term adaptation in auditory nerve responses, *Hear. Res.*, 15, 249-260.

Yost, W.A., Grantham, D.W., Lutfi, R.A., and Stern, R.M. (1982). The phase angle of addition in temporal masking for diotic and dichotic listening conditions, *Hear. Res.*, 7, 247-259.

Zwislocki, J. (1960). Theory of temporal auditory summation, *J. Acoust. Soc. Am.*, 32, 1046-1060.

Preadaptations in the Auditory System of Mammals for Phoneme Perception

Günter Ehret
Department of Comparative Neurobiology
University of Ulm
D-7900 Ulm
Federal Republic of Germany

1. Introduction

Many auditory physiologists concerned with human hearing and speech perception study auditory processes in birds and mammals or at least accept and consider data and models from animals as relevant for the understanding of human auditory mechanisms. The general philosophy behind this comparative approach may sometimes be guided not so much by an interest in the diversity of auditory specialization and ecological adaptation, but by the search for the otherwise inaccessible parts and functions of the human auditory system in animals. The structural and, as far as we know, functional congruence of the peripheral auditory systems of mammals and man is the basis for the numerous successful predictions of human peripheral auditory mechanisms by animal studies and for the well-founded hopes that sound processing in the human outer, middle, and inner ear, auditory nerve, and brainstem may be explained by research on animals.

On these foundations we may ask at what levels and by what mechanisms human auditory functions may become species-specific, especially with regard to speech perception. Do we have animal models for the study of perceptual features that have been thought to be speech-specific, such as categorical perception, perceptual constancy despite of variability in many acoustic dimensions, perception of the formant structure in multi-tone complexes, phoneme perception, and left hemisphere dominance for semantic processing?

In the following, I shall review evidence from mammals demonstrating that such features have been found in sound perception of several species and may therefore be general preadaptations for the analysis and recognition of communication sounds in mammals, including humans.

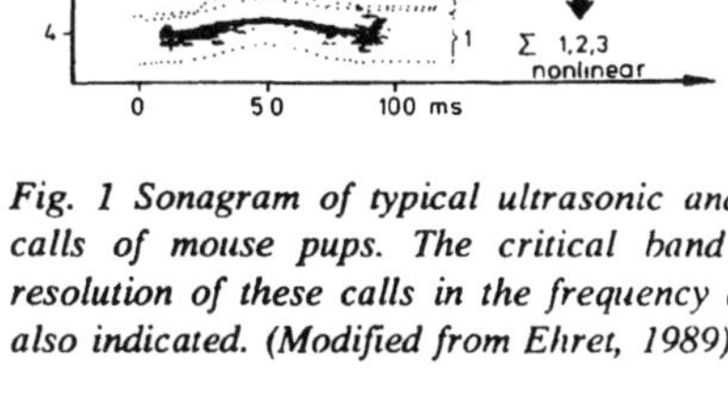

Fig. 1 Sonagram of typical ultrasonic and wriggling calls of mouse pups. The critical band filters for resolution of these calls in the frequency domain are also indicated. (Modified from Ehret, 1989)

2. Categorical Perception

Young pups of house mice (Mus musculus) produce pure ultrasonic calls mainly when they are in an uncomfortable situation outside the nest (e. g. Zippelius and Schleidt, 1956; Okon, 1972; Ehret, 1975; Sales and Smith, 1978). The calls alarm the mother or another caretaker, who search and find the pup by phonotaxis, pick it up and carry it back to the nest (e.g. Noirot, 1972; Smotherman et al., 1974; Haack et al., 1983). The calls are frequency-modulated single tones with durations between 30 and 120 ms, located in a frequency band usually between 40 and 80 kHz (Fig. 1; see also e. g. Ehret, 1975; Sales and Smith, 1978). Since the calls release a stereotyped phonotaxic search and pup retrieval, this unconditioned instinctive parental behaviour can be used to test what features of the ultrasounds (US) are important for recognition.

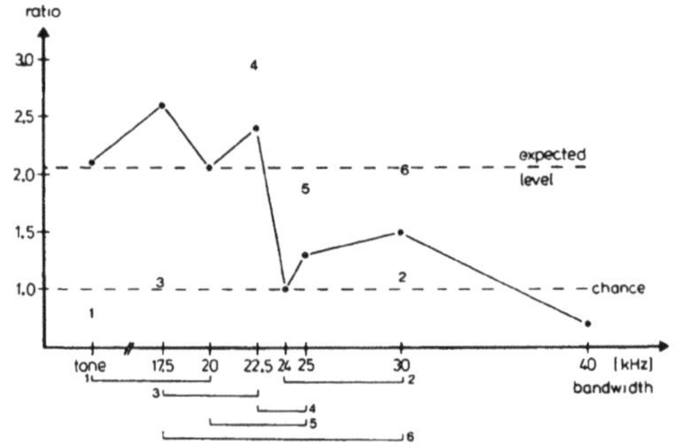

Fig. 2 Categorical perception of mouse pup ultrasounds in the frequency domain. The labelling function is derived from a continuum of noise bandwidths centered at 50 kHz (ultrasound models) and labelled against a neutral non-preferred 20 kHz stimulus. In addition, the outcome of discrimination tests between the ultrasound models indicated is shown by numerals. The ordinate gives the ratio of the numbers of responses to the ultrasound models and the 20 kHz tone (labelling tests) or the ratio of the number of responses to two ultrasound models (discrimination tests). The expected level shows the ratio obtained from a comparison of preferred natural ultrasounds versus 20 kHz tone bursts. tone = tone of 60 kHz frequency. (Data from Ehret and Haack, 1981, 1982).

In a two-alternative choice test we varied the bandwidths of synthetized US systematically and found that the mice formed two perceptual categories (Fig. 2; Ehret and Haack, 1981, 1982; Ehret, 1987 b). Sounds centered around about 50 kHz with bandwidths less than 24 kHz were preferred releasers with a preference level very similar to that of natural calls; sounds of 24 kHz bandwidth and larger all appeared to be little attractive. These labelling tests demonstrated a clear boundary in the bandwidths continuum close to 23 kHz (Fig. 2). Categorical perception was verified by additional discrimination tests that showed within-category non-discrimination and across-category discrimination (Fig. 2).

The auditory mechanism underlying this type of categorical perception most probably is the critical band filter (Fig. 1). Critical bandwidths determined psychophysically with a narrow-band noise masking procedure equal 23 kHz at a center frequency of 50 kHz (Ehret, 1976), which is just the critical noise bandwidth of a preferred releaser of parental behaviour. Additional tests confirmed the relationship between the bandwidths of the auditory filters and stimulus recognition (Ehret and Haack, 1982; Ehret, 1983).

Ultrasounds are not only categorically perceived in the frequency domain but also in the temporal domain. Labelling and discrimination tests on a continuum of call durations showed (Fig. 3) that 50 or 60 kHz tones of 25 ms and shorter belong to a non-preferred category if compared with a long-duration (> 80 ms) preferred sound, while tone durations of 30 ms and longer are labelled same as the comparison tones with long durations (Ehret and Haack, 1982; Ehret, 1991). Remarkably, sounds taken from the two categories are discriminated across the category border close to 25 ms only if the duration difference is at least 20 - 25 ms (Fig. 3). Although belonging to different categories, sounds with less than 20 ms absolute duration difference are not discriminated. Thus, the category boundary may be established on the basis of a natural time constant or a threshold of duration discrimination in the auditory system. A threshold or a time constant of about 20 ms in the temporal domain has been observed in several psychophysical studies in man including the perception of temporal order (Summerfield, 1982), the detection of a gap between a noisy sound onset and a buzz-like stimulus continuation (Stevens and Klatt, 1974), the perception of a temporal gap in noise (Penner, 1975), the perception of tone-onset differences between two frequencies (Pisoni, 1977), and the detection of amplitude modulation as a function of modulation frequency (de Boer, 1985). In addition, studies on the perception of voice-onset times of speech phonemes in man and animals are in harmony with a basic 20 - 25 ms critical duration of processing in the mammalian auditory system, since the shortest boundary on the continuum of voice-onset-time occurs at about 25 ms for the /ba/-/pa/ discrimination both in man and chinchilla (Pisoni and Lazarus, 1974; Kuhl and Miller, 1978).

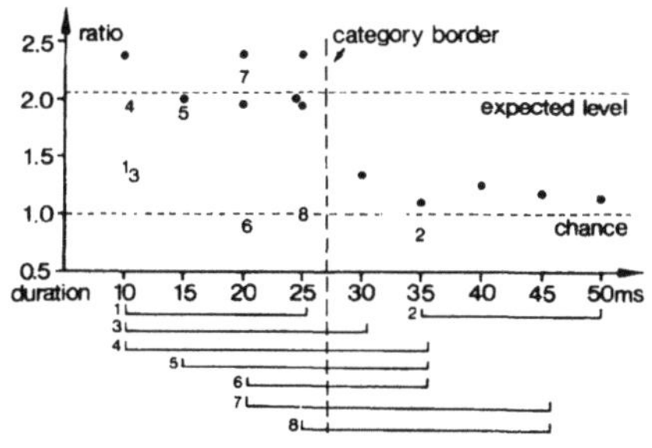

Fig. 3. Categorical perception of mouse pup ultrasounds in the temporal domain. The labelling function (filled circles) is derived from 50 kHz tone bursts that varied along a continuum of sound duration and were labelled against a preferred comparison stimulus of 50 kHz and at least 85 ms duration. In addition, the outcome of discrimination tests between the sounds of different duration as indicated by numerals is presented. The ordinate gives the ratio of the number of responses to the long comparison stimulus and the test stimuli of the shorter durations (10 - 50 ms, labelling tests) or the ratio of the number of responses to two stimuli of different durations (discrimination tests). Expected level as in Fig. 2. (Data from Ehret and Haack, 1982 and Ehret, 1991).

These experiments on ultrasound perception in mice clearly demonstrate the phenomenon of categorical perception in the case of a non-primate species-specific call. Category boundaries seem to be set and can be explained by general auditory mechanisms. The ascription of meaning to the categories, however, needs higher innate or learned strategies that become evident in the correct or biologically adaptive responding to stimuli from the different categories.

A further case of categorical perception of species-specific communication calls has been described. Japanese macaque monkeys produce two types of frequency modulated contact calls ("coo" sounds), one in which the frequency maximum is reached early in the call (early high), the other with a late frequency maximum (late high; Green, 1975). The two types convey different information about the sender. Early-high calls are typical of isolated animals, while late-high calls are emitted by a subordinate to a dominant animal. May et al. (1989) showed that Japanese macaques label a synthetized continuum of calls with different positions of frequency peaks into two categories. Discrimination tests under high-uncertainty conditions confirmed the category border of the position of the frequency peak close to 125 ms after the beginning of the call.

The physiological mechanisms of the auditory system for this kind of categorization are not yet clear. The critical parameter could be the relative duration of an upward compared to a downward frequency sweep in the call or the duration after call onset until the maximum frequency is reached. Since neurons selectively sensitive to upward or downward frequency sweeps and to the speed of frequency modulation have been found in the inferior colliculus and auditory cortex of mammals (e. g. Whitfield and Evans, 1965; Nelson et al., 1966; Suga, 1973; Mendelson and Cynader, 1985), the neuronal basis for categorization, in terms of encoding the relevant sound parameter, is present in the auditory system.

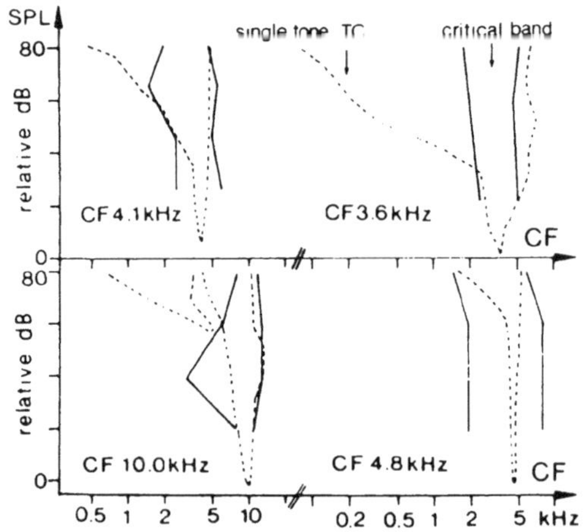

Fig. 4 Comparison of single-tone tuning curves (TC) (dashed lines) and tuning curves for complex sound analysis = critical bands measured in a narrow-band masking paradigm (solid lines) for four neurons of the inferior colliculus of the cat. CF = characteristic frequency, SPL = sound pressure level. (Modified from Ehret and Merzenich, 1988).

3. Perceptual Constancy

Perceptual constancy for speech sounds across various speakers and in a wide range of intensities is an absolute must if speech is going to be used as a reliable vehicle for the transfer of semantic information without ambiguities introduced by intonation- or intensity-dependent processing in the auditory system. The most suitable way to establish perceptual constancy in the frequency domain is to use the outputs of the critical band filters of the auditory system as a basis for decisions about the spectral composition of a sound.

Many psychophysical tests have shown that critical bands are spectral filters of constant bandwidth over a broad range of sound intensities within which sound energy is integrated into units of perception (e. g. Fletcher, 1940; Zwicker und Feldtkeller, 1967; Scharf, 1970; Scharf and Meiselman, 1977; Moore, 1982; Ehret, 1988). Thus, the output of the whole bank of critical band filters provides an instantaneous picture of the spectral energy distribution of a sound characterized by an emphasis on spectral peaks and, for a given sound spectrum, by a constant relationship between the output amplitudes of single filters independent of sound intensity. Vowels in speech, for example, can be identified by the frequency ratios of their formants largely independently of the pitch of the voice and its intensity (Flanagan, 1972).

We found that the key-features of the critical band filters as they are established in psychophysical tests are realised by a spike-rate code in single neurons of the auditory midbrain (inferior colliculus) of the cat (Ehret and Merzenich 1985, 1988). In Fig. 4, examples of critical band filter shapes are shown for four neurons together with the conventional frequency tuning curves. It is evident that the "tuning curves for complex sound analysis" (critical band filters) have rather constant bandwidths and can differ substantially in shape from the single-tone tuning curves, so that conventional tuning curves seem to be inadequate predictors of frequency resolution at the level of the inferior colliculus. Further, we have shown that not only spectral filtering is independent of sound intensity but also spectral integration within the critical bands. In Fig. 5, the signal-to-noise ratio at the masked tonal threshold (tone level minus noise spectral level) is shown for many neurons in the inferior colliculus of the cat as a function of the neurons' characteristic frequencies (CF) and of the sound pressure level (SPL) of the masked CF-tone. Since statistically significant relationships did not occur, we find that spectral integration within critical band filters is, on the average, the same for neurons in the whole frequency range and independent of sound intensity.

These data on the physiology of critical bands show that this central mechanism of hearing in mammals, being responsible for spectral sound analysis, becomes manifest in neuronal response characteristics at the midbrain level and thus serves as an essential prerequisite for perceptual constancy in the frequency domain and for evaluation of spectral features of animal calls and speech in higher brain centers. Hence, the physiological mechanisms underlying critical band filtering in mammals can be regarded as a preadaptation for speech analysis in the spectral domain of the human auditory system.

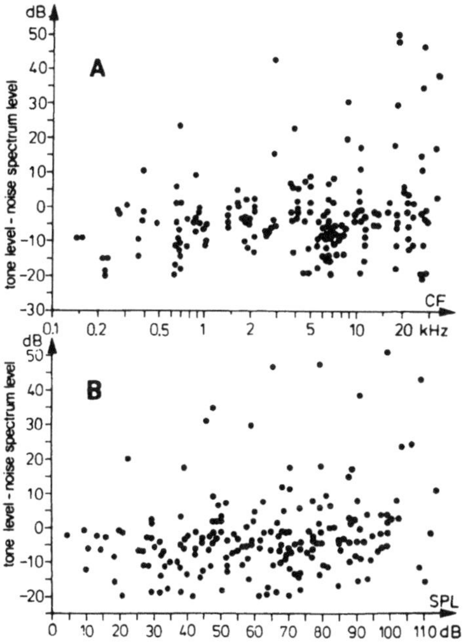

Fig. 5 Signal-to-noise ratios at the masked tonal thresholds (tone level minus noise spectrum level) for noise bandwidths equal to the critical bandwidths of neurons in the inferior colliculus of the cat. The frequency of the tone to be masked was equal to the characteristic frequency (CF) of the neuron. The critical bandwidth was determined in a narrow-band masking paradigm. Signal-to-noise ratios are shown as a function of CF (A) and sound pressure level (SPL; B). (Modified from Ehret and Merzenich, 1988).

4. Perception of Formant Structure

In harmonically structured sounds like vowels certain harmonics are often stressed by resonances of the vocal tract. These resonances are called formants. Each vowel in human speech has a characteristic formant composition which, however, does not form a seperate perceptual category, but can change gradually into that of another vowel.

Mouse pups struggling for their mother's nipples when she is lying in a lactating position on the pups, produce low-frequency harmonically structured calls, the "wriggling calls" (Fig. 1; Ehret, 1975; Ehret and Bernecker, 1986). These calls are of communicative significance and stimulate maternal care, namely licking of pups, changing lactation position, and nest building. We were interested in the question of how the mothers perceive the wriggling-call structure and whether the harmonics have a formant character (Ehret and Riecke, unpublished). Fig. 6 shows data from a series of tests in which the synthesized wriggling calls were presented in a lactation situation, while the mother could also be stimulated by natural wriggling calls from her own pups. A quality coefficient (Q) was calculated, indicating the relative effectiveness of response release by a call model compared with that of natural calls in the same lactation period. Thus, influences of general motivation, attention, and arousal were eliminated, so that the responsiveness to the call models became comparable among the animals.

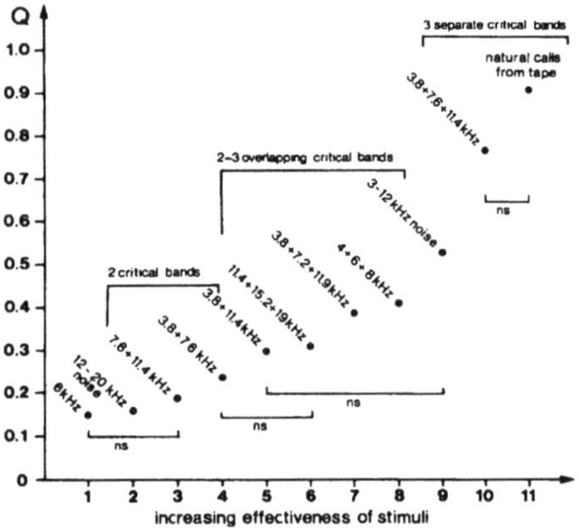

Fig. 6 The effectiveness of various synthesized stimuli as models of wriggling calls for the release of maternal behaviour. The effectiveness is expressed by a quality coefficient (Q) calculated from the relative number of responses to a given call model divided by the relative number of responses to natural calls of pups produced in the test situation. Q can vary between zero (no response to call model) and 1 (equal relative responsiveness to call model and natural calls). Each data point is the mean of tests with five animals. The results of some statistical comparisons of the means are shown to give an idea of which stimuli are not different (ns) in releasing responses. It is also shown how the stimuli could be resolved by the critical band filters of the mouse (bandwidths from Ehret, 1976).

In Fig. 6, average Q-values (n = 5 for each call model) are shown, and the call models are ordered for increasing effectiveness in releasing maternal behaviour. Playbacks of natural calls from tape are almost as effective as the calls produced by pups in the test situation. A high releasing potential not significantly different from that of natural calls was recorded in response to a three-component call resembling the main formants of natural wriggling calls: 3.8 + 7.6 + 11.4 kHz. All the other call models including noise bands and three-, two-, and one-component sounds were significantly less efficient releasers. The quality coefficient decreased with decreasing number of formants in the frequency range of about 3 - 12 kHz (the main range of natural calls, Fig. 1). It is interesting that 1. the first formant of 3.8 kHz, which is the fundamental of the harmonic complex, is more important in its contribution to the response release than the other two formants; 2. the phenomenon of hearing of the missing fundamental (3.8 kHz) seems to occur in the 11.4 + 15.2 + 19 kHz complex, which is as good a releaser as the 3.8 + 11.4 kHz complex; 3. the formants should fall into three critical bands with little overlap (bandwidths about 4 kHz between 3 and 10 kHz; Ehret, 1976) in the low frequency range between about 3 and 12 kHz (Fig. 6).

These results show that wriggling calls seem to be recognised mainly on the basis of their formant structure, which is represented by the output of three neighbouring critical band filters. These outputs are summed in a nonlinear way to generate optimum call recognition (Fig. 1). This strategy of wriggling call perception in mice, which obviously is linked to the summation of outputs of critical bands, seems to be comparable of the summation of formant energies for vowel perception in human speech and may again be regarded as a preadaptation in the auditory system of mammals that later became useful in speech sound recognition.

5. Phoneme Perception

Phonemes may be defined as the smallest acoustical units on the basis of which speech syllables or words are discriminated. Four features seem to be most important (e. g. Liberman et al., 1956; Liberman and Pisoni, 1977): the formant structure of vowels (the constant frequency parts of the formant complexes), formant transitions (frequency-modulated parts at the beginnings and ends of the formants), noise bursts characterising many consonants, and temporal gaps between consonants and vowels (e. g. voice-onset-time). Suga (1988), in comparing the acoustical features of speech that are used for information coding with the respective features of echolocation sounds of the mustached bat, uses the term "information-bearing element" for the constant-frequency and frequency-modulated parts of vowels and for the noise bursts, and the term "information-bearing parameter" for factors characterizing relationships between the elements such as, for example, voice-onset-time. By the work of Suga and his colleagues (reviews see Suga et al., 1981; Suga, 1988), the mustached bat has become the best studied mammal with regard to encoding biologically significant information by information-bearing elements, parameters, and combinations of them, and representing this information in parametric maps in the auditory cortex.

This example demonstrates that formant composition, formant transitions, and temporal relationships among sound elements are perceived as separate acoustical units and used for the extraction of different aspects of meaning of the sound. Hence, mechanisms comparable to phoneme perception are present in the auditory system of this bat, and indicate that this level of analysis is reached in a non-primate mammal.

As far as I know, echolocation sound is the only case of a species-specific call for which associations of various sound parameters with certain meanings has been demonstrated so far. As explained before, however, the preadaptation for the perception of the four types of above-mentioned features are present in mechanisms of sound analysis in the auditory system of mammals, so that we can predict more cases of phoneme-like perception of species-specific calls to be found by further studies.

Examples of categorical perception of speech phonemes by chinchillas and macaque monkeys with the same category boundaries as determined by human listeners (e. g. Kuhl and Miller, 1975, 1978; Kuhl, 1987; Waters and Wilson, 1976) clearly demonstrate the potential of mammals for speech phoneme perception, which, therefore, must have evolved long before our primate ancestors spoke the first word. Obviously, auditory mechanisms of speech analysis preceded the production of speech. This is reflected by responses of neurons in the medial geniculate body of cats and the auditory cortex of macaque monkeys, which show rather selective responsiveness to phonemes of human speech (e. g. Keidel, 1974; Steinschneider et al., 1990).

6. Left Hemisphere Dominance for Semantic Processing

In most people the left hemisphere of the forebrain is dominant for the processing of the semantic content of speech, which means mainly a dominance for processing and recognition of phonemes that characterize syllables and words and sequences of them (e. g. Kimura, 1961; Cutting, 1974; Bradshaw and Nettleton, 1981; Molfese et al. 1983). Since this left hemisphere advantage occurs already in newborn infants (e. g. Molfese and Molfese, 1979; Woods, 1983; Bertoncini et al. 1989), it seems to be an inborn preadaptation which might have a long evolutionary history.

Studies on the recognition of species-specific coo calls in Japanese macaques (Beecher et al. 1979; Petersen et al., 1984) showed a left hemisphere advantage for the perception of the information-bearing element (position of the frequency peak) that was decisive for the categorical perception of these calls (see before). Ablation of the left-side auditory cortex temporarily impaired coo call discrimination, while a similar ablation of the right side had no effect (Heffner and Heffner, 1986). This shows that macaque monkeys recognize calls and particular call features important for communication preferentially with the left hemisphere.

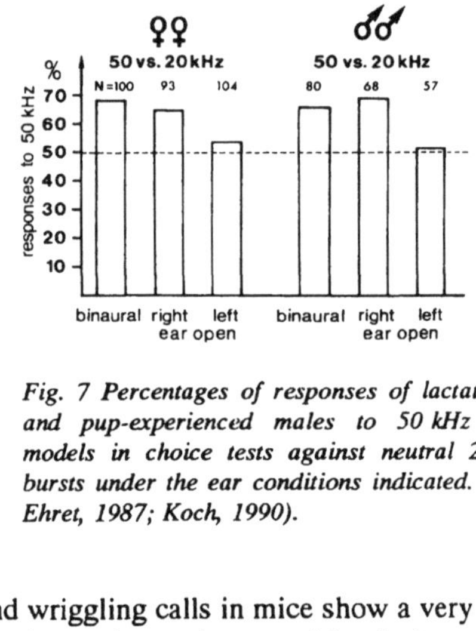

Fig. 7 Percentages of responses of lactating females and pup-experienced males to 50 kHz ultrasound models in choice tests against neutral 20 kHz tone bursts under the ear conditions indicated. (Data from Ehret, 1987; Koch, 1990).

Our studies on hemisphere lateralization of the perception of ultrasounds and wriggling calls in mice show a very close correspondence with lateralized semantic processing and speech recognition in humans (Ehret, 1987 a, and unpublished; Haase and Ehret, 1990; Koch, 1990). Lactating mothers and fathers, the latter only after achieving experience with pup care, prefer models of pup ultrasounds (50 kHz tone bursts) compared to a neutral sound (20 kHz tone bursts) under binaural and right ear (left hemisphere) listening conditions (Fig. 7). This preference for the ultrasound is lost if they hear only with their left ear (right hemisphere). Further tests showed that the right ear (left hemisphere) advantage occurs only in a situation in which the ultrasounds are of communicative significance and can initiate an instinctive maternal response. If female mice without pup experience are conditioned with an operant-reward procedure to prefer 50 kHz tone bursts over 20 kHz tones and are tested under the same experimental setting with the same behavioural task and the same stimuli as the mothers with pups, they do not show a hemisphere advantage. They are able to discriminate the 50 and 20 kHz tone bursts and prefer 50 kHz under all ear conditions (binaural, only right ear or left ear open; Ehret,

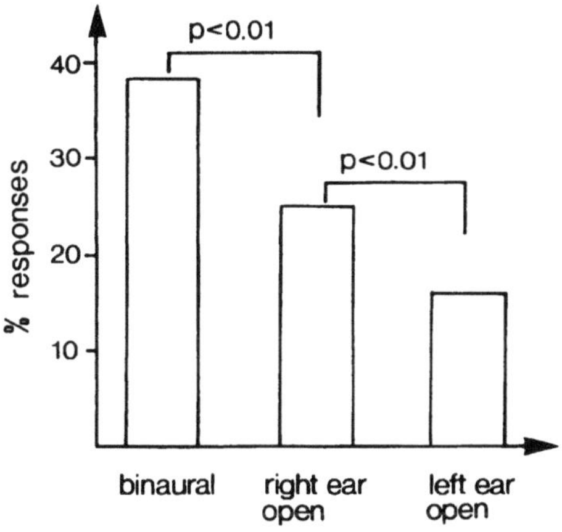

Fig. 8 Percentages of responses to natural wriggling calls of females in a lactation situation under the ear conditions indicated. (modified from Haase and Ehret, 1990).

1987 a). These data show that both hemispheres can do sound discrimination, take a decision about what sound is important, and release the appropriate response equally well. The left hemisphere advantage comes into play only in a communicative situation in which ultrasound can release an instinctive behaviour or, in other words, conveys a message that fits into innate releasing mechanisms for the extraction of meaning.

The right ear (left hemisphere) advantage is also visible in the perception of wriggling calls of mouse pups by the mother in a situation of lactation (Fig. 8). We also used some of the synthetized call models shown in Fig. 6 to test whether a right ear advantage occurs with good releasers only or also with sub-optimum sounds. Fig. 9 gives a clear answer. Call models of little behavioural relevance (6 kHz and 3.8 + 11.4 kHz, compare Fig. 6) do not lead to a differential processing in the left and right hemisphere. The three-component call model (3.8 + 7.6 + 11.4 kHz) that released maternal responses almost equally well as the natural calls is perceived with a large and statistically significant right ear advantage (Fig. 9). This is a very interesting result because it shows that for a distorted signal, which lacks important information-bearing elements and consequently semantic content, also the left hemisphere advantage of perception and recognition is lost. A very similar effect of loss of lateralisation has been shown with synthetized speech phonemes that are either heard as speech (left hemisphere advantage) or not (no lateralization; Cutting, 1974).

These results on the left hemisphere advantage for semantic processing and species-specific call recognition in mice demonstrate no basic differences with left hemisphere dominance of human speech perception. The mechanisms responsible for lateralization may be the same in both species and related to gating mechanisms in the left ventrolateral thalamus (e. g. Ojemann, 1975; Mateer and Ojemann, 1983; Hugdahl et al., 1990). In this view, the left hemisphere advantage for species-specific call recognition in a communicative context could be mediated by general mechanisms of selective attention that are not special for humans.

7. Conclusions

My review on preadaptations in the auditory system of mammals for processing complex sounds like speech phonemes may be condensed into four essential points: 1. Most information about mechanisms of speech perception will be obtained from studies using stimuli that are complex in the spectral and/or temporal and/or spectro-temporal domain. 2. In speech perception, mechanisms and strategies of analysis - including categorical perception, perceptual constancy, formant and phoneme perception, left hemisphere advantage for semantic processing - are found that are general characteristics of mammalian auditory systems. 3. On a perceptual level, speech seems not to be handled in a special way in the human brain or basically differently from communication calls in the brains of other mammals. Mammalian auditory pathways, therefore, are adequate systems for testing hypotheses about mechanisms of human speech perception, provided that species-specific calls are used as stimuli, not human speech. 4. Fundamental differences between human and mammalian speech and complex sound perception may first occur at the recognition or language level, that is, in the *interpretation* of the semantic content of speech sounds. Animals can perceive and analyse speech, but they do not know what we mean.

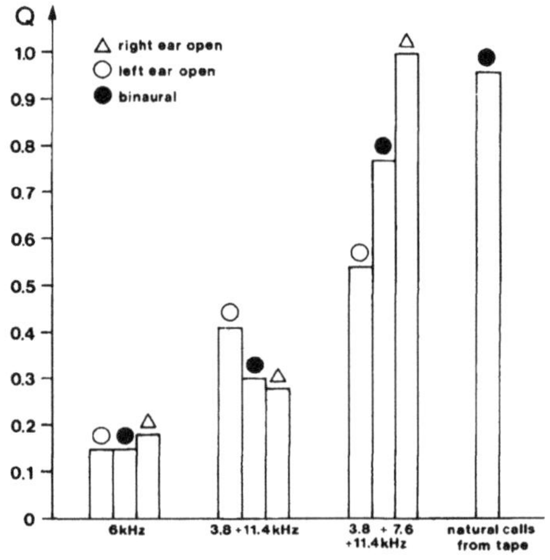

Fig. 9 Average (n = 5) relative effectiveness of various models of wriggling calls for the release of maternal behaviour. The quality coefficient (Q, same as in Fig. 6) is obtained for the ear conditions indicated. A large right ear advantage is visible only in the case of the three component call model (Ehret, unpublished).

Acknowledgements

Our original studies on sound perception in the mouse where supported by several grants of the Deutsche Forschungsgemeinschaft.

References

Beecher, M.D., Petersen, M.R., Zoloth, S.R., Moody, D.B., and Stebbins, W.C. (1979). Perception of conspecific vocalizations by Japanese macaques, *Brain Behav. Evol.*, 16, 443 - 460.

Bertoncini, J., Morais, J., Bijeljac-Babic, R., McAdams, S., Peretz, J., and Mehler, J. (1989). Dichotic perception and laterality in neonates, *Brain Lang.*, 37, 591 - 605.

de Boer, E. (1985). Auditory time constants: a paradox?, in: *Time Resolution in Auditory Systems,* (A. Michelsen, ed.), Springer, Berlin, 141 - 158.

Bradshaw, J.L. and Nettleton, N.C. (1981). The nature of hemispheric specialization in man, *Behav. Brain Sci.*, 4, 51-91.

Cutting, J.E. (1974). Two left-hemisphere mechanisms in speech perception, *Percept. Psychophys.*, 16, 601 - 612.

Ehret, G. (1975). Schallsignale der Hausmaus (**Mus musculus**), *Behaviour*, 52, 38 - 56.

Ehret, G. (1976). Critical bands and filter characteristics in the ear of the house mouse (**Mus musculus**), *Biol. Cybernet.*, 24, 35 - 42.

Ehret, G. (1983). Auditory processing and perception of ultrasound in house mice, in: *Advances in Vertebrate Neuroethology* (J.-P. Ewert, R.R. Capranica, D.J. Ingle, eds.), Plenum Press, London, 911 - 918.

Ehret, G. (1987 a). Left hemisphere advantage in the mouse brain for recognizing ultrasonic communication calls, *Nature*, 325, 249 - 251.

Ehret, G. (1987 b). Categorical perception of sound signals: facts and hypotheses from animal studies, in: *Categorical Perception* (S. Harnad, ed.), Cambridge University Press, Cambridge, 301 - 331.

Ehret, G. (1988). Frequency resolution, spectral filtering, and integration on the neuronal level, in: *Auditory Function. Neurobiological Bases of Hearing* (G.M. Edelman, W.E. Gall, W.M. Cowan, eds.), Wiley, New York, 363 - 384.

Ehret, G. (1989). Hearing in the mouse, in: *The Comparative Psychology of Audition. Perceiving Complex Sounds* (R.J. Dooling, S.H. Hulse, eds.), Erlbaum, Hillsdale, 3 - 32.

Ehret, G. (1992). Categorical perception of mouse pup ultrasounds in the temporal domain, *Anim. Behav.*, 43, 409-416.

Ehret, G. and Bernecker, C. (1986). Low-frequency sound communication by mouse pups (**Mus musculus**): wriggling calls release maternal behaviour, *Anim. Behav.*, 34, 821-830.

Ehret, G. and Haack, B. (1981). Categorical perception of mouse-pup ultrasounds by lactating females, *Naturwissenschaften*, 68, 208.

Ehret, G. and Haack, B. (1982). Ultrasound recognition in house mice: key-stimulus configuration and recognition mechanism, *J. Comp. Physiol. A.*, 148, 245 - 251.

Ehret, G. and Merzenich, M.M. (1985). Auditory midbrain responses parallel spectral integration phenomena, *Science*, 227, 1245 - 1247.

Ehret, G. and Merzenich, M.M. (1988). Complex sound analysis (frequency resolution, filtering and spectral integration) by single units of the inferior colliculus of the cat, *Brain Res. Revs.*, 13, 139-163.

Flanagan, J.L. (1972). *Speech Analysis, Synthesis, and Perception*, Springer, Berlin.

Fletcher, H. (1940). Auditory patterns, *Rev. Modern Phys.*, 12, 47 - 65.

Green, S. (1975). Variation of vocal pattern with social situation in the Japanese monkey (**Macaca fuscata**): a field study, in: *Primate Behavior*, Vol. 4 (L.A. Rosenblum, ed.), Academic Press, New York, 1-102.

Haack, B., Markl, H., and Ehret, G. (1983). Sound communication between parents and offspring, in: *The Auditory Psychobiology of the Mouse* (J.F. Willott, ed.), Thomas, Springfield, 57 - 97.

Haase, H. and Ehret, G. (1990). Lateralization of sound perception in the brain of the mouse (**Mus musculus**), in: *Brain-Perception-Cognition* (N. Elsner, G. Roth, eds.), Thieme, Stuttgart, 150.

Heffner, H.E. and Heffner, R.S. (1986). Effect of unilateral and bilaterial auditory cortex lesions on the discrimination of vocalizations by Japanese macaques, *J. Neurophysiol.*, 56, 683 - 701.

Hugdahl, K., Wester, K., and Asbjφrnsen, A. (1990). The role of the left and right thalamus in language asymmetry: dichotic listening in Parkinson patients undergoing stereotactic thalamotomy, *Brain Lang.*, 39, 1 - 13.

Keidel, W.D. (1974): Information processing in higher parts of the auditory pathway, in: *Facts and Models in Hearing* (E. Zwicker, E. Terhardt, eds.), Springer, Berlin, 216-226.

Kimura, D. (1961). Cerebral dominance and the perception of verbal stimuli, *Canad. J. Psychol.*, 15, 166 - 171.

Koch, M. (1990). Neuroendokrinologische Aspekte des Jungeneintrageverhaltens bei der Hausmaus (**Mus musculus**), *Konstanzer Dissertationen*, Vol. 265. Hartung-Gorre, Konstanz.

Kuhl, P.K. (1987). The special-mechanisms debate in speech research: categorization tests on animals and infants, in: *Categorical Perception* (S. Harnad, ed.), Cambridge University Press, Cambridge, 355 - 386.

Kuhl, P.K. and Miller, J.D. (1975). Speech perception by the chinchilla: voiced-voiceless distinction in alveolar plosive consonants, *Science*, 190, 69 - 72.

Kuhl, P.K. and Miller, J.D. (1978). Speech perception by the chinchilla: Identification functions for synthetic VOT stimuli, *J. Acoust. Soc. Am.*, 63, 905 - 917.

Liberman, A.M., Delattre, P.C., Gertman, L.J., and Cooper, F.S. (1956). Tempo of frequency change as a cue for distinguishing classes of speech sounds, *J. Exp. Psychol.*, 52, 127-137.

Liberman, A.M. and Pisoni, D.B. (1977). Evidence for a special speech-perceiving subsystem in the human, in: *Recognition of Complex Acoustic Signals* (T.H. Bullock, ed.), Abakon Verlagsgesellschaft, Berlin, 59 - 76.

Mateer, C.A. and Ojemann, G.A. (1983). Thalamic mechanisms in language and memory, in: *Language Functions and Brain Organization* (S.J. Segalowitz, ed.), Academic Press, New York, 171 - 191.

May, B., Moody, D.B., and Stebbins, W.C. (1989). Categorical perception of conspecific communication sounds by Japanese macaques, **Macaca fuscata**, *J. Acoust. Soc. Am.*, 85, 837-847.

Mendelson, J.R. and Cynader, M. S. (1985). Sensitivity of cat primary auditory cortex (AI) neurons to the direction and rate of frequency modulation, *Brain Res.*, 327, 331 - 335.

Molfese, D.L. and Molfese, V.J. (1979). Hemisphere and stimulus differences as reflected in the cortical responses of newborn infants to speech stimuli, *Dev. Psychol.*, 15, 505 - 511.

Molfese, V.J., Molfese, D.L., and Parsons, C. (1983). Hemisphere processing of phonological information, in: *Language Functions and Brain Organization* (S.J. Segalowitz, ed.), Academic Press, New York, 29 - 49.

Moore, B.C.J. (1982). *An Introduction to the Psychology of Hearing*, 2nd Ed., Academic Press, New York.

Nelson, P.G., Erulkar, S.D., and Bryan, J.S. (1966). Responses of units of the inferior colliculus to time-varying acoustic stimuli, *J. Neurophysiol.*, 29, 834 - 860.

Noirot, E. (1972). Ultrasound and maternal behavior in small rodents, *Dev. Psychobiol.*, 5, 371 - 387.

Ojemann, G.A. (1975). Language and the thalamus: object naming and recall during and after thalamic stimulation, *Brain Lang.*, 2, 101 - 120.

Okon, E.E., (1972). Factors affecting ultrasound production in infant rodents, *J. Zool. Lond.*, 168, 139 - 148.

Penner, M.J. (1975). Persistence and integration: two consequences of a sliding integrator, *Percept. Psychophys.*, 18, 114 - 120.

Petersen, M.R., Beecher, M.D., Zoloth, S.R., Green, S., Marler, P.R., Moody, D.B., and Stebbins, W.C. (1984). Neural lateralization of vocalizations by Japanese macaques: communicative significance is more important than acoustic structure, *Behav. Neurosci.*, 98, 779 - 790.

Pisoni, D.B. (1977). Identification and discrimination of the relative onset time of two component tones: implications for voicing perception in stops. *J. Acoust. Soc. Am.*, 61, 1352 - 1361.

Pisoni, D.B. and Lazarus, J.H. (1974). Categorical and noncategorical modes of speech perception along a voicing continuum, *J. Acoust. Soc. Am.*, 55, 328 - 333.

Sales, G.D. and Smith, J.C. (1978). Comparative studies of the ultrasonic calls of infant murid rodents, *Dev. Psychobiol.*, 11, 595 - 619.

Scharf, B. (1970). Critical bands, in: *Foundations of Modern Auditory Theory*, Vol. 1 (J. V. Tobias, ed.), Academic Press, New York, 159 - 202.

Scharf, B. and Meiselman, C.H. (1977). Critical bandwidths at high intensities, in: *Psychophysics and Physiology of Hearing* (E.F. Evans, J.P. Wilson, eds.), Academic Press, London, 221 - 232.

Smotherman, W.P., Bell, R.W., Starzec, J., Elias, J., and Zachman, T.A. (1974). Maternal responses to infant vocalizations and olfactory cues in rats and mice, *Behav. Biol.*, 12, 55 - 66.

Steinschneider, M., Arezzo, J.C., and Vaughan, H.G. (1990). Tonotopic features of speech-evoked activity in primate auditory cortex, *Brain Res.*, 519, 158 - 168.

Stevens, K.N. and Klatt, D.H. (1974). Role of formant transitions in the voiced-voiceless distinction for stops, *J. Acoust. Soc. Am.*, 55, 653 - 659.

Suga, N. (1973). Feature extraction in the auditory system of bats, in: *Basic Mechanisms in Hearing* (A.R. Møller, ed.), Academic Press, New York, 675 - 744.

Suga, N. (1988). Auditory neuroethology and speech processing: complex-sound processing by combination-sensitive neurons, in: *Auditory Function. Neurobiological Bases of Hearing* (G.M. Edelman, W.E. Gall, W.M. Cowan, eds.), Wiley, New York, 679 - 720.

Suga, N., Kuzirai, K., and O'Neill, W.E. (1981). How biosonar information is represented in the bat cerebral cortex, in: *Neuronal Mechanisms of Hearing* (J. Syka, L. Aitkin, eds.), Plenum Press, New York, 197 - 219.

Summerfield, Q. (1982). Differences between spectral dependencies in auditory and phonetic temporal processing: relevance to the perception of voicing in initial stops, *J. Acoust. Soc. Am.*, 72, 51 - 61.

Waters, R.S. and Wilson, A. (1976). Speech perception by rhesus monkeys: the voicing distinction in synthesized labial and velar stop consonants, *Percept. Psychophys.*, 19, 285-289.

Whitfield, I.C. and Evans, E.F. (1965). Responses of auditory cortical neurons to stimuli of changing frequency, *J. Neurophysiol.*, 28, 655 - 672.

Wood, B.T. (1983). Is the left hemisphere specialized for language at birth? *Trends Neurosci.*, 6, 115 - 117.

Zippelius, H.M. and Schleidt, W.M. (1956). Ultraschall-Laute bei jungen Mäusen, *Naturwissenschaften*, 53, 502

Zwicker, E. and Feldtkeller, R. (1967). *Das Ohr als Nachrichtenempfänger*, Hirzel, Stuttgart.

Chapter 2
Separation of Simultaneous Signals

Segregation of the Responses to Paired Vowels in the Auditory Nerve of the Guinea-Pig Using Autocorrelation

A.R. Palmer
MRC Institute of Hearing Research
University Park
Nottingham NG7 2RD
U.K.

1. Introduction

Sachs et al. (this volume) state that the spectra of speech sounds may be represented in either a simple place code with peaks of activity in frequency regions corresponding to highest stimulus amplitude, or a code which depends on both the place and the temporal patterning of the activity. Given the strict topographical organization of auditory nuclei, place codes represent an intuitively obvious means of representing variations in spectra. However, for a simple place code to be utilized at all stimulus levels, some form of selective listening seems to be required to overcome the dynamic range limitations of the different groups of afferent fibres and this, as Sachs and his colleagues have demonstrated (see Blackburn and Sachs, 1990), may be accomplished by the chopper population in the cochlear nucleus.

The simple place code does not, however, appear adequate under all circumstances. For example, psychophysical studies have demonstrated that listeners are better able to distinguish the members of a pair of vowels (simultaneously present) when their voice pitch (F_0) is different (Scheffers, 1983; Assmann and Summerfield, 1990). Modelling of these results (Scheffers, 1983; Assmann and Summerfield, 1990) suggests that this improvement in detectability is unlikely to be possible on the basis of the change in the place representation of the simultaneous vowels. It appears, therefore, that this task requires access to information in the timing of the nerve fibre discharges.

The fine timing of the discharges of auditory nerve fibres provides a robust representation of the spectrum and the voice pitch of vowels (e.g. Sachs et al., 1983) and has sufficient information for the segregation of the responses to a pair of simultaneously presented vowels on different voice pitches (Palmer, 1990). In these studies, the activity synchronized to different stimulus components was estimated after fourier transforming the time-locked histograms into the frequency domain.

I present here the application of a model directly using the timing information, to the activity of cochlear nerve fibres. The model, originally proposed by Licklider (1951), was recently implemented for psychophysical data by Meddis and Hewitt (1988, 1991) and is illustrated in Fig. 1. The time waveforms at the output of a bank of bandpass filters are autocorrelated and displayed as an autocorrelogram which maintains a 'place' representation i.e. sequentially in order of centre frequency of the channel (Fig. 1a). In each channel there is a peak at the F_0 and other peaks separated by the period of the channel centre frequency (i.e. by 1 ms in the 1 kHz channel). This progressive decrease in peak spacing with channel

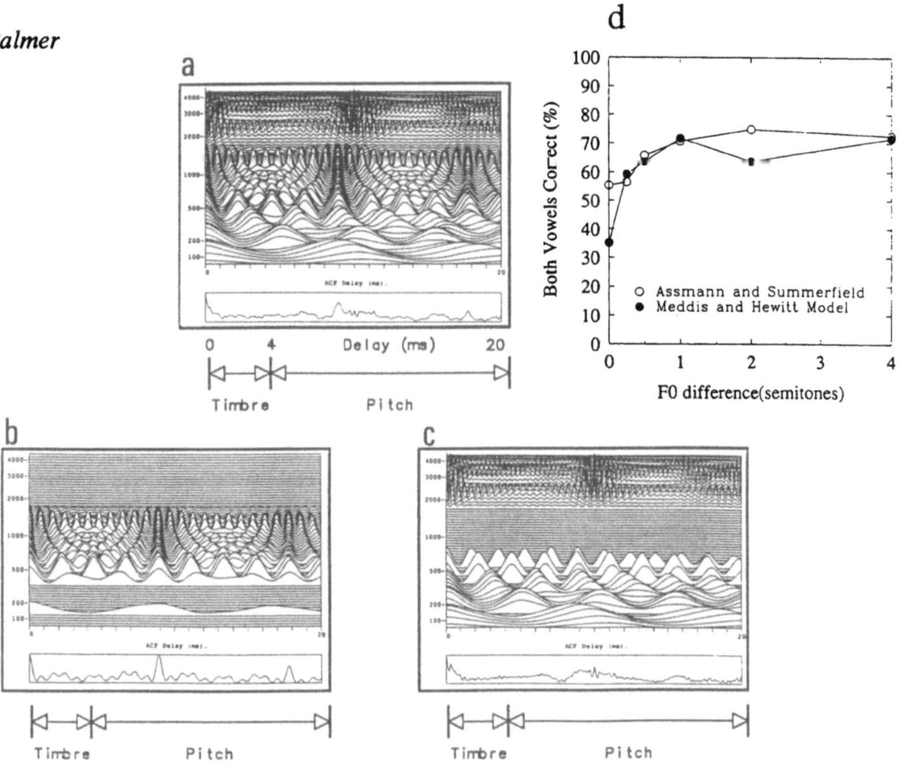

Fig. 1 Meddis and Hewitt's implementation of Licklider's autocorrelation model. (a) Autocorrelogram of the responses to the pair of vowels /i/, F_0 100 Hz and /3/, F_0 112 Hz. Insets in a-c show the pooled autocorrelogram. (b) channels with a peak at 8.9 ms: the delay of the largest peak of the pooled autocorrelogram in (a). (c) all channels without a peak at 8.9 ms. (d) predicted (filled circles) and measured (unfilled circles, from Assmann and Summerfield, 1990) performance in identification of the constituents of a pair of vowels.

centre frequency leads to a characteristic "tree-like" pattern in the autocorrelogram with a straight vertical line of peaks at the F_0 and a series of buttresses or arches which is repeated at each period of the F_0. The autocorrelation functions in each channel are then summed across frequency and the dominant voice pitch is estimated from the delay of the largest peak (8.9 ms in Fig. 1a) in the function obtained (the pooled autocorrelation). If less than 80% of channels have a peak at this delay a second pitch is deemed to be present, and all channels with a peak at this delay (Fig. 1b) are then separated from the rest (Fig. 1c). One highly desirable feature of this method (pointed out by Licklider, 1951) is that the estimate of the voice pitch is made both from resolved responses to single harmonics and from unresolved harmonics which produce activity strongly modulated at the voice pitch. The channels not characterized by a peak at the dominant pitch are considered to reflect activity due to the second vowel. The final step in Meddis and Hewitt's implementation used a template derived from the low-time region of the pooled autocorrelogram for single vowels to identify the vowels in the segregated channels. This led to a good fit to the psychophysical data of Assmann and Summerfield (1990) as shown in Fig. 1d. Application of these analyses to the physiological data achieved a good segregation of the neural activity due to the constituents of the pairs of vowels.

2. METHODS

The data in this paper were obtained from microelectrode recordings of the responses of single auditory nerve fibres from the anaesthetized guinea pig. The methods used to obtain these recordings were conventional and full details may be found in Palmer et al. (1986) and Palmer (1990). The stimuli were vowel sounds produced with a software cascade synthesizer (Klatt, 1980). Steady-state approximations to the vowels /a/, /i/ and /ɔ/, for which the synthesis parameters are shown in Table 1, were presented either alone or in pairs. The pairs of vowels /a(100), i(125)/ (i.e. a stimulus consisting of the simultaneous presentation of the vowel /a/ with F_0 of 100 Hz and the vowel /i/ with a F_0 of 125 Hz) and /ɔ/ (100), i(125)/ were presented at 85 and 83 dB SPL respectively, and the single vowels /a/, /i/ and /ɔ/ at 84, 77 and 79 dB SPL. At these high levels a good place representation in the majority of cochlear nerve fibres no longer persists (see Sachs et al, 1991).

Table I. Frequency (Freq.) and bandwidth (BW) in Hertz of the formants F1-F5 of the synthetic single vowels /i/, /a/ and /ɔ/

		F1		F2		F3		F4		F5	
	f_0	Freq.	BW	Freq.	BW	Freq.	BW	Freq.	BW	Freq.	BW
/i/	125	270	90	2290	110	3010	170	3300	250	3850	200
/a/	100	730	90	1090	110	2440	170	3300	250	3850	200
/ɔ/	100	450	90	750	110	2850	170	3300	250	3850	200

The times at which discharges occurred in response to the vowels were measured and used to compute the autocorrelation function for each fibre. In the first instance this was done by taking the intervals between each spike and subsequent spikes occurring up to 40 ms later. This form of discrete autocorrelation function has a disadvantage for the present purposes because it cannot register any intervals shorter than the refractory period of the fibre (approximately 1 ms). Since the low-time part of the autocorrelation function is essential for Meddis and Hewitt's model, the functions used here are autocorrrelations computed from 80-ms wide period histograms of the fibre response. Examples, for a single fibre, of the discrete autocorrelation function and that computed from the period histogram are shown in Fig. 2. The function computed from the period histogram (Fig. 2b) is much smoother, but apart from the lack of a refractory gap at the onset is very similar to the discrete autocorrelation (Fig. 2a) computed from the intervals. The discrepancy between the two functions at long time delays is probably a result of adaptation of the neural discharge which does not affect the interval-based analysis.

To obtain the autocorrelograms shown in Figs. 2-4 the frequency axis from 200 Hz to 4000 Hz was divided into 71 1/16 octave channels. The autocorrelation functions of all fibres whose best frequency fell within the limits of each frequency channel were averaged and plotted at equal separations along the ordinate. This yields an autocorrelogram showing the timing of impulses in each of the 71 frequency (place) ordered channels.

3. Results

Fig. 3 shows autocorrelograms derived from the responses of auditory nerve fibres to the single vowels /a/ (Fig. 3a) /i/ (Fig. 3b) and /ɔ/ (Fig. 3c). In all three cases the features previously described using other analyses (such as the ALSR of Young and Sachs, 1979; or the average fourier spectra of Delgutte and Kiang, 1984) are readily visible. In the first panel, for example, the first formant of /a/ at 730 Hz dominates a wide range of frequency channels from below its frequency up to the frequency of the second formant. The second formant (1090 Hz) then dominates channels from its frequency upwards. In contrast to strictly linear models such as Meddis and Hewitt (1991) and Assmann and Summerfield (1990), in which the response to the centre frequency component of each channel is always visible forming "tree" structures, these physiological autocorrelograms contain wide regions in which the peaks have the same time separation and thus form straight vertical lines. In the instance of /i/ (Fig. 3b), in which the first and second formants are widely separated in frequency, the fibres between the formants do respond to the centre frequency component and in this region the "tree" structure can be discerned. The amplitude of the peak at 8 ms in individual frequency channels in Fig. 3b is little different whether that peak is due to a single harmonic near the first formant (in the lowest frequency channels) or due to the interaction of several components which beat at the F_0 (in the region between F1 and F2). This is probably as a result of saturation of the fibre discharge as these data were collected at a relatively high sound level (77 dB SPL). When the autocorrelations in the individual frequency channels are pooled (summing all channels across each vertical bin) the curves shown in Fig. 3d-f are obtained. The large well-defined peak in these figures (excluding the zero time peak) is in each case at the delay corresponding to the F_0 of the single vowel (10 ms for /a/ and /ɔ/ which have a F_0 of 100 Hz and 8 ms for /i/ which has a F_0 of 125 Hz). Channels responding to a single harmonic of the vowel near a formant and

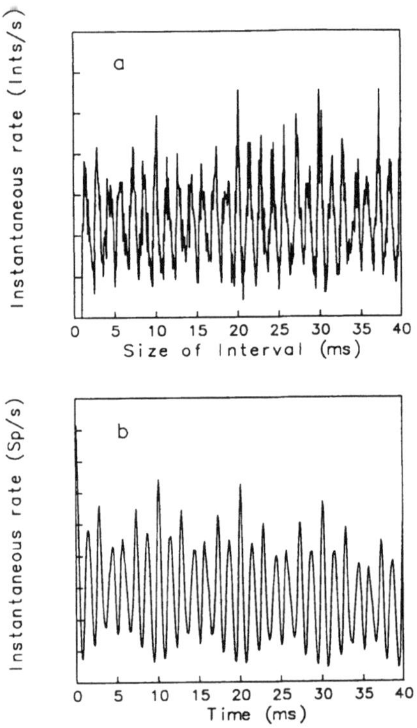

Fig. 2 (a) Discrete autocorrelation function obtained by binning the intervals between each spike and successive spikes (up to 40 ms later). (b) Autocorrelation function obtained from the same spike train by true autocorrelation of the "time waveform" computed as a post stimulus time histogram. The characteristic frequency of this fibre was 0.86 kHz and the stimulus was the vowels /a/ (F_0 100 Hz) and /i/ (F_0 125 Hz) simultaneously presented.

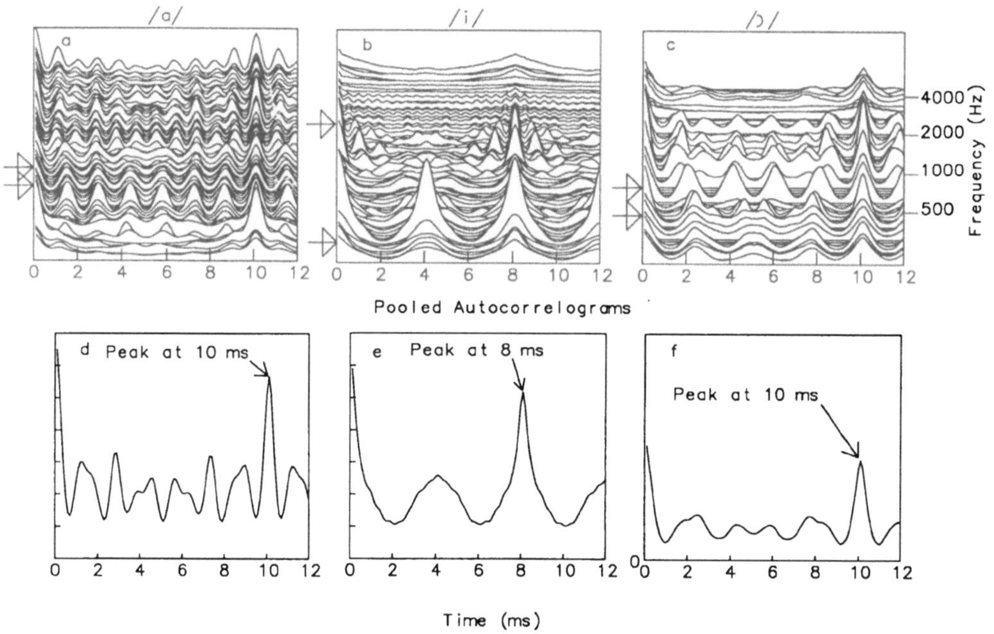

Fig. 3 (a) Autocorrelogram of the responses of auditory nerve fibres to the vowel /a/, F_0 100 Hz. (d) Pooled autocorrelogram obtained by summing each vertical bin across all frequency channels in (a). (b,c,e,f) Show the same analyses for the vowels /i/, F_0 125 Hz and , F_0 100 Hz. Arrows in Figs a-c show the position of the formants.

those which beat at the F_0 frequency contribute strongly to the F_0 peak in the pooled autocorrelogram.

Fig. 4a shows the autocorrelogram to the double vowel /a(100),i(125)/. Some features which were evident in the autocorrelogram to the single vowels alone are still evident. In the lowest frequency channels the response is to the first formant of /i/, while the middle frequency regions are dominated by responses to the first and second formants of the /a/. The pooled autocorrelogram (Fig. 4d) shows a well-defined peak at 10 ms, but no peak at 8 ms corresponding to the 125 Hz F_0 of the /i/. (Indeed, the nearest feature to 8 ms in this pooled autocorrelogram is a dip.) This is because many of the channels which contributed to the 8 ms peak in the response to the /i/ alone, including those which produced beating at the F_0, are now completely dominated by the responses to the formants of the /a/. The remaining panels of Fig. 4 show the segregation of the channels on the basis of whether they show a peak at the same delay (10 ms) as that in the pooled autocorrelogram in Fig. 4d. Meddis and Hewitt (1991) defined a peak as a single point higher than its neighbours. In the physiological data even channels responding to the F2 of /i/ still showed some response to the /a/ and a

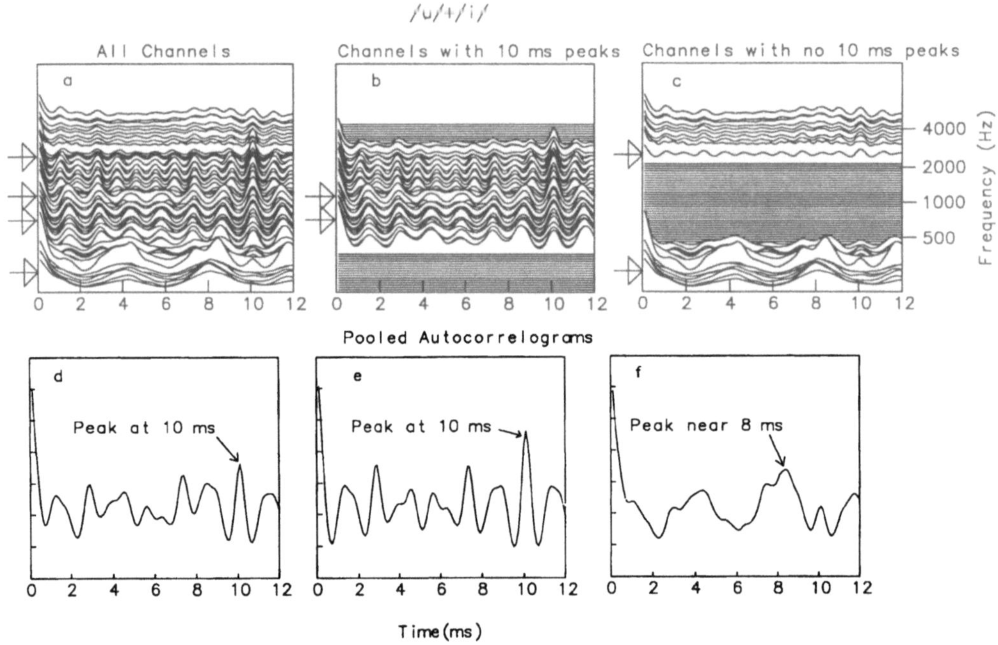

Fig. 4 (a), (d) Autocorrelograms and pooled autocorrelograms of the responses to the vowels /a/, F0 100 Hz and /i/, F_0 125 Hz played simultaneously. (c-f) show the segregation of the channels on the basis of the presence (b),(e) or absence (c),(f) of a peak at 10 ms. Arrows in Figs a-c show the position of the formants.

small peak was present at 10 ms. For this reason, an entirely arbitrary threshold value was used for the inclusion of a peak. With suitable choice of this threshold an acceptable segregation of the channels responding to the /a/ was achieved, as can be seen in Fig. 4b and 4e. The final panels (Fig. 4c,f) show those channels which did not contain a peak at 10 ms greater than the threshold value. The channels in Fig. 4c,f are those which were responding to the /i/. In this case, the pooled autocorrelogram of Fig. 4f shows a broad peak near 8 ms.

Fig. 5 shows a similar analysis of the responses to the double vowel /ɔ/ (100), i(125)/. At 1/16 octave intervals there were some frequency channels (shown by straight lines in Fig. 5) for which no data was collected for this pair of vowels. Nevertheless, channels responding to one or other of the vowels can be distinguished in Fig. 5a. The peak in the pooled autocorrelogram (Fig. 5d) is at 8 ms, which corresponds to the F_0 of the /i/, the stronger vowel of the pair, and is only marginally larger than that at 10 ms. Segregation based on the presence of a peak at 8 ms is shown in Figs. 5b,c,e,f. A problem with this vowel pair is that with 100 and 125 Hz as the F_0s the harmonic at 500 Hz is shared by both vowels and is also the closest to the first formant of the /ɔ/. The very strong response to the 500 Hz harmonic is therefore mainly due to the /ɔ/, but results in a peak at 8 and 10 ms and therefore appears in Fig 5b (as the 8 ms peaks were extracted first). Indeed, as can be seen by the position of

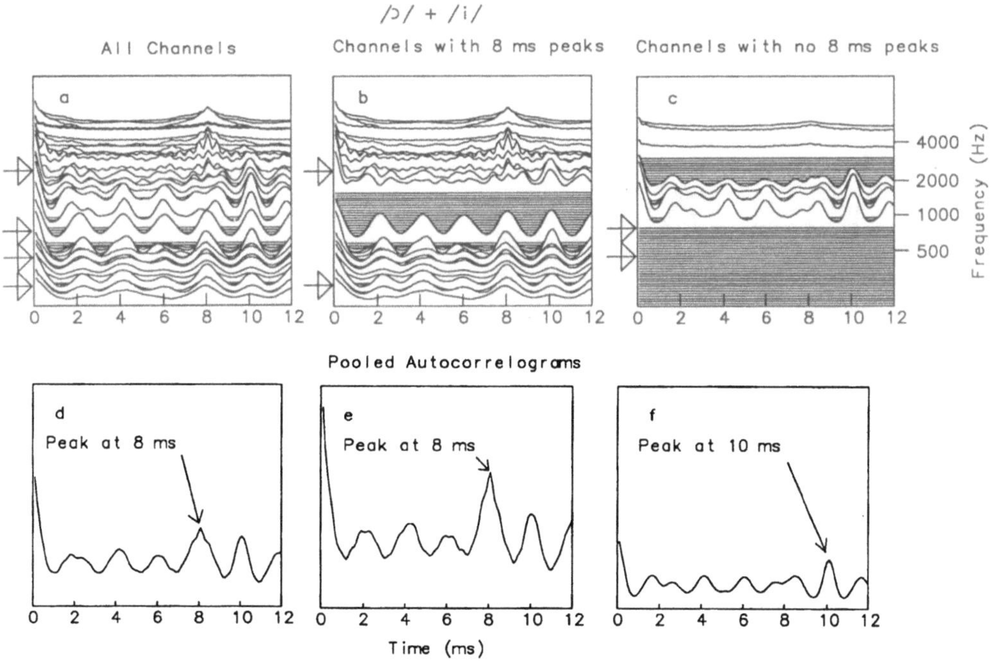

Fig. 5 Analyses in the same format as Fig. 4 for the responses to the vowels , F_0 100 Hz and /i/, F_0 125 Hz. Segregation in this instance was on the basis of the presence or absence of a peak at 8 ms.

the arrows in Fig. 5c, the channels around the first formant of the /ɔ/ have not been correctly segregated and appear in Fig. 5b. The channels at the first formant of the /ɔ/ have peaks at both 8 and 10 ms and will be segregated according to whichever is extracted first. It was not possible to adjust the threshold value for the peak to segregate the channels correctly, since 8 and 10 ms peaks near the first formant of the /ɔ/ were of comparable amplitude. The channels at and above the second formant of the /ɔ/ were generally correctly segregated from the rest, but some channels in this region were also segregated on the basis of a peak at 8 ms which was smaller than a 10 ms peak.

The final stage in Meddis and Hewitt's model was the identification of the segregated vowels and comparison of the performance of the model with the psychophysical results obtained with these stimuli. To do this they first obtained a template for each single vowel using the low-time (below 4.5 ms) part of the pooled autocorrelogram. The low-time parts of the pooled autocorrelograms from the segregated vowels were then compared with the set of templates and the most similar template taken as the vowel most likely to be chosen by a subject. Clearly, the physiological data for the limited vowel combinations shown here are not extensive enough to provide any kind of adequate test of this part of the model. However, we can compare the low-time regions of the single-vowel and segregated vowel autocorrelograms

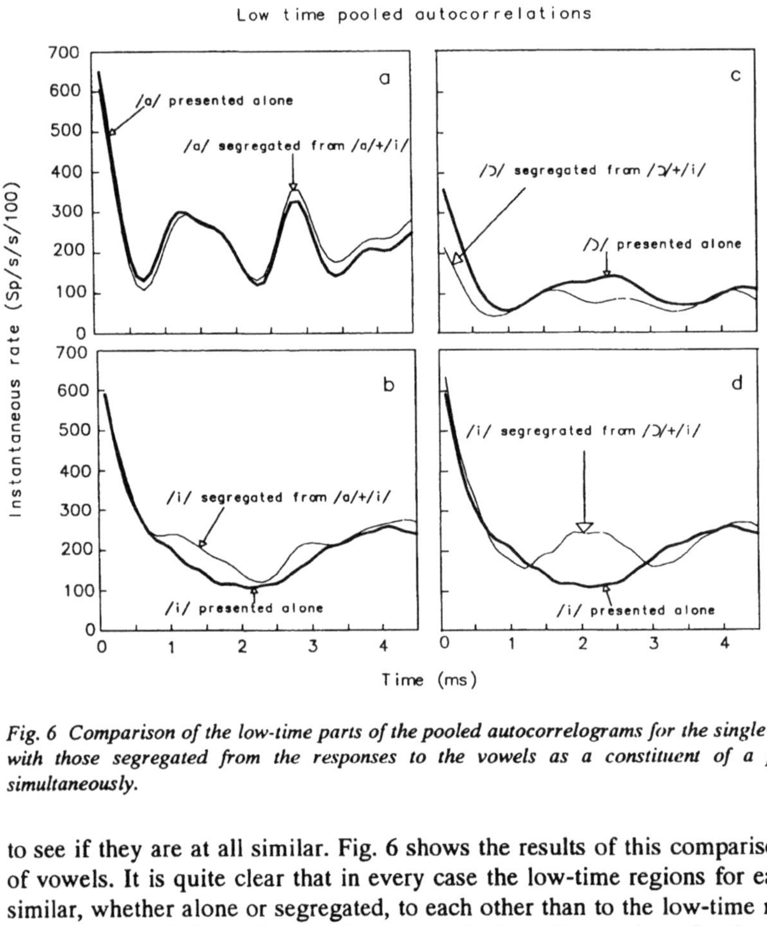

Fig. 6 Comparison of the low-time parts of the pooled autocorrelograms for the single vowels presented alone with those segregated from the responses to the vowels as a constituent of a pair of vowels played simultaneously.

to see if they are at all similar. Fig. 6 shows the results of this comparison for the two pairs of vowels. It is quite clear that in every case the low-time regions for each vowel are more similar, whether alone or segregated, to each other than to the low-time regions of any other of the vowels. Indeed, the match between the low-time regions for the vowels is generally rather good. The largest mismatch is shown in Fig. 6d and is caused by the very strong response to the 500 Hz harmonic being wrongly assigned to the /i/ rather than the /ɔ/.

4. DISCUSSION

Even in the absence of a difference in F_0 listeners are still able to identify members of a pair of vowels at performance levels much better than chance (chance performance in Fig. 1d is about 7%). This indicates that template matching is taking place comparing the "spectrum" of the responses with some stored representations of the spectra of the vowels and this has been modelled by both Assmann and Summerfield (1989, 1990) and Meddis and Hewitt (1991). The addition of a difference in F_0 acts as a guide for this matching process and thereby improves performance. The segregation demonstrated here depends on the recognition of a common cadence in the discharges in different input channels. Grouping these channels together (or selectively attending to these channels) separates the responses to the vowels on the different F_0s, allowing a template matching less influenced by spurious contribution from the second vowel. It is immaterial here whether the final internal representation is in terms of a rate/place or temporal/place code once the timing information has indicated which channels to include. The final stage in the model involves the identification of the vowel on the basis of the timing information. On the basis of a very small sample it appears that such identification would also be possible in the physiological data. It is noticeable however, that the shape of the low-time part of the autocorrelation function for the single vowels, in the physiological data, is mainly a result of summation across a limited frequency region. For the /a/ and /i/, whether alone or segregated from the vowel pair, the low-time region appears to reflect activity near the first formant, while the low-time region of the /ɔ/ autocorrelograms is due to activity near the second formant. Identification is therefore mainly an assessment of differences in the frequency region of strong spectral components, usually the first formant. This final identification step, based entirely on timing, seems to be inconsistent with psychophysical studies which indicate that vowel identification is based upon the frequency of both the first and second formants (e.g. Peterson and Barney, 1952; Carlson et al., 1975). It also seems to be somewhat beyond the minimum processing needed for segregation and association of activity peaks with common voice pitch. If the timing information alone is used in vowel identification, a scheme such as that of Secker-Walker and Searle (1990), in which the formant frequencies are computed directly from the peak spacing in the segregated channels, would probably give acceptable results for these physiological data.

Acknowledgements

I thank Padma Moorjani for technical assistance and A. Lea, I.M. Winter, R. Meddis and A.Q. Summerfield for helpful discussions and reading this manuscript.

References

Assmann, P. and Summerfield, A.Q. (1989). Modeling the Perception of Concurrent Vowels: Vowels with the Same Fundamental Frequencies, *J. Acoust. Soc. Am.*, 85, 327-338.

Assmann, P. and Summerfield, A.Q. (1990). Modeling the Perception of Concurrent Vowels: Vowels with Different Fundamental Frequencies, *J. Acoust. Soc. Am.*, 88, 680-697.

Blackburn, C.C. and Sachs, M.B. (1990). The Representation of the Steady-State Vowel /eh/ in the Discharge Patterns of Cat Anteroventral Cochlear Nucleus Neurons, *J. Neurophysiol.*, 63, 1191-1212.

Carlson, R., Fant, G. and Granstrom, B. (1975). Two-formant Models, Pitch and Vowel Perception, in *Auditory Analysis and Perception of Speech*, G. Fant and M.A.A. Tatham (eds.), Academic, London, 55-82.

Delgutte, B. and Kiang, N.Y.S. (1984). Speech Coding in the Auditory Nerve: I Vowel-like Sounds, *J. Acoust. Soc. Am.*, 75, 866-878.

Klatt, D.H. (1980). Software for a Cascade/Parallel Formant Synthesizer, *J. Acoust. Soc. Am.*, 67, 971-995.

Licklider, J.C.R. (1951). A Duplex Theory of Pitch Perception, *Experientia*, 7, 128-133.

Meddis, R. and Hewitt, M.J. (1988). A Computational Model of Low Pitch Judgement, in: H. Duifhuis, J.W., Horst, and H.P. Wit (eds.), *Basic Issues in Hearing*, Academic, London, 148-153.

Meddis, R. and Hewitt, M.J. (1992) Modelling the identification of concurrent vowels with different fundamental frequencies, *J. Acoust Soc. Am.*, 91, 233-245.

Palmer, A.R. (1990). The Representation of the Spectra and Fundamental Frequencies of Steady-state Single- and Double-vowel sounds in the Temporal Discharge Patterns of Guinea Pig Cochlear-Nerve Fibers, *J. Acoust Soc. Am.*, 88, 1412-1426.

Palmer, A. R., Winter, I. M., and Darwin, C. J. (1986). The Representation of Steady-state Vowel Sounds in the Temporal Discharge Patterns of the Guinea Pig Cochlear Nerve and Primarylike Cochlear Nucleus Neurons, *J. Acoust. Soc. Am.*, 79, 100-113.

Peterson, G.E. and Barney, H.L. (1952). Control Methods Used in the Study of Vowels, *J. Acoust. Soc. Am.*, 24, 175-184.

Secker-Walker, H.E. and Searle, C.L. (1990). Time-domain analysis of auditory-nerve-fibre firing patterns. *J. Acoust. Soc. Amer.*, 88, 1427-1436.

Scheffers, M. T. M. (1983). *Sifting Vowels: Auditory Pitch Analysis and Sound Segregation*, Doctoral Thesis, University of Groningen.

Young, E.D. and Sachs, M.B. (1979). Representation of Steady-state Vowels in the Temporal Aspects of the Discharge Patterns of Populations of Auditory Nerve Fibers, *J. Acoust. Soc. Am.*, 66, 1381-1403.

Modelling Sound Source Separation

Martin Cooke
Department of Computer Science
University of Sheffield
Sheffield, UK

1. MOTIVATION

It is possible to cast the main role of early audition as a search for meaningful organisation in the signal reaching the ears. The theoretical foundations for this notion have been cogently expressed in Bregman's book on auditory scene analysis (Bregman, 1990). This area is an attractive and potentially fertile one for modellers since it provides an explanatory basis for signal pre-processing in tasks such as speech recognition in complex, multi-source listening conditions.

However, modelling auditory scene analysis presents certain difficulties. First, there is a representational mismatch between the vocabulary of the psychoacoustician and that of the modeller. Whilst experimental descriptions of auditory grouping effects are generally couched in terms of **objects** (e.g. formants, tones) and their properties (e.g. time of onset, amplitude modulation rate), the modeller has to contend with quasi-continuous **signals** in which these objects exist implicitly, if at all. As a consequence, it is difficult to apply grouping notions such as harmonicity, common amplitude modulation and onset/offset synchrony without an adequate representational basis.

A second problem for the modeller is the complexity of search implied by some aspects of auditory scene exploration. For example, any cross-channel comparison of properties of the kind proposed in Brian Moore's descriptions of CMR and ACM (this volume) is likely to be computationally expensive, particularly at the data-rates suggested by the analysis in Roy Patterson's paper (this volume).

The model outlined here addresses these difficulties by employing an object-based, time-frequency representation of the data flowing from a model of the auditory periphery. This representation - synchrony strands - makes explicit the temporal evolution of similar responses in frequency-specific channels and is sufficiently expressive to allow an effective search for organisation in the auditory scene. Synchrony strands appear to fulfil much the same role as the 'primary auditory contours' discussed in Ernst Terhardt's paper (this volume).

2. A BRIEF, ILLUSTRATED GUIDE TO THE MODEL

The model is described in some detail in Cooke (1991). Here, I have chosen to depict its action on a stimulus used in the experiments of Gardner, Gaskill, and Darwin (1989), which Chris Darwin refers to in his contribution (a schematic of the stimulus appears as Fig. 1 in his paper). The synthetic 4-formant syllable has F1, F3, and F4 synthesised on a fundamental of 110 Hz, whilst its F2 has a fundamental of 174 Hz. If listeners were to hear all formants excited by the same fundamental, the predominant percept would be the syllable /ru/, whilst if F2 were omitted, the main response would be /li/. I'll refer to this as the "ru-li" stimulus.

2.1 The Representational Basis: Synchrony Strands

Synchrony strands are formed via two stages of grouping applied to the outputs of a gammatone auditory filterbank (Patterson and Holdsworth, in press). The first process groups channels of the filterbank which appear to be dominated by the same stimulus component. Since channels have overlapping frequency-selectivity, responses in neighbouring channels often show similarities. At 1 ms time intervals, the instantaneous frequency, amplitude, and amplitude-modulation rate of each filter output are calculated. The instantaneous frequency is median-smoothed to extract a single dominant frequency in each channel. Motivated by the DOMIN scheme of Carlson and Granstrom (1982), it is possible to apply an ordering constraint to estimate which channels are responding to the same stimulus component. This operates by examining the difference between a channel's instantaneous frequency and its centre frequency. In the (spectral) locality of a resolved stimulus component, we will find groups of channels for which this difference is first positive, then zero, then negative, as responses are pulled either upwards or downwards towards the locally dominant stimulus frequency. This pattern of responses provides a powerful constraint for grouping such collections of channels together. A single frequency, amplitude, and amplitude-modulation rate is calculated for the group.

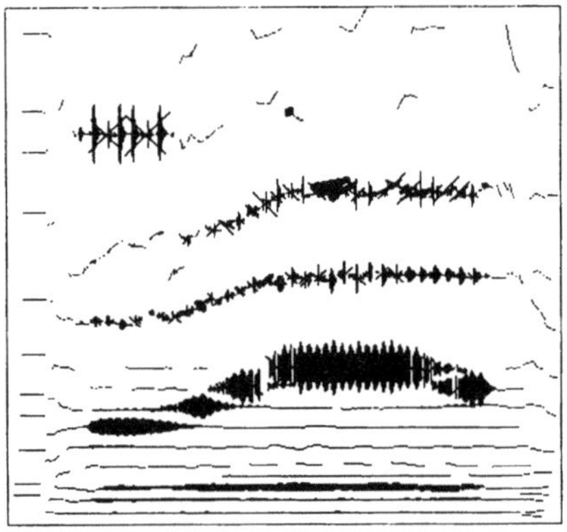

Fig. 1 Synchrony strands analysis of a four-formant synthetic syllable. The syllable has formants F1, F3, and F4 generated on a fundamental of 110 Hz, while F2 has a fundamental of 174 Hz. The data come from the study of Gardner, Gaskill, and Darwin (1989), and a schematic of the stimulus is shown in Fig. 1 of that paper. Each strand sweeps out a contour in time and frequency, and has an amplitude which is represented by the instantaneous width of the contour, displayed orthogonally to the direction of strand movement. Harmonics of 110 Hz are resolved in the F1 region, while a wider harmonic spacing of 174 Hz is seen in the F2 region. Significant amplitude modulation is also displayed, particularly on the second and higher formants, and the rate of modulation in the F2 region can be seen to differ from that on the third and fourth formants.
Time axis: 0-370ms / Freq axis: 0-4500 Hz (linear in Hz)

The second stage in synchrony strand formation aims to track the evolution of these groups in time. A first-order continuity constraint is applied to collections of groups in successive time-frames in order to define a potential existence region for groups in the current frame. It is also necessary to cater for onsets and offsets in this tracking process. The motivation for such a constraint comes from experimental work on the sequential organisation of tones (e.g. Ciocca and Bregman, 1987) and to some extent from studies of spectral continuity (e.g. Cole and Scott, 1973) and pitch contour continuity (e.g. Darwin and Bethell-Fox, 1977).

The resulting representation is depicted in Fig. 1, which shows the synchrony strands (and their instantaneous amplitude) for the "ru-li" stimulus. Note that the first 5 or 6 harmonics in the first formant region are resolved, and that the second formant is also split into harmonics, albeit with a different harmonic spacing. Also visible in this representation is amplitude modulation. Again, two rates of AM are clear. There are thus two ways in which F2 might be perceptually segregated from the remaining formants, though, as Darwin notes in his paper, there is no evidence that phonetic segregation can be achieved solely by the difference in amplitude modulation rate (i.e. when only unresolved harmonics specify the formant).

2.2 Exploring the Auditory Scene

The computational problem of auditory scene exploration faced by the model may be posed as follows: how do we find those subsets of a collection of synchrony strands such that members of a subset belong together ? An exhaustive search of all solution states is out of the question, since, for a set of n objects, there are $k = 2^n$ different groups, and 2^k different collections of groups ! Instead, a seed-driven exploration is used, motivated by the following observations:

1. All the evidence in the auditory scene should be accounted for, i.e. associated with some or other group. However, objects should be allowed to be members of more than one group, since there is ample experimental evidence that the principle of disjoint allocation (Bregman, 1990, chapter 7) does not apply to early stages of grouping (e.g. Darwin, this volume).
2. It should be possible to build similar groups from different seeds, thus rendering the choice of seed non-critical.
3. If we start with the most dominant objects in the scene, they are likely to attract significantly larger numbers of adherents than if we were to choose brief, low amplitude seeds.

Scene exploration starts with the selection of the most dominant strand (here, dominance corresponds roughly to the number of channels which contributed data to the group multiplied by the length of the strand). From this, the set of strands which overlap in time with the seed is computed, and a similarity metric is applied to each strand in that set to determine whether it might be grouped with the seed. Once this stage of simultaneous grouping has finished, it is possible to exploit the time-frequency nature of strands to examine whether any of the new group recruits have extended the temporal basis of the group. If so, further stages of simultaneous grouping are possible. Once this process is complete, the next most dominant ungrouped strand is chosen as a seed, and the interleaved stages of simultaneous grouping and temporal extension are applied. The process terminates when all strands are members of one or more groupings.

So far, the description says nothing about the similarity metric which is applied in group formation. It is possible to cast any simultaneous grouping principle in the computational

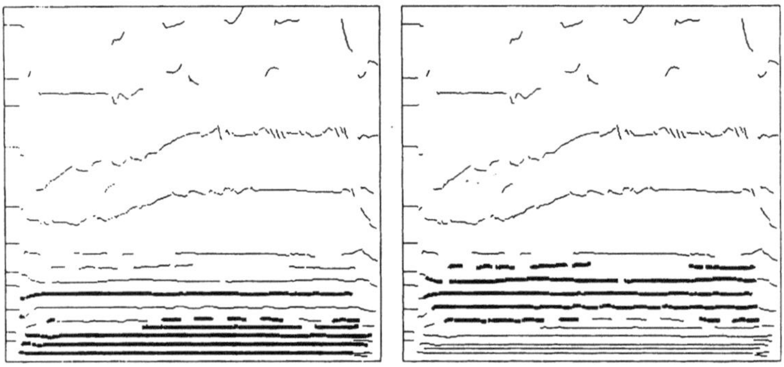

Fig.2 Two harmonic groups discovered in the strands analysis depicted in Fig. 1. Strands in the group are shown as thick lines. No amplitude information is displayed in this figure.

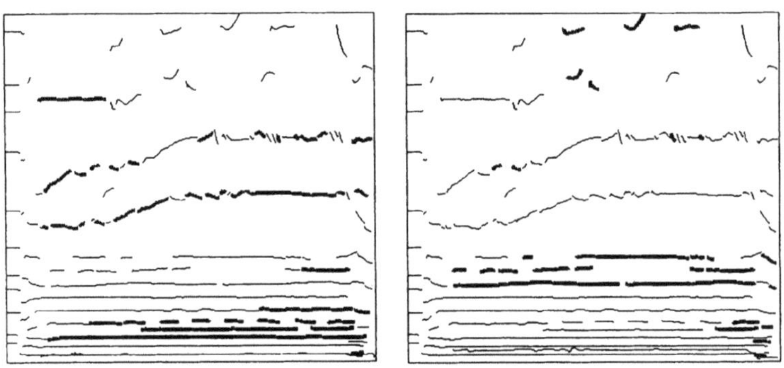

Fig. 3 Two amplitude modulation groups discovered in the strands analysis of Fig. 1.

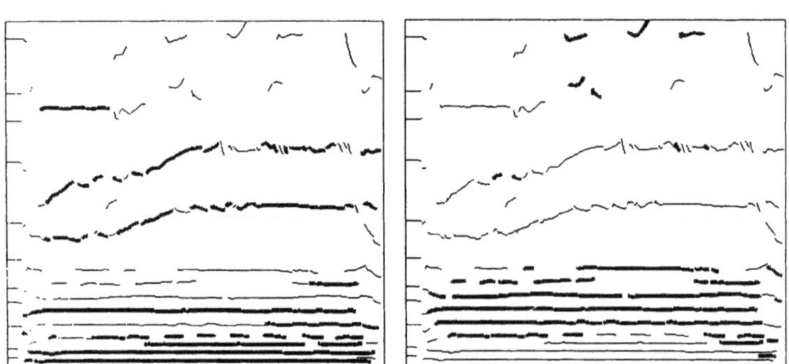

Fig. 4 Two combined groups resulting from the second level of grouping.

framework expressed above. Currently, we have implementations of harmonicity, common amplitude modulation and common frequency movement, though the evaluation results are based solely on the first two of these. Fig. 2 shows two of the harmonic groups discovered in the "ru-li" stimulus. These correspond to the first and second formants, although one of the F2 harmonics is sufficiently harmonically-related to the lower harmonic series to be a member of both groupings. Fig. 3 illustrates two amplitude modulation groups discovered in the same stimulus. One point of note here is that there is sufficient amplitude modulation on some strands in the F1 region to cause their grouping with strands corresponding to F3 and F4.

The first stage of auditory scene exploration applies grouping principles independently; there is little experimental data on the interaction of such forces for organisation. Further stages of grouping are necessary, however, in order to link, for example, harmonic groups in the lower frequencies to amplitude modulation groups in higher frequencies. Ultimately, higher-level processes will have to resolve competition for elements, and may employ schema-driven processes (Bregman, 1990) for this task. The current model is limited to primitive grouping processes.

A second stage of grouping is implemented in the model, based on the similarity of properties derived from each first-level grouping. Specifically, an estimate of the pitch contour over the time interval which each group occupies is derived from both harmonic and amplitude modulation groups (this estimate is displayed in figures 2 and 3 and, for the 174 Hz fundamental, is visible between the lowest pair of strands in the figures). Next, precisely the same search algorithm as was used to explore the strand collection is used to search the set of first-level groups - the only difference is that similarity is now based on derived properties of groups rather than primitive properties of strands. The results of this second grouping stage are depicted in Fig. 4, illustrating that the model is capable of segregating information in the F2 region from that in the locality of F1, F3 and F4.

3. EVALUATION

The model's ability to segregate speech from a variety of other sources has been evaluated, and results are reported in Cooke (1991). The evaluation first required a solution to the following mixture correspondence problem: given a collection of strands resulting from an analysis of the mixture of two sources, is it possible to identify which strands resulted from which source ? Fortunately, the answer appears to be 'yes', leading to quantitative estimates of such things as the degree to which the second source infiltrated groups representing the first source. Such estimates are only meaningful, however, when compared with the result of selecting groups at random. The following table illustrates the percentage intrusion from the second source for both grouped and random conditions:

type of second source	*% intrusion*	
	grouped	***random***
1 KHz tone	4	8
white noise	9	39
noise burst sequence	1	2
student laboratory noise	9	34
music	18	46
synthetic FM tone (siren)	6	7
telephone-ringing	13	27
female speaker	11	22
male speaker	8	13

The main advantage of this direct, numeric indication of performance is that it will allow a rapid assessment of the effect of incorporating other grouping rules (e.g. onset/offset synchrony) into the system.

4. Issues for Models of Grouping

This paper has outlined a model of sound source separation. The system is far from complete, but it does provides a framework within which any principle for simultaneous organisation can be embodied. Planned extensions include an enrichment of the representational basis to make onsets and offsets explicit in order to support grouping by onset/offset synchrony; a model for the sequential organisation of groups; conflict-resolution strategies to enable competition for elements to be resolved; integration of top-down (schema-driven) processes.

There are some significant problems and issues which future grouping systems must tackle. One such is the precision with which auditory grouping effects have been quantified. For example, in invoking any similarity principle, the question of just how similar two objects have to be in order for them to belong to the same perceptual group must be tackled. In some cases a usable similarity metric is available in the experimental literature (e.g. the mistuning function for harmonicity of Moore, Glasberg, and Peters, 1985), but generally the experimental data are too sparse to be interpreted in this way.

A further issue is the choice of an appropriate representational basis for models of source separation. Whilst autocorrelogram-like analyses are a popular starting point (Weintraub, 1987; Assman and Summerfield, 1990; Meddis and Hewitt, 1992; Duda, Lyon and Slaney, 1990), such representations do not make explicit features such as onsets, harmonics, and formants. Such auditory images are, as Patterson et al. (this volume) point out, rich in **data**. However, it is debatable whether such analyses carry sufficient **representational** power to serve as the basis for models of auditory scene analysis. Of course, data-rich analyses have the potential to become representationally-rich, and devising appropriate signal-to-symbol transformations is one of the great challenges for auditory modelling research.

The system described in this paper purchases most of its computational power from the strand representation, which attempts to make explicit the information upon which grouping may be based. I believe it is crucial to get away from the artificial time-frequency graticule which has dominated modelling work, in much the same way as work in computational vision abandons the bitmap at an early stage of analysis. In addition to the computational benefits for auditory scene exploration engendered by an object-centred viewpoint, it also becomes clear how results such as those thrown up by Darwin's onset asynchrony studies (reported in this volume) might be modelled. The important new result from that work is that a component's onset asynchrony can reduce the contribution which that component makes to the pitch calculation. Any scheme which operates by determining pitch in a frame-by-frame manner will need to revise its decisions when the segregated component is removed.

A consideration of this leads to the following question: which comes first, an estimate of pitch or some group from which it is possible to derive a pitch ? Put another way, is it necessary to make organisation explicit first, then derive properties from such groups, or vice versa ? Segregation systems such as that of Assman and Summerfield (1990) first derive a pitch estimate, then use it to select a subset of channels which are compatible with that estimate. By contrast, the system described here first discovers organisation, then derives a pitch contour.

Another issue is whether the default condition for auditory scene analysis is segregation or fusion. In the model described here, objects will remain segregated unless a reason can be found for fusing them with any existing organisation. However, Bregman (1990, p. 334) has suggested that the default condition in the auditory system appears to be fusion. For example, he argues that we do not perceive large numbers of separate sources for white noise stimuli, even though there are no obvious attributes on which they might be fused. It is not clear, however, how this approach could be implemented computationally in a manner which makes it distinct from the current search framework. For example, to segregate an inharmonic component from a harmonic series, it seems necessary to first detect the harmonic organisation, which is precisely what happens in the current model.

Finally, it is of interest to consider the relationship between models and experiments in auditory grouping. Whilst models, by definition, begin life as parasites, there will be a stage in their development when they possess sufficient predictive power to enable their use as tools in experimental design. In particular, the assumptions made in creating complex stimuli might be checked (e.g. is F2 really resolved into constituent harmonics ?). Auditory scene analysis is a complex area for experimentation, particularly if the many possible ways in which two or more grouping principles might interact are considered. This has in the past led to the use of simple stimuli whose relevance to sources such as speech is questionable. The availability of computational models of auditory scene analysis promises to liberate experimenters from some of these constraints.

Acknowledgements

Thanks to Malcolm Crawford for useful discussions and proof-reading. This work was supported in part by a research grant from the SERC Image Interpretation Initiative.

References

Assman, P.F. and Summerfield, A.Q. (1990). Modelling the perception of concurrent vowels: Vowels with different fundamental frequencies, *J. Acoust. Soc. Am.*, 88, 680-697.

Bregman, A.S. (1990). *Auditory Scene Analysis*, MIT Press.

Carlson, R. and Granstrom, B. (1982). Towards an auditory spectrograph, in: *The representation of speech in the peripheral auditory system*, R. Carlson and B. Granstrom (eds), Elsevier.

Ciocca, V. and Bregman, A.S. (1987). Perceived continuity of gliding and steady-state tones through interrupting noise, *Perception and Psychophysics*, 42, 476-484.

Cole, R.A. and Scott, B. (1973). Perception of temporal order in speech, *Can. J. Psych.*, 27, 441-449.

Cooke, M.P. (1991). *Modelling auditory processing and organisation*, Ph.D. Thesis, University of Sheffield.

Darwin, C.J. and Bethell-Fox, C.E. (1977). Pitch continuity and speech source attribution, *J. Exp. Psych. Human Perception and Performance*, 3, 665-672.

Duda, R.O., Lyon, R.F., and Slaney, M. (1990). Correlograms and the separation of sounds, *Proc. Asilomar Annual Conf. on Signals, Systems and Computers*.

Gardner, R.B., Gaskill, S.A., and Darwin, C.J. (1989). Perceptual grouping of formants with static and dynamic differences in fundamental frequency, *J. Acoust. Soc. Am.*, 85, 3, 1329-1337.

Meddis, R. and Hewitt, M. (1992). Modelling the identification of concurrent vowels with different fundamental frequencies, *J. Acoust. Soc. Am.*, 91, 233-245.

Moore, B.C.J., Glasberg, B.R., and Peters, R.W. (1985). Relative dominance of individual partials in determining the pitch of complex tones, *J. Acoust. Soc. Am.*, 77, 1853-1860.

Patterson, R.D. and Holdsworth, J. (in press). A functional model of neural activity patterns and auditory images, in: *Advances in Speech, Hearing and Language Processing*, (W.A. Ainsworth, ed.), Vol. 3. JAI Press, London. (in press)

Weintraub, M. (1987). Sound separation and auditory perceptual organisation, in: *The psychophysics of speech perception*, M.E.H. Schouten (ed), Martinus Nijhoff.

Listening to two Things at Once

C.J. Darwin
Experimental Psychology
University of Sussex
Brighton BN1 9QG
U.K.

1. INTRODUCTION

Our auditory system allows us to listen to a particular sound source, largely unperturbed by the presence of other sounds. Understanding how it does this is a major challenge. At present, we know rather little of the mechanisms responsible for this ability, although there have been a number of demonstrations of factors that are important. This paper will outline different types of mechanism that might contribute and then describe some new experimental data aimed at illuminating the relationship between mechanisms of pitch perception and those used in auditory grouping.

2. MECHANISMS FOR SOURCE SEPARATION

Albert Bregman's recent book "Auditory Scene Analysis" (Bregman, 1990, p. 408) distinguishes two types of mechanism that can be used to organise sound from more than one source. On the one hand the listener might use primitive grouping mechanisms that partition the input on the basis of simple stimulus properties. On the other hand, the listener might use schema-governed mechanisms that select an array of data that meets certain criteria. The primitive grouping mechanisms use simple general properties of a single sound source (such as common onset time or frequency continuity) to which the listener may be innately attuned and so do not depend on specific experience. The schemata that govern the second mechanism on the other hand are learned and so depend on the listener's specific experience. The first mechanism could be caricatured as bottom-up, the second as top-down.

Bregman's distinction has a parallel in computational approaches to speech processing. Primitive grouping mechanisms based on pitch have been used with some success to segregate the voices of different speakers (Parsons, 1976; Stubbs et al., 1988; Weintraub, 1987), but they are limited to the voiced portions of speech and have difficulty maintaining source continuity across silent or voiceless intervals. This failure highlights the basic problem with the purely bottom-up grouping approach for speech segregation: there are no simple properties that distinguish the components of one speaker's voice from those of another.

The alternative, top-down, schemata-based approach has been used in speech processing to recognise two simultaneous sounds by Roger Moore and his colleagues at the RSRE in Malvern (Moore et al., 1991). They have taken the interesting step of extending the Hidden Markov Model (HMM) approach in speech recognition to the case where there are two (known) sounds present at the same time. An HMM contains stochastic templates: the program must first be trained on a representative selection of sounds that might occur, to allow it to develop a statistical model of each possible sound category. In recognition, there are a variety of algorithms that find which sound's model is most likely to have generated the presented sound. The RSRE group have extended the normal 'Viterbi' decoding algorithm to provide the correct 'maximum likelihood' recognition and optimal decomposition of the signal into two contributing sound sources. The algorithm is capable of performing speech recognition on two speakers simultaneously and shows substantial improvements in recognition accuracy for a single speaker against a background sound (such as a machine gun!) for which the program has a model.

The two approaches complement each other. The top-down approach produces good separation of speech from known sounds but fails on novel sounds that do not come close to any of the stored templates. It would gain rather little benefit from the presence of primitive grouping cues. By contrast, the bottom-up approach is agnostic as to the identity of the sounds that it is separating. It will work well if there are primitive grouping cues, and will fail if they are absent.

It is reasonably clear that both types of mechanism operate in human speech perception. Primitive grouping cues substantially improve recognition of one voice against a background of another (Brokx et al., 1982; Scheffers, 1983) and they also limit the possible interpretations that the listener makes of multiple sound-source data (Darwin, 1981; Darwin, 1991; Gardner et al., 1989). On the other hand, there is experimental evidence for a schema-driven mechanism that we use for selecting components that form possible speech sounds. Listeners can overcome inappropriate grouping cues to gain a clear speech percept (Cutting, 1976; Remez, 1987; Remez et al., 1981) and can identify remarkably well simultaneous pairs of known speech sounds which cannot be separated by primitive grouping cues (Scheffers, 1983). It is perhaps worth noting in passing that this schema-driven mechanism might not be learned (Mattingly et al., 1991).

3. Pitch Perception and Source Segregation

Difference in fundamental frequency is the best-documented primitive cue for the separation of different speech sound sources. The auditory system can exploit the fact that a periodic sound consists of frequency components that are integer multiples of the fundamental. Simultaneous speech sounds on different fundamentals are more easily identified than those on the same fundamental (Assmann et al., 1989; Assmann et al., 1990; Brokx et al., 1982; Scheffers, 1983); a single formant may be perceptually removed from a syllable if it is on a different fundamental from the rest of the syllable (Darwin, 1981; Darwin, 1991; Gardner et al., 1989) and a single harmonic may be perceptually removed from a steady vowel if it is not sufficiently close in frequency to a harmonic of the fundamental (Darwin et al., 1986).

Although the effect of fundamental frequency on speech sound source separation is indisputable, the mechanism or mechanisms by which fundamental frequency exercises its influence is less clear. Do similar mechanisms operate in the perception of the pitch of two simultaneous tones and in the perceptual segregation of two simultaneous voiced speech sounds?

I will first summarise previous experimental evidence on this question and then present new data that we have recently obtained at Sussex, both on speech source separation and on pitch perception.

We have previously argued that the harmonic sieve (Duifhuis et al., 1982) might operate in sound source separation as well as in pitch peception (Moore et al., 1985) on the grounds that similar amounts of mistuning are necessary for a harmonic to make a reduced contribution to both pitch and vowel quality (Darwin et al., 1986). The sieve (partly) blocks the (sufficiently) mistuned harmonic from both the subsequent pitch and the subsequent vowel classifiers.

The harmonic sieve, by definition, can only operate on resolved harmonics, and so is ineffective at separating unresolved harmonics. Harmonics may be unresolved because they are too close in frequency either to the next harmonic in the same series, or to a harmonic from a different series. High-numbered harmonics (above say the 8th) are excluded on the first criterion, so any source segregation that takes place for them must be occurring by some mechanism other than the harmonic sieve. Two periodic sounds whose fundamentals are very close together will also have (low-numbered) harmonics that are close together in frequency and so are unresolved from each other. For this reason the harmonic sieve cannot explain the improvement that occurs in identification scores for pairs of vowels when fundamental frequency differences of a semitone or less are imposed on them.

Although the harmonic sieve cannot segregate unresolved harmonics, it is clear that sounds which have no harmonic structure (Burns et al., 1981) or consist only of unresolved harmonics (Houtsma et al., 1990) can give a sensation of pitch. The pitch sensation produced by these sounds is less clear and pitch discrimination is much poorer for these sounds than for sounds that contain resolved components (Houtsma, 1984; Houtsma et al., 1990; Patterson et al., 1977). This weaker sensation of pitch is likely to be carried by the temporal pattern of amplitude modulation of the auditorially filtered waveform. Pitch discrimination becomes even poorer for sounds that consist only of unresolved components when the phase of these components is altered to reduce the depth of amplitude modulation of the auditorially filtered waveform (Houtsma et al., 1990).

At Sussex, we have recently carried out an experiment to see whether the distinction between resolved and unresolved harmonics affects formant segregation in a similar way to pitch discrimination. Is it harder to segregate a formant when it only contains unresolved harmonics than when it contains resolved harmonics?

To address this question we used the "ru-li" experimental paradigm (Darwin, 1981; Gardner et al., 1989). The basic sound used in these experiments is represented schematically in Fig. 1. A three-formant "base" syllable /li/ has added to it an extra (second) formant which is the F_2 of /ru/ to produce a composite four-formant syllable. When all four formants are excited by the same fundamental listeners report hearing /ru/, but if the second formant is excited by a sufficiently different fundamental then listeners can hear the syllable /li/ with the second formant emerging as a separate sound source. With smaller differences in fundamental frequency between the second and the other formants subjects report a "duplex" percept of a separate second formant but still /ru/. There are thus two stages in the segregation of a formant. With small F_0 differences the formant stands out as a separate sound source but is still phonetically integrated into the syllable to maintain the /ru/ percept; this stage corresponds to "duplex" perception. With larger F_0 differences the formant phonetically segregates and the syllable is heard as /li/.

In our earlier experiments (Darwin, 1981; Gardner et al., 1989), the second formant generally had some resolved harmonics. The base syllable - formants 1,3&4 - was excited at 110 Hz and the second formant was excited over a range of values from 110 to 174 Hz. The second formant frequency varied between 780 and 1400 Hz. 780 Hz corresponds roughly to the 7th harmonic of 110 Hz and the 4th harmonic of 174 Hz, whereas 1400 Hz corresponds roughly to the 13th harmonic of 110 Hz and the 8th harmonic of 174 Hz.

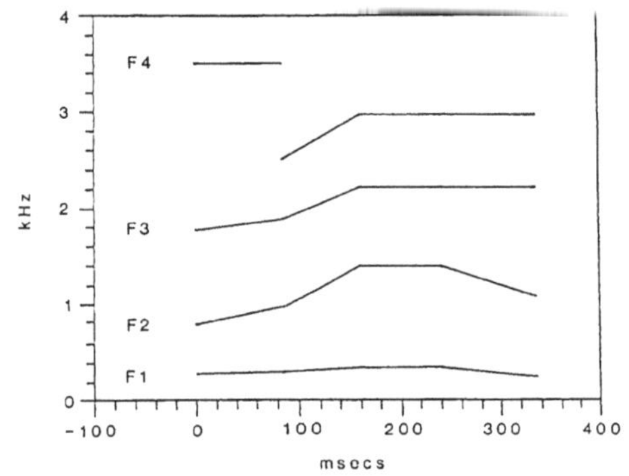

Fig. 1 Schematic spectrogram of formant tracks for a composite /ru/-/li/ syllable. Formants 1, 2 & 3 make /ru/ and formants 1, 3 & 4 make /li/. The percept of the whole syllable changes from /ru/ to /li/ when the fundamental frequency difference between the second formant and the rest is increased.

In this new experiment we used three different fundamentals for the base syllable: 80, 120 and 200 Hz, and then made the F_0 of F_2 either 0, 2.5, 5, 10, 20, 40 or 80% higher than the F_0 of the base. The experiment was run as a student project by Charles Edwardes on a variety of listeners - naive undergraduates and more experienced lab members. About half of the 12 listeners (all naive undergraduates) heard almost no /li/ sounds in the experiment and their data has been excluded. The remaining 5 more experienced listeners (though not more experienced in this task) gave very clear data which is shown in Fig. 2. The subject was given the choice of four responses to each stimulus. In each response category (except /li/ alone which we would expect to be almost never heard) there was a substantial effect of the F_0 of the base syllable. The pattern of results follows from the hypothesis that segregation is harder for unresolved than for resolved harmonics.

Fig. 2 shows the percentage of trials on which a particular response was given as a function of the percent F_0 difference between F_2 and the base syllable, with the base syllable's F_0 as parameter. In the top left panel the decline of "/ru/" responses with increasing F_0 difference is more rapid for the two higher base F_0s (200 and 120 Hz) than for the lowest F_0 (80 Hz). The decline in "/ru/" responses is complemented by an increase in both "/ru/+buzz" and in "/li/+buzz" responses. Here "buzz" refers to the sound of F_2.

With a base F_0 of 200 Hz, an increase of only 2.5% for the F_0 of F_2 is sufficient to give clear phonetic segregation with almost 100% "/li/+buzz" responses. Here the second formant frequency range corresponds to harmonics 4 through 7, all of which are clearly resolved.

With a base F_0 of 120 Hz, a more complex picture emerges. For small (2.5 and 5%) F_0 differences, the dominant response is a "duplex" one: subjects hear "/ru/+buzz". A difference of around 10% is needed before the phonetic segregation occurs and "/li/+buzz" becomes the dominant response. At an F_0 of 132 Hz (120+10%) the second formant frequency range corresponds to harmonics 6 through 11, so there will be a mixture of resolved and unresolved harmonics.

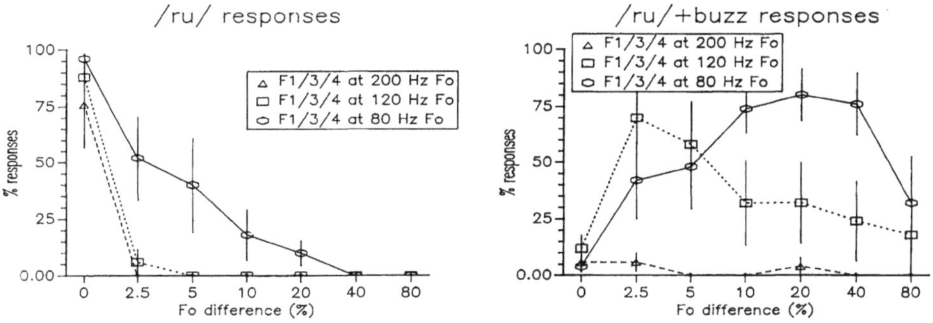

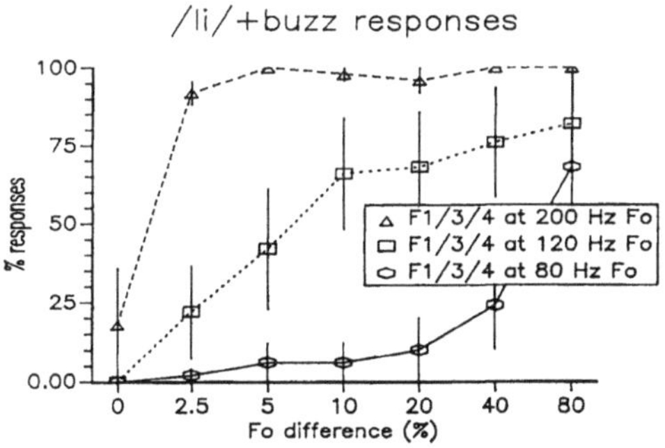

Fig. 2 Responses given to the composite /ru/-/li/ syllable shown in Figure 1. The different panels show different response categories; the abscissa is % F_0 difference between F2 and the other formants; the parameter is the F_0 of formants 1,3&4. The data are from 5 experienced listeners.

With a base F_0 of 80 Hz the pattern of results is similar to that at 120 Hz, but larger F_0 differences are needed to give both types of segregation. Now the "/ru/+buzz" response does not dominate until there is a 10% F_0 difference, and the "/li/+buzz" response requires a full 80%. At 88 Hz (80+10%) the second formant frequency range corresponds to harmonics 9 through 16 and so none would be resolved. However, at 144 Hz (80+80%) the second formant frequency range corresponds to harmonics 6 through 10, so again there will be a mixture of resolved and unresolved harmonics.

In summary, phonetic segregation of a formant can be achieved with a much smaller F_0 difference when the segregated formant contains resolved harmonics than when it only contains unresolved harmonics. In fact there is no evidence from our experiment that phonetic segregation of a formant *can* be achieved at all when only unresolved harmonics specify the formant. Identification of a formant as a separate sound (i.e. "/ru/+buzz" responses) *can* be achieved with only unresolved harmonics (as we have shown previously for F_4 segregation). The experiment thus extends to sound segregation the auditory system's greater sensitivity to F_0 differences for resolved harmonics found by Houtsma & Smurzynski.

A consequence of this conclusion is that when two speech sounds have only a small F_0 difference, segregation should be much clearer in the first formant region than in the higher formants. Such a difference has in fact already been found by John Culling. Culling started from the observation (Scheffers, 1983) that identification of pairs of vowels improves when there is a small (0.5 or 1 semitone) F_0 difference between the two vowels. In a series of experiments (Culling, 1990; Culling, 1991; Darwin et al., 1990) Culling demonstrated that this improvement in identification over the first semitone is due entirely to the first formant region. Higher formants only contribute to vowel separation when the F_0 difference is around 4 semitones.

In summary, we have shown that speech segregation shares with pitch perception sensitivity to the difference between resolved and unresolved harmonics. This common influence could arise because both pitch perception and speech segregation are subject to the same limitations of auditory coding, or it could arise because the process of sound segregation uses mechanisms common to pitch processing or even the results of pitch processing.

Carrying out experiments on the effect of fundamental frequency differences on speech segregation brought home to me how little work had been done on the perception of the pitch of simultaneous complex sounds. In particular we know almost nothing of how auditory primitive grouping cues influence pitch perception when there are multiple sound sources. Apart from the pioneering work of Beerends and Houtsma (Beerends, 1989; Beerends et al., 1986; Beerends et al., 1988; Beerends et al., 1989; Houtsma et al., 1984) and McAdams (McAdams, 1980; McAdams, 1984) some preliminary experiments by Elisabeth Cohen (Cohen, 1980) and work on the harmonic sieve (Duifhuis et al., 1982; Moore, 1987; Moore et al., 1985) neither pitch theorists nor experimenters have addressed the issue of how we perceive multiple pitches in complex sounds. The field is potentially a very rich one since it has important implications in both speech and music perception.

4. Auditory Grouping and Pitch Perception

Is pitch perception influenced by auditory grouping? How does the pitch perception mechanism determine which of the frequency components that are present at a particular time (or indeed across different times (Hall et al., 1981)) should contribute to a particular pitch percept? Over the last year or so Valter Ciocca and I (together with Roel Smits, Antonio Buffa, and Deirdre Williams) have investigated these questions exploiting a paradigm introduced by Brian Moore and his colleagues (Moore et al., 1985). We have asked the following questions:

1. Can a difference in onset time prevent a harmonic from contributing to the pitch of a complex sound?
2. Can a difference in amplitude modulation reduce a harmonic's contribution to the pitch of a complex sound?
3. Are sounds which arrive at the same ear (or from the same direction in space) more likely to contribute to a common pitch than those that do not?
4. Can a particular harmonic contribute only to the pitch of one of a number of simultaneous sounds? Alternatively: Does the Principle of Disjoint Allocation hold for pitch perception?

The paradigm allows the experimenter to measure the contribution that a particular harmonic makes to the pitch of a complex sound. The subject's task is to adjust the pitch of the second of two consecutive sounds until it matches the pitch of the first. The second sound is always strictly harmonic. The first sound typically is based on a harmonic series, but may have one of its components mistuned. The mistuned component may alter the pitch of the complex, and this alteration will be apparent in the fundamental frequency of the matched harmonic sound. The original work with this paradigm (Moore et al., 1985) demonstrated that a component mistuned by up to about 3% of its harmonic frequency made a full contribution to the pitch of the complex, but that above that its contribution declined until by about 8% mistuning it no longer made any contribution. The pitch shift produced by a mistuned component is thus a measure of the extent to which it is integrated into the pitch percept.

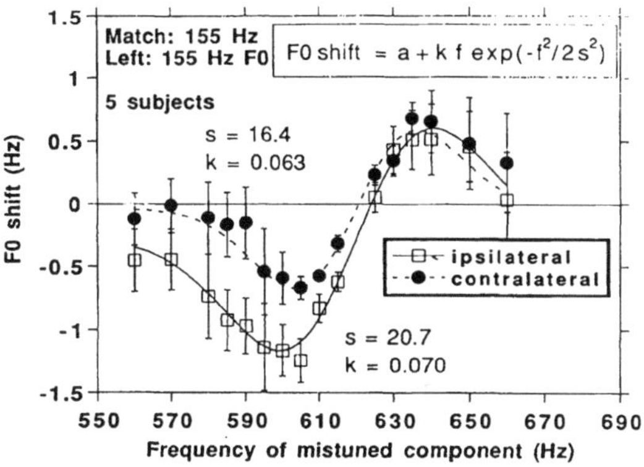

Fig. 3 Pitch shift produced by mistuning the fourth harmonic of a 5-harmonic complex presented either to the same or opposite ear as the rest of the complex.

We have replicated Moore's results with more values of mistuning than used by Moore (Darwin et al., 1991). Fig. 3 shows a subset of that data, using the first five harmonics of a 155-Hz fundamental, with the fourth harmonic mistuned and presented either ipsi- or contralaterally to the other harmonics. Here we have modelled the pitch shift by assuming that the contribution that a harmonic makes is reduced according to a Gaussian curve as its frequency deviates from harmonic. The measured pitch shift from the in-tune value (ΔF_0) is thus:

$$\Delta F_0 = a + k\ \Delta f \exp(-\Delta f^2/2s^2)$$

where Δf is the deviation of the mistuned component from harmonic, s is the standard deviation of the Gaussian (proportional to the width of the sieve's hole), k is a measure of the maximum contribution the harmonic makes, and a allows for inaccuracy in measuring the zero baseline for ΔF_0. This equation gives a good fit to our data. It would be difficult to distinguish the fit of this equation from one that was linear for small mistunings.

4.1 Grouping by Onset Asynchrony

To illustrate the use of the paradigm let us look first at an experiment that Valter Ciocca and I recently carried out at Sussex. We were interested in whether a component that started before the others in a complex would make less of a contribution to the pitch of the complex than if it started simultaneously. We already know that onset time differences are a powerful cue for segregating an individual harmonic from a vowel percept (Darwin, 1984; Darwin et al., 1984) and for hearing out an individual component in a complex (Rasch, 1981; Rasch, 1984), but it is not clear whether they preclude a component from the pitch calculation.

In this experiment we used two different durations (80 ms and 410 ms) of a basic 12-harmonic complex on a fundamental frequency of 155 Hz. We used two different durations since Moore (Moore, 1987) found that a mistuned harmonic was more likely to be incorporated into the pitch of a short (50 ms) than a long (410 ms) complex (200 Hz F_0) tone. For each of the two durations we allowed the fourth harmonic to vary both in onset time and in frequency. The nominally 620-Hz component was mistuned by ± 0, 10, 20, 50 Hz, and could start 0, 30 or 300 ms before the remaining 12 harmonics. 6 subjects performed 5 matches to each of these stimuli, making their adjustments with a Rollerball attached to a MacII. The sounds were generated from the MacII in real time, using specially developed 56001 assembler code (Russell et al., 1991) running on a Digidesign Audiomedia™ card.

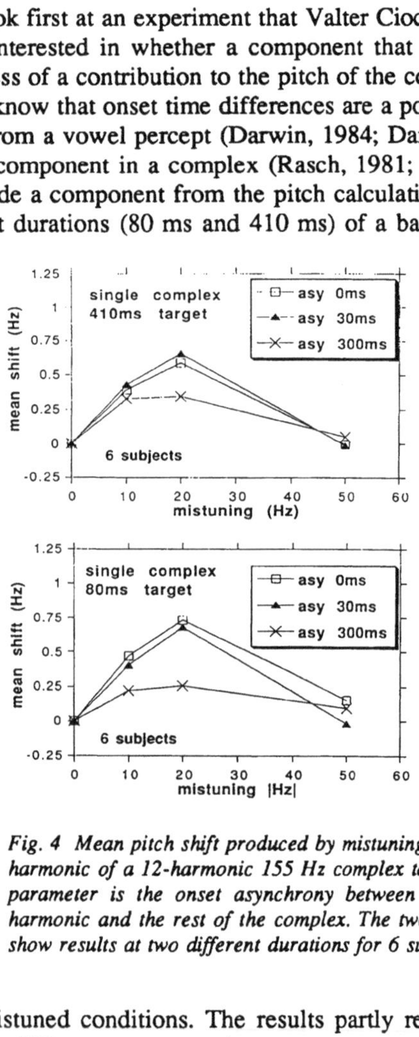

Fig. 4 Mean pitch shift produced by mistuning the 4th harmonic of a 12-harmonic 155 Hz complex tone. The parameter is the onset asynchrony between the 4th harmonic and the rest of the complex. The two panels show results at two different durations for 6 subjects.

The results of the experiment are shown in Fig. 4 as the mean matched pitch shift for each absolute amount of mistuning. This mean shift is calculated as half the difference between the matched pitches to the upward and the downward mistuned conditions. The results partly replicate Moore's findings and show a clear effect of a 300 ms onset asynchrony.

For both the 80 and 410 ms durations there is a large and statistically reliable pitch shift for the 0 and 30 ms asynchrony conditions which is greatest at 20 Hz (3%) mistuning, and has returned to zero at 50 Hz (8%). The 0 and 30 ms conditions do not differ at all from each other, and rather little across the two durations. There is very little evidence for the mistuned component being more integrated into the shorter than the longer sound as found by Moore (Moore, 1987).

300 ms onset asynchrony shows a clear effect. Pitch shifts are less with 300 ms than with 0 or 30 ms asynchrony at both durations, but the reduction in pitch shift is greater for 80 ms than for 410 ms duration.

In summary, a 300 ms onset asynchrony reduces the contribution that a mistuned harmonic makes to the pitch of a complex tone. The reduction is greater for an 80 ms than for a 410 ms tone. The pitch of a complex tone, like the quality of a vowel, is not simply determined by the frequency components that are present at a particular time. It also depends on the time at which the sounds started.

Our results are compatible with experiments done using a different paradigm by Vos (1991). He found no effect of a 20 ms onset asynchrony on the perceptual separation of two simultaneous complex tones. Since natural musical instruments show quite substantial differences in onset time of different harmonics (Risset et al., 1982) it is reassuring that the system is tolerant of some asynchrony between components.

We cannot say whether or not primitive auditory grouping mechanisms are operating before the pitch perception mechanism on the basis of these results, since they are also compatible with an explanation in terms of the rapid adaptation that occurs in the auditory response to a tone over its first few tens of milliseconds (Summerfield et al., 1987).

4.2 Grouping by Amplitude Modulation

There has been considerable and justified interest in the possible role that common amplitude modulation might play in auditory grouping, particularly in the context of comodulation masking release (Hall et al., 1990) and other across-channel masking phenomena (Moore et al., 1990; Yost et al., 1989). We have recently investigated whether a common pattern of amplitude modulation might provide a primitive grouping principle for components that belong to the same complex tone.

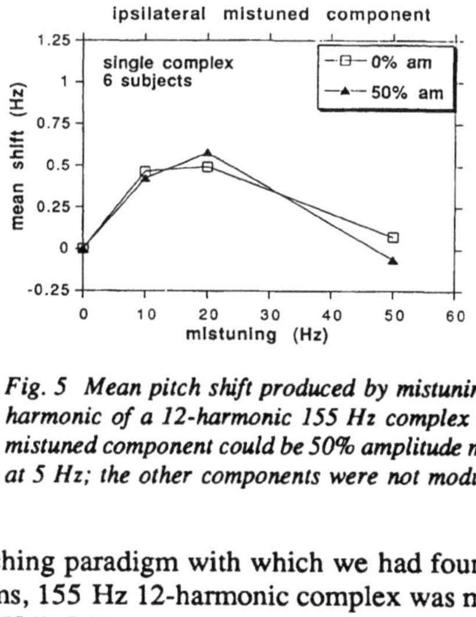

Fig. 5 Mean pitch shift produced by mistuning the 4th harmonic of a 12-harmonic 155 Hz complex tone. The mistuned component could be 50% amplitude modulated at 5 Hz; the other components were not modulated.

Our experiment used the same pitch matching paradigm with which we had found onset asynchrony effects. One component of a 410 ms, 155 Hz 12-harmonic complex was mistuned and given either no amplitude modulation or 50% 5 Hz AM. The remaining 11 components were not amplitude modulated.

The results for 6 subjects are shown in Fig. 5. Amplitude modulating the mistuned component does not reduce its contribution to the pitch of a complex whose other components are not amplitude modulated.

4.3 Grouping by Ear

Although the classical selective attention literature (Broadbent, 1958) showed that listeners can selectively attend more easily to spatially separated voices, spatial separation has not proved to be an overwhelming primitive grouping principle. Specifically, for identification of the pitch of two simultaneous 2-tone complexes, Beerends and Houtsma concluded that "Identification performance is only weakly dependent on the manner of distributing partials between the ears" (Beerends et al., 1989).

We have investigated the importance of ear of presentation in the mistuning paradigm. The simplest case is where all the in-tune components of a complex go to one ear, and the mistuned either to the same ear (ipsilateral) or the opposite ear (contralateral). We can then measure the extent of the pitch shift produced by the mistuned component as a function of the degree of mistuning and the distribution of the components across the ears. Fig. 3 shows the results of such an experiment conducted by Valter Ciocca and myself for a 5-component 155-Hz, 410 ms complex. There is a clear effect of ear: the mistuned component makes less of a contribution to the pitch of the complex when it goes to the opposite ear than when it goes to the same ear as the other, harmonic components. Although contralateral presentation clearly reduces the contribution of the mistuned component, it does still make a significant contribution to the perceived pitch.

4.4 Disjoint Allocation

In all the pitch matching experiments that I have described so far, there has been but a single basic harmonic complex. There has been no other complex sound competing for the mistuned component. We now turn to the more complex question of how we decide whether a particular component belongs to one or the other or even both of two possible complex tones. The basic design of the following experiments was conceived with Roel Smits (Darwin et al., 1990) and has since been extended with Valter Ciocca.

In these experiments we have set up the following situation: the listener is presented with two simultaneous complex tones, with fundamentals at, say, 155 Hz and 200 Hz. These two fundamentals have been chosen so that the third harmonic of 200 Hz (600Hz) and the fourth harmonic of 155 Hz (620 Hz) are separated by 3%. These two components, however, are replaced with a single component whose frequency can be varied. We then ask the listeners to match the pitch of either the 155 Hz or the 200 Hz complex as a function of the frequency of the single mistuned component.

The single mistuned component could potentially contribute to the pitch of either or both of the complex tones. To help clarify the issues here let us oppose two extreme hypotheses.

First, decisions about the pitches of the two complexes might be taken independently; all the available data is used for both decisions. This hypothesis predicts that the pattern of pitch matches to either complex tone is the same as we would expect if the other complex were absent. That is, the pitch shift should reach a maximum at 3% and decline to around zero at around 8%.

Second, decisions might be taken dependently; for example, if a particular component is exactly in tune with one harmonic series, it might be "captured" by that series and prevented from contributing to the pitch of the other series. This hypothesis follows the Principle of Disjoint Allocation (Bregman et al., 1975). The particular frequencies that we have used were chosen with this hypothesis in mind. When the mistuned component is exactly in tune with the 200 Hz complex (at 600 Hz), it is potentially able to produce the largest pitch shift in the other complex. But if it is captured by the 200 Hz complex then it cannot contribute to the 155 Hz.

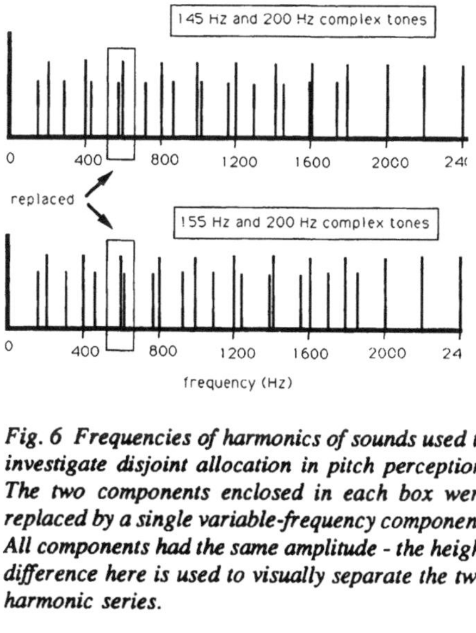

Fig. 6 Frequencies of harmonics of sounds used to investigate disjoint allocation in pitch perception. The two components enclosed in each box were replaced by a single variable-frequency component. All components had the same amplitude - the height difference here is used to visually separate the two harmonic series.

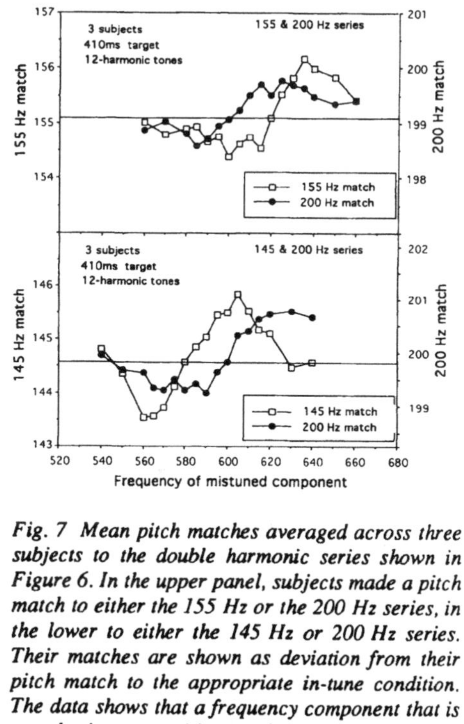

Fig. 7 Mean pitch matches averaged across three subjects to the double harmonic series shown in Figure 6. In the upper panel, subjects made a pitch match to either the 155 Hz or the 200 Hz series, in the lower to either the 145 Hz or 200 Hz series. Their matches are shown as deviation from their pitch match to the appropriate in-tune condition. The data shows that a frequency component that is exactly in tune with one harmonic series still contributes to the pitch of another harmonic series even though it is mistuned by 3% from this second series.

Our experiment in fact used two different pairs of fundamentals, 155 & 200 Hz as described above, and also 145 & 200 Hz (Fig. 6). The same design principles apply to this second pair of fundamentals. Our results clearly support the first hypothesis: decisions about the pitches of the two tones appear to be taken independently. In Fig. 7 we show the mean pitch matches for three subjects. The results are displayed differently from those in the preceding figures in that we are not averaging the upward and downward pitch shifts. The graphs are all aligned to the pitch match for the appropriate in tune condition. It is clear from the data that a component that is precisely in-tune with one harmonic series can still make a full (mistuned) contribution to the pitch of another simultaneous complex. So for instance in the 145 & 200 Hz results, a 600 Hz mistuned component, though perfectly in tune with the 200 Hz complex, is producing a maximal pitch shift in the 145 Hz complex.

5. Conclusions

In this paper we have explored the relationship between pitch perception and speech separation. We have presented new experimental evidence that grouping for speech categorisation can take place on the basis of common harmonicity, and have extended previous findings by showing that this grouping is considerably less sensitive to F_0 differences when it is based on unresolved rather than on resolved harmonics. We have also presented new experimental evidence on auditory grouping in pitch perception itself. We have shown that both onset time and ear of presentation can be used as grouping cues for pitch. A mistuned component that starts at a different time from the rest of a sound makes less of a contribution to the pitch of that sound than if it had started at the same time. Similarly, a mistuned component that arrives at a different ear makes less of a contribution to the pitch of a complex than does one that arrives at the same ear. Amplitude modulation, by contrast, does not appear to act as a grouping cue for pitch. We have also demonstrated that the principle of Disjoint Allocation does not apply to pitch perception.

Acknowledgments

This research was supported by the Image Interpretation and Computational Science Initiatives of the S.E.R.C. through grants GR/F 34060 and GR/F 45356.

References

Assmann, P.F. and Summerfield, A.Q. (1989). Modelling the perception of concurrent vowels: Vowels with the same fundamental frequency, *J. Acoust. Soc. Am.*, 85, 327-338.

Assmann, P.F. and Summerfield, A.Q. (1990). Modelling the perception of concurrent vowels: Vowels with different fundamental frequencies, *J. Acoust. Soc. Am.*, 88, 680-697.

Beerends, J.G. (1989). The influence of duration on the perception of pitch in single and simultaneous complex tones, *J. Acoust. Soc. Am.*, 86, 1835-1844.

Beerends, J.G. and Houtsma, A.J.M. (1986). Pitch identification of simultaneous dichotic two-tone complexes, *J. Acoust. Soc. Am.*, 80, 1048-1055.

Beerends, J.G. and Houtsma, A.J.M. (1988). The influence of duration on the perception of single and simultaneous two-tone complexes, in *Basic Issues in Hearing*, edited by H. Duifhuis, J.W. Horst, and H.P. Wit, Academic, London.

Beerends, J.G. and Houtsma, A.J.M. (1989). Pitch identification of simultaneous diotic and dichotic two-tone complexes, *J. Acoust. Soc. Am.*, 85, 813-819.

Bregman, A.S. (1990). *Auditory Scene Analysis: the perceptual organisation of sound*, Bradford Books, MIT Press, Cambridge, Mass.

Bregman, A.S. and Rudnicky, A. (1975). Auditory segregation: stream or streams?, *J. Exp Psychol: Hum. Perc. & Perf.*, 1, 263-267.

Broadbent, D.E. (1958). *Perception and Communication*, Pergamon, London.

Brokx, J.P.L. and Nooteboom, S. G. (1982). Intonation and the perceptual separation of simultaneous voices, *J. Phonetics*, 10, 23-36.

Burns, E.M. and Viemeister, N.F. (1981). Played again SAM: Further observations on the pitch of amplitude-modulated noise, *J. Acoust. Soc. Am.*, 70, 1655-1660.

Cohen, E.A. (1980). *The influence of nonharmonic partials on tone perception*, Stanford University. Ph.D.

Culling, J.F. (1990). Exploring the conditions for perceptual separation of concurrent voices using F_0 differences, *Proc. I.O.A.*, 12, 559-566.

Culling, J.F. (1991). *The perceptual separation of concurrent vowels*, University of Sussex. DPhil thesis.

Cutting, J.E. (1976). Auditory and linguistic processes in speech perception: inferences from six fusions in dichotic listening, *Psych Rev*, 83, 114-140.

Darwin, C.J. (1981). Perceptual grouping of speech components differing in fundamental frequency and onset-time, *Q Jl exp Psychol*, 33A, 185-208.

Darwin, C.J. (1984). Perceiving vowels in the presence of another sound: constraints on formant perception, *J. Acoust. Soc. Am.*, 76, 1636-47.

Darwin, C.J. (1991). The relationship between speech perception and the perception of other sounds, in *Modularity and the motor theory of speech perception*, edited by I.G. Mattingly and M.G. Studdert-Kennedy, Erlbaum, Hillsvale, N.J., pp. 239-259.

Darwin, C.J., Buffa, A., and Smits, R.L.H.M. (1990). Pitch of simultaneous complex tones with a single mistuned frequency component, *Proc. I.O.A.*, 12, 499-506.

Darwin, C.J., Buffa, A., Williams, D., and Ciocca, V. (1991). Pitch of dichotic complex tones with a mistuned frequency component, in *Auditory physiology and perception*, edited by Y. Cazals, L. Demany, and K. Horner, Pergamon, Oxford.

Darwin, C.J. and Culling, J.F. (1990). Speech perception seen through the ear, *Speech Comm.*, 9, 469-475.

Darwin, C.J. and Gardner, R.B. (1986). Mistuning a harmonic of a vowel: grouping and phase effects on vowel quality, *J. Acoust. Soc. Am.*, 79, 838-45.

Darwin, C.J. and Sutherland, N.S. (1984). Grouping frequency components of vowels: when is a harmonic not a harmonic?, *Q Jl Exper Psychol*, 36A, 193-208.

Duifhuis, H., Willems, L.F., and Sluyter, R.J. (1982). Measurement of pitch in speech: an implementation of Goldstein's theory of pitch perception, *J. Acoust. Soc. Am.*, 71, 1568-1580.

Gardner, R.B., Gaskill, S.A., and Darwin, C.J. (1989). Perceptual grouping of formants with static and dynamic differences in fundamental frequency, *J. Acoust. Soc. Am.*, 85, 1329-1337.

Hall, J.W. and Grose, J.H. (1990). Comodulation masking release and auditory grouping, *J. Acoust. Soc. Am.*, 88, 119-125.

Hall, J.W. and Peters, R.W. (1981). Pitch from nonsimultaneous successive harmonics in quiet and noise, *J. Acoust. Soc. Am.*, 69, 509-513.

Houtsma, A.J.M. (1984). Pitch salience of various complex sounds, *Music Percepn.*, 1, 296-307.

Houtsma, A.J.M., Canning, J.M., and Beerends, J. (1984). A preliminary study of identification of harmonic intervals made by simultaneous complex tones, in: *Computational models of hearing and vision*, edited by Estonian Academy of Sciences, Tallinn, pp. 19-23.

Houtsma, A.J.M. and Smurzynski, J. (1990). Pitch identification and discrimination for complex tones with many harmonics, *J. Acoust. Soc. Am.*, 87, 304-310.

Mattingly, I.G. and Studdert-Kennedy, M.G. (Ed) (1991). *Modularity and the motor theory of speech perception*, Erlbaum, Hillsvale, N.J.

McAdams, S. (1980). The effects of spectral fusion on the perception of pitch for complex tones, *J. Acoust. Soc. Am.*, 68 S1, 109.

McAdams, S. (1984). *Spectral fusion, spectral parsing and the formation of auditory images*, Stanford University. unpublished Ph.D. dissertation.

Moore, B.C.J. (1987). The perception of inharmonic complex tones, in *Auditory processing of complex sounds*, edited by W.A. Yost and C.S. Watson (Erlbaum, Hillsdale, N.J.), pp. 180-189.

Moore, B.C.J., Glasberg, B.R., Gaunt, T., and Child, T. (1990). Across-channel masking of changes in modulation depth for amplitude- and frequency-modulated signals, *Q. Jl exp. Psychol.*

Moore, B.C.J., Glasberg, B.R., and Peters, R.W. (1985). Relative dominance of individual partials in determining the pitch of complex tones, *J. Acoust. Soc. Am.*, 77, 1853-60.

Moore, R.K., Varga, A.P., and Kadirkamanatha, M. (1991). *Automatic separation of speech and other complex sounds using hidden Markov model decomposition*, Institute of Acoustics Speech Group Meeting; February 1991, Brighton, Sussex.

Parsons, T.W. (1976). Separation of speech from interfering speech by means of harmonic selection, *J. Acoust. Soc. Am.*, 60, 656-60.

Patterson, R.D. and Johnson-Davies, D. (1977). Detection of a change in the pitch of AM noise, in *Psychophysics and physiology of hearing*, edited by E.F. Evans and J.P. Wilson, Academic Press, London.

Rasch, R. (1981). *Aspects of the perception and performance of polyphonic music*, Drukkerij Elinkwijk BV, Utrecht.

Rasch, R.A. (1984). The perception of simultaneous notes such as in polyphonic music, *Acustica*, 40, 22-33.

Remez, R.E. (1987). Units of organization and analysis in the perception of speech, in *The psychophysics of speech perception*, edited by M.E.H. Schouten, Martinus Nijhoff, Dordrecht, pp. 419-432.

Remez, R.E., Rubin, P.E., Pisoni, D.B., and Carrell, T.D. (1981). Speech perception without traditional speech cues, *Science*, 212, 947-950.

Risset, J.-C. and Wessel, D.L. (1982). Exploration of timbre by analysis and synthesis, in *The Psychology of Music*, edited by D. Deutsch, Academic, New York, pp. 25-58.

Russell, P. and Darwin, C.J. (1991). Real-time synthesis of complex sounds on a Mac II with 56001 DSP chip, *Brit. J. Audiol.*, 25, 59-60.

Scheffers, M.T. (1983). *Sifting vowels: Auditory pitch analysis and sound segregation*, Groningen University, The Netherlands. Ph.D.

Stubbs, R.J. and Summerfield, A.Q. (1988). Evaluation of two voice-separation algorithms using normally-hearing and hearing-impaired listeners, *J. Acoust. Soc. Am.*, 84, 1236-1249.

Summerfield, A.Q. and Assmann, P. (1987). Auditory enhancement in speech perception, in *The psychophysics of speech perception*, edited by M.E.H. Schouten, Martinus Nijhoff, Dordrecht, pp. 140-150.

Vos, J. (1991). *Perceptual separation in musical intervals with simultaneous complex tones: the effect of slightly asynchronous onsets*, Abstract submitted to Institute of Acoustics Speech Group Meeting; February 1991, Brighton, Sussex.

Weintraub, M. (1987). Sound separation and auditory perceptual organisation, in *The psychophysics of speech perception*, edited by M.E.H. Schouten, Martinus Nijhoff, Dordrecht, pp. 125-134.

Yost, W.A. and Sheft, S. (1989). Across-critical-band processing of amplitude-modulated tones, *J. Acoust. Soc. Am.*, 85, 848-857.

Detecting F_0 Differences and Pitch-Pulse Asynchronies

Robert P. Carlyon
Laboratory of Experimental Psychology
Sussex University
Brighton BN1 9QG
England.

1. INTRODUCTION

One of the most demanding tasks facing the auditory system is the perceptual separation of concurrent complex sounds. The level of performance which listeners can achieve is impressive: for example, listeners can correctly identify pairs of vowels which are both presented to the same ear, have identical onsets and offsets, and have spectra which overlap (Assmann and Summerfield, 1990; Scheffers, 1983). In such "double vowel" experiments, listeners not only have to identify the formants in the spectrum, but also assign each formant to the appropriate vowel. To do this, they use differences in fundamental frequency (F_0) between the two vowel sounds to be identified. A great deal of theoretical effort has gone into modelling the way in which listeners process such F_0 information (Assmann and Summerfield, 1990; Meddis and Hewitt, 1991). However, most relevant psychoacoustical experiments have measured the detection of *successive* differences in F_0, whereas speech tasks require the listener to make *simultaneous* comparisons. As a first step towards providing a psychoacoustical basis for perceptual models, the experiments reported here measured thresholds for the detection of differences in F_0 between pairs of simultaneous formant-like sounds occupying different spectral frequency regions. We were also interested in how sensitive listeners are to another potential cue to monaural separation of concurrent sounds, termed "pitch-pulse asynchrony" (Summerfield and Assmann, 1991).

Pitch-pulse asynchrony refers to a situation in which two groups of components can have identical F_0s, but in which the peaks in the waveform of one group are delayed slightly with respect to those in the other group. Such a situation might occur if two speakers each pronounced a vowel at the same F_0, but had started speaking at a different time. A listener might use this asynchrony to perceptually separate two formants which, had they been synchronous, he would have grouped together. Listeners are largely insensitive to phase differences between individual components that are filtered into separate frequency channels by the peripheral auditory system (Zwicker, 1952), so the asynchrony cue is probably strongest in high spectral frequency regions, where auditory filters are widest, and at low F_0s, where component spacing is narrowest. It is precisely under such conditions that F_0 information is most degraded (Hoekstra, 1979; Houtsma and Smurzynski, 1990) and where large F_0 differences are required for concurrent sound segregation (Culling, 1990).

It is worth noting that two groups of components with different F_0s will always produce a pitch-pulse asynchrony at some point throughout their waveforms: even if their pitch pulses start out as synchronous, the difference between their periods will cause pitch pulses in one group to "lag behind" those in the other. To be more precise, when the F_0s of two component groups differ by *x* Hz, the offset between adjacent peaks (the "group phase disparity") rotates through 360° every 1/*x* seconds. For small mistunings, where the group phase disparity rotates through less than 360° throughout the signal, we would expect performance to increase monotonically with increases in mistuning, even if listeners were in fact detecting the resulting asynchrony.

The experiments reported here asked whether, at low F_0s, listeners do indeed detect mistunings from the resulting asynchrony. At least three previous studies measured the detection of across-frequency timing differences (Strickland et al., 1989; Wakefield and Edwards, 1987; Yost and Sheft, 1989) . Those studies measured thresholds for the detection of envelope disparities between pairs of amplitude-modulated sinusoids. They showed that threshold measured in degrees was roughly independent of modulation frequency (equal to F_0) in the range between about 6 and 64 Hz. As we shall see, this finding did not occur for the multi-component stimuli of the present study.

2. EXPERIMENT 1

2.1 Method and rationale

Experiment 1 measured five-point psychometric functions for the detection of mistunings and of asynchronies, at F_0s of 20 Hz and 125 Hz, using a 2I, 2AFC task. The two (simultaneous) component groups had centre frequencies (CFs) of 1500 Hz and 3500 Hz respectively, with triangular (48 dB/octave) spectral envelopes. The stimuli were generated digitally by summing sinusoids whose amplitudes had been calculated to fit under the constant spectral envelope. Only sinusoids with amplitudes within 15 dB of the component at CF (45 dB SPL) were included. The stimulus duration was 200 ms with 5- ms raised-cosine ramps, and stimuli were played out at a sampling frequency of 15 625 Hz with 12-bit resolution, and presented monaurally to three normal listeners. In both conditions, the standard stimulus consisted of the two groups with identical F_0s and pitch pulses in synchrony. For the signals in the "asynchrony" condition, the group with a CF of 3500 Hz was delayed relative to the lower group on half the trials, and advanced on the other half. Delaying and advancing waveforms was done by generating versions of each group with durations longer than 200 ms, advancing one group, and then windowing. For the signals in the "mistuning" condition both groups started out in synchrony, but the F_0 of the upper group was shifted up and that of the lower group shifted down on half the trials, and the converse was true for the other half. In each condition, data were averaged over the two directions of mistuning or delay, and each point was derived from 200 trials. For all stimuli, the overall starting point was randomised by an amount common to both groups over a duration equal to one period, and the overall F_0 was randomised by varying the playback rate by +/- 10%. This was done to prevent listeners from responding on the basis of the starting phase or F_0 of either group in isolation. All stimuli were presented in a background of pink noise, with noise energy around 1500 and 3500 Hz filtered out[1]. At the higher F_0 we included mistunings so large (> 5 Hz, = 4%) that the group phase disparity rotated more than once throughout the 200-ms stimulus. Thus, if listeners were detecting mistuning on the basis of pitch-pulse asynchronies, then we would not expect performance at 125 Hz to increase monotonically with increases in mistuning beyond 4%.

2.2 Results

Fig. 1 shows psychometric functions in the asynchrony condition for the two F_0s. Only the data for listener GC are shown, but data for the other two listeners are similar. In the asynchrony condition, d' increases monotonically as a function of the envelope phase delay between the two groups. In contrast to the data at 20 Hz, performance at 125 Hz was essentially at chance for all but the largest asynchrony.

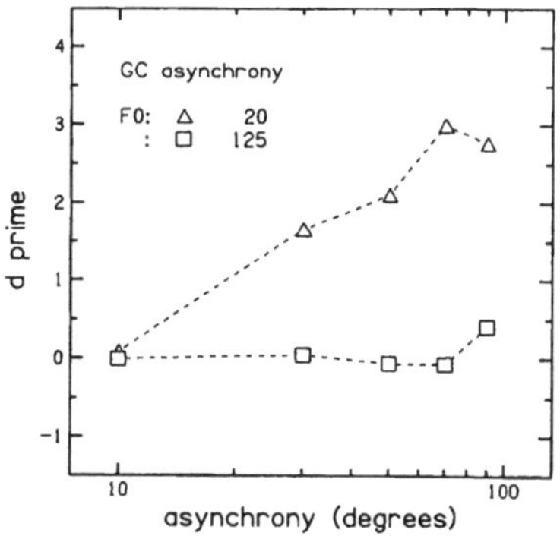

Fig. 1 Listener GC's psychometric functions for the detection of asynchrony in expt. 1.

Data for the mistuning condition are shown by the symbols in Fig. 2. Performance is better at 20 Hz than at 125 Hz, but the difference is not as marked as for the asynchrony condition. The solid lines show the sensitivity (d') for each mistuning that would be predicted from the listener's sensitivity to the mean asynchrony caused by that mistuning. (Recall that for mistunings < 5 Hz, the mean asynchrony caused by a mistuning is proportional to the amount of mistuning). The predictions, based on the data in Fig. 1, show that the data for an F_0 of 20 Hz are consistent with the idea that listeners were detecting mistuning on the basis of the asynchrony that it caused. This was not the case at 125 Hz, where listeners could detect mistuning but not asynchrony. Furthermore, performance for all three listeners continued to improve monotonically with increases in mistuning beyond 5 Hz (4% at this F_0), despite the absence of a similar monotonic increase in mean asynchrony.

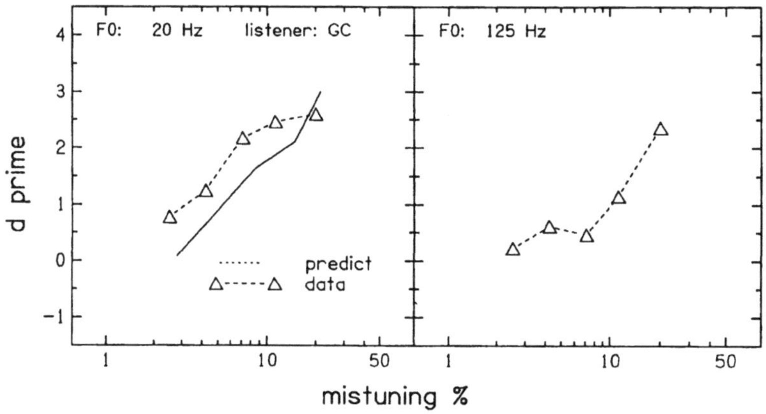

Fig. 2 Listener GC's psychometric functions for the detection of mistuning in expt. 1.

The conclusion to be drawn from experiment 1 is that listeners may detect mistuning on the basis of asynchrony when the F_0 is 20 Hz, but not when it is 125 Hz.

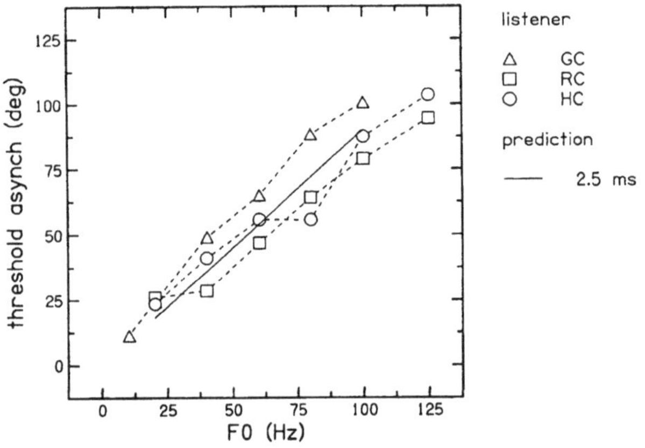

Fig. 3 Adaptive thresholds for the detection of asynchrony in expt. 2.

3. EXPERIMENT 2

Experiment 2 repeated experiment 1 using an adaptive procedure, and measured thresholds for F_0s of 20, 40, 60, 80, 100, and 125 Hz. Data for the asynchrony condition are shown in Fig. 3, and correspond to a constant time difference of approximately 2-3 ms for all three listeners, as indicated by the solid line. The increase in thresholds measured in degrees with increases in F_0 is consistent with the findings of Summerfield and Assmann (1991), who reported that pitch-pulse asynchrony aided the identification of double vowels with F_0s of 50 but not of 100 Hz. Data for the mistuning condition are shown by the symbols in Fig. 4, and show that thresholds (% mistuning) also increase with increases in CF. However, this does not mean that the same mechanisms underly the detection of mistuning and of asynchrony: the solid lines at the bottom of each plot are the "mean asynchrony" predictions based on the data in Fig. 3, and show that the predictions underestimate thresholds for F_0s at and above 40 Hz. An interesting finding is that thresholds at F_0s above 40 Hz are significantly higher than frequency DLs for groups of unresolved components in tasks requiring successive frequency comparisons (Hoekstra, 1979; Houtsma and Smurzynski, 1990). This suggests that such tasks may overestimate our sensitivity to the simultaneous differences in F_0 that occur in speech (and in the present study).

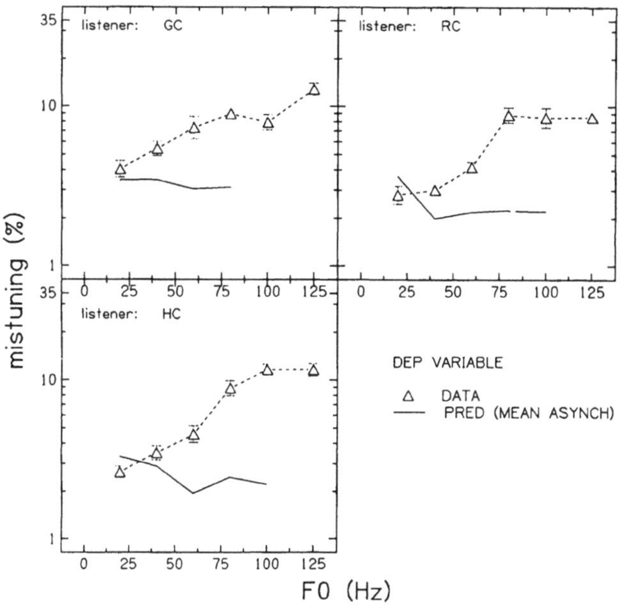

Fig. 4 Adaptive thresholds for the detection of mistuning in expt. 2.

4. Discussion and Further Experiments

4.1 Detecting asynchrony

Experiment 2 showed that asynchrony thresholds corresponded to constant time differences for F_0s between 20 and 100 Hz, in contrast to the constant number of degrees reported by Wakefield (1987) and by Yost (1989). There are two possible explanations for this effect.

One possibility is that listeners were simply detecting onset disparities between the first pitch pulse in each group. This explanation was supported by an additional experiment in which thresholds were compared at signal durations of 50 and 450 ms, with abrupt signal onsets and offsets occurring at least a quarter of a period away from pitch peaks. Thresholds differed by a mean factor of less than 1.2 for both F_0s (20 and 80 Hz) tested, considerably lower than the factor of 3 predicted from optimal combination of independent observations[2]. This is consistent with listeners comparing mainly the first pulse in each group. However, two findings lead us to qualify this conclusion. First, when 150-ms ramps were imposed on the 450-ms stimuli, thresholds did not change markedly. Therefore, if listeners were using onset cues, they were able to do so for stimuli with gradual onsets. Second, we repeated the experiment at an F_0 of 20 Hz, but this time comparing threshold for a 50-ms segment with that for a 200-ms sound generated by repeating the 50 ms segment four times. We then tried to "persuade" the listener to treat the first and second halves of the 200-ms signal as separate entities, by introducing long (up to 180 ms) silent intervals between them, and in some conditions by inserting brief "resetting" sounds in the silent interval (Hafter et al., 1988). The resetting sounds included 10-ms 500-Hz tone pips, 1-kHz square waves, and were presented either to the contralateral or ipsilateral ear. None of these manipulations resulted in a threshold reduction re the regular 200-ms condition, and the threshold reduction re the 50-ms condition was always less than the $\sqrt{2}$ predicted from the optimum combination of two observations. Thus, if listeners do attend only to the first pulse in each group, they do so in a particularly stubborn and ecologically disadvantageous manner. An alternative possibility is that there is a lower bound on the threshold that listeners can achieve. This might occur due to the temporal smearing caused by the auditory filters through which the stimuli pass. This explanation could account for the difference between the present data and those obtained with amplitude-modulated sinusoids. In those studies (Strickland et al., 1989; Wakefield and Edwards, 1987; Yost and Sheft, 1989), the envelope waxes and wanes very gradually, and so the modulation depth at the output of an auditory filter is limited by the input waveform. For our stimuli, which had many more components and much more abrupt envelopes, the limitation is caused by the temporal response of the filter, and is largely independent of F_0. However, signal detection theory would still predict a $\sqrt{2}$ drop in threshold with a doubling of duration, provided that the psychometric functions have unity slope, which was true for the range of asynchronies tested in experiment 1 (see footnote 2). In order for this explanation to account for the small effect of signal duration, psychometric functions would have to drop steeply towards zero for asynchronies less than 2-3 ms. Unfortunately, the functions measured in experiment 1 did not include such small asynchronies.

4.2 Detection of mistuning as a function of F_0

Experiment 2 showed that mistuning thresholds increased monotonically with increases in F_0. However, Carlyon (1991) reported that thresholds for detecting mistuning of two groups of resolved harmonics were lower (about 1%) than when one of the groups was unresolved (7%). It is therefore likely that if experiment 2 could have been extended to include F_0s sufficiently high for both groups to become resolved, then thresholds would have dropped again. Unfortunately, this was not possible because the spectral envelopes were too narrow to ensure that enough components of a sufficiently high F_0 would fall under each envelope.

5. CONCLUSION

Two experiments investigated the detection of mistuning and pitch-pulse asynchronies between pairs of formant-like sounds. The results indicate that listeners can detect mistunings from the resulting pitch-pulse asynchrony when the F_0 is 20 Hz, but not for higher F_0s. Thresholds for the detection of asynchronies corresponded to a constant time delay for F_0s between 20 and 100 Hz, suggesting that the cue is most useful at low F_0s. This conclusion is consistent with the "double vowel" data of (Summerfield and Assmann, 1991)

Notes

1. 3-dB down points 1208-1862 Hz and 2818-4346 Hz, lowpass slopes 96 dB/octave, highpass 135 dB/octave; N0 at 500 Hz = 17.8 dB SPL.
2. Signal detection theory predicts $\sqrt{n}$ change in d' for every *n* independent observations, and this results in a corresponding change in threshold if d' is proportional to asynchrony. We fitted the data from experiment 1 with a straight line relating log asynchrony to log d', and obtained slopes close to the predicted value of unity.

Acknowledgments

This research was supported by a Royal Society University Research Fellowship and an MRC project grant to the author. I thank Dr. Valter Ciocca for comments on an earlier version of the article, and the British Council for travel support.

References

Assmann, P. and Summerfield, Q. (1990). Modeling the perception of concurrent vowels: Vowels with different fundamental frequencies, *J. Acoust. Soc. Am.*, 88, 680-697.

Carlyon, R.P., Demany, L., and Semal, C. (1991). Detection of across-frequency differences in F_0, *J. Acoust. Soc. Am.*, submitted.

Culling, J. (1990). Perceptual separation of concurrent vowels: effects of across-formant inconsistencies in F_0, *Brit. J. Audiol.*, in press.

Hafter, E.F., Buell, T.N., and Richards, V.M. (1988). Onset-coding in lateralization: its form, site, and function, in: *Auditory Function: Neurobiological Bases of Hearing*, edited by G.M. Edelman, W.E. Gall, and M.W. Cowan, (Wiley, New York), 647-676.

Hoekstra, A. (1979). *Frequency discrimination and frequency analysis in hearing*, Institute of Audiology, University Hospital, Groningen, Netherlands, PhD Thesis.

Houtsma, A.J.M. and Smurzynski, J. (1990). J.F. Schouten revisited: pitch of complex tones having many high-order harmonics, *J. Acoust. Soc. Am.*, 87, 304-310.

Meddis, R. and Hewitt, M. (1991). Modeling the identification of concurrent vowels with different fundamental frequencies, *J. Acoust. Soc. Am.*, submitted.

Scheffers, M.T.M. (1983). *Sifting vowels: auditory pitch analysis and sound segregation*, Univ. Groningen, Netherlands. Doctoral dissertation.

Strickland, E., Viemeister, N.F., Fantini, D.A., and Garrison, M.A. (1989). Within- versus cross-channel mechanisms in detection of envelope phase disparity, *J. Acoust. Soc. Am.*, 86, 2160-2166.

Summerfield, A.Q. and Assmann, P.F. (1991). Perception of concurrent vowels: Effects of pitch-pulse asynchrony and harmonic misalignement, *J. Acoust. Soc. Am.*, 89, 1364-1377.

Wakefield, G.H. and Edwards, B. (1987). Discrimination of envelope phase disparity, *J. Acoust. Soc. Am.*, 82, S41.

Yost, W.A. and Sheft, S. (1989). Across-critical-band processing of amplitude-modulated tones, *J. Acoust. Soc. Am.*, 85, 848-857.

Zwicker, E. (1952). Die Grenzen der Hörbarkeit der Amplitudenmodulation und der Frequenzmodulation eines Tones, *Acustica*, 4, 415-420.

Roles of Harmonicity and Coherent Frequency Modulation in Auditory Grouping.

Quentin Summerfield
MRC Institute of Hearing Research
University Park
Nottingham NG7 2RD
U.K.

1. Introduction

When two talkers speak at the same time, the instantaneous values of the fundamental frequencies (F_0s) of their voices are generally different, even if the long-term mean values of F_0 are the same. As Chris Darwin emphasises (this volume), the resulting difference in harmonicity is a powerful cue that helps listeners to segregate competing voices and to attend selectively to one or other of them (e.g. Broadbent and Ladefoged, 1957; Assmann and Summerfield, 1991; see Darwin, 1990, for a review). When the F_0 of a voice changes, its harmonics change in frequency coherently; all rise or fall by the same percentage of their starting frequency. Can this coherent frequency modulation (CFM) of the components of a voice provide an additional basis for grouping?

Modulating the F_0 of a voice increases its *prominence* in a mixture of voices (McAdams, 1989; Marin and McAdams, 1991). However, studies that have investigated whether CFM provides a basis for *grouping* have concluded either that it plays no role (Gardner and Darwin, 1986; Gardner et al., 1989) or that it plays only a small role (Chalikia and Bregman, 1985; Demany and Semal, 1990). Two explanations have been offered. Carlyon (1991) demonstrated that listeners cannot distinguish coherent from incoherent FM among a small set of inharmonic tones. Fig. 1 shows two of the conditions that his listeners could not distinguish. He concluded that there can be no mechanism for detecting CFM as such, so CFM cannot provide a basis for grouping. Carlyon's result is compatible with the summary description of across-channel masking in Brian Moore's key paper: "modulation in one frequency region may make it more difficult to detect or discriminate modulation in another frequency region". Possibly, modulation detection interference prevents listeners from using CFM to segregate competing voices.

An alternative explanation that might apply to speech sounds, where many components are modulated together, is that listeners *can* use CFM but harmonicity is such a powerful basis for grouping that it permits (nearly) all the segregation that can occur, leaving little extra for CFM to contribute. The results of an experiment by Chalikia and Bregman (described in Bregman, 1990) support this view. They synthesised vowels whose components were placed randomly in frequency rather than harmonically. The vowels were mixed in pairs. In one condition, the same pattern of CFM was given to both vowels. In another condition, different patterns of CFM were given to the two vowels. Listeners identified the constituent vowels more accurately in the second condition. Thus, CFM played a role when effects of harmonicity were prohibited.

Two limitations of Chalikia and Bregman's experiment were that the effect of CFM was small (an additional 3% correct) and listeners identified different stimuli in different conditions. Thus, differences in "phonetic goodness" may have exaggerated, or diminished, effects of CFM (c.f. Terhardt, 1987). The experiments described below sought to corroborate Chalikia and Bregman's result using a procedure that avoids these problems. The minimum level was measured at which a set of "target" vowels could be identified in the presence of "masking" vowels. The easier a target is to segregate from a masker, the lower its masked threshold will be. Confounding effects of phonetic goodness were avoided by using the same targets in different conditions.

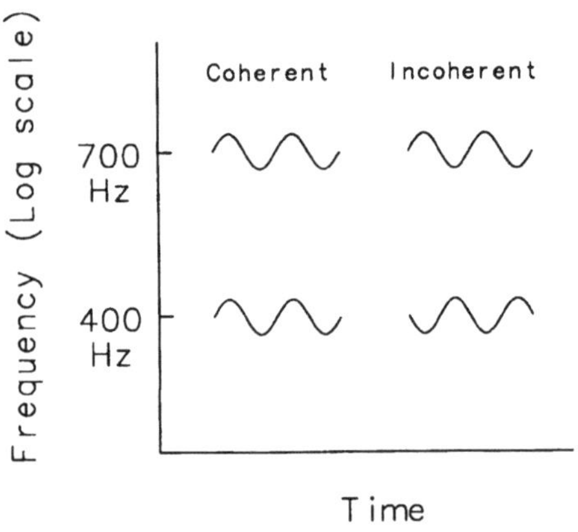

Fig. 1 Schematic spectrograms of stimuli used by Carlyon (1991). Listeners cannot distinguish coherent FM (left) from incoherent FM (right) among a set of inharmonic tones.

2. Psychophysical Procedure

The experiments used a 2-interval 5-alternative forced-choice task developed from procedures described by Demany and Semal (1990) and Summerfield and Assmann (1991). Each trial involved two observation intervals. Maskers were presented in both intervals. A target was presented in one interval, chosen randomly. Maskers and targets were 5-formant synthetic vowel-like sounds. Targets were exemplars of the five vowels, /a/, /i/, /ɜ/, /u/, and /ɔ/. Fig. 2 shows an F1/F2 plot of the maskers and targets. Subjects attempted to indicate which interval contained the target and what its identity was. Both aspects had to be corrected for the response to be scored as correct. The levels of targets relative to maskers were controlled by an adaptive rule which estimated the relative level giving 71%-correct responses. Trials from

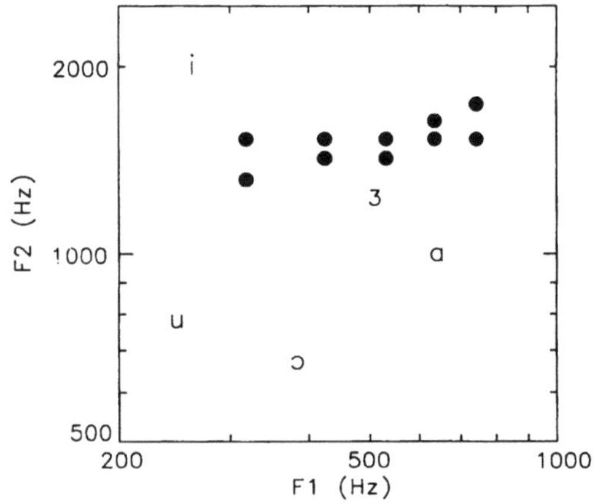

Fig. 2 F1/F2 plot of maskers (filled circles) and targets (phonetic symbols).

five adaptive staircases, one for each vowel, were randomly interleaved, giving five masked thresholds. They were averaged to provide one overall threshold at the end of each run.

To prevent listeners from using unintended cues, four parameters were varied randomly. (i) Overall level was roved over an 11-dB range between the two intervals, so that absolute level could not be used to locate the interval containing the target. (ii) Different maskers with different F_0s, chosen randomly from a small set, were presented in each interval, so that the target could not be recovered by subtracting the spectral profile of the masker from the profile of the masker+target. (iii) The F_0 of the target was chosen randomly from four values: 100, 112, 126, and 141 Hz. Thus, listeners could not locate targets by listening for a sound on a particular pitch. (iv) Where maskers had different F_0s from targets, the difference could be either positive or negative. Thus, listeners could not locate targets by listening consistently for either the lower- or higher-pitched member of the pair. From the listener's perspective, therefore, each trial involved two snippets of speech, one composed of one voice, the other of two. Listeners knew that the second voice would say one of the five target vowels. They had to identify the snippet which contained two voices, and indicate which of the five vowels had been spoken by the second voice.

3. CONDITIONS

Experiments which seek a role for CFM must control for effects of harmonicity. Fig. 3 illustrates the problem. In condition A, the F_0s of Voice 1 and Voice 2 are modulated incoherently and achieve a maximum difference of N semitones (STs). In B, they are modulated coherently with a constant difference of N STs. A role for CFM, independent of harmonicity, is confirmed only if it is easier to segregate the voices in A than B. These conditions were included along with several others.

The relationship between the F_0s of maskers (M) and targets (T) in the different conditions is schematised in Fig. 4. The traces illustrate the F_0 contours used in conditions with static targets (left) and modulated targets (right). Maskers and targets were 400 ms in duration. When the F_0 was modulated, the modulation rate was 2.5 cycles/s and the modulation depth (zero-peak) was 2 STs.

Consider first the conditions with static targets. In condition (1), maskers and targets had the same fixed F_0. In (2), their F_0s differed by 2 STs (12%). In (3), the difference was 4 STs (26%). In (4), the F_0 of the masker was modulated around the F_0 of the target so that the maximum difference in F_0 was 2 STs. In (5), the mean F_0 of the masker differed by 2 STs from the F_0 of the target, so the maximum difference was 4 STs. In (8), thresholds were measured in absence of maskers.

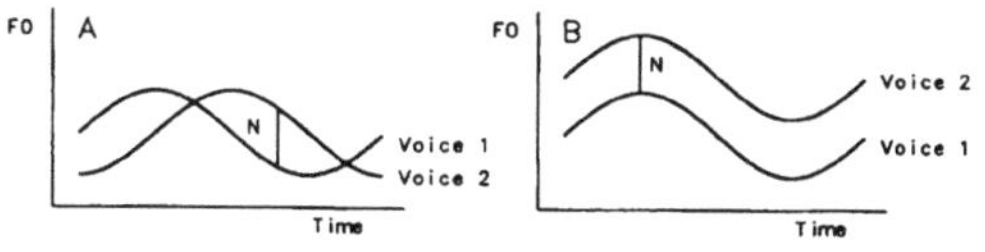

Fig. 3 (A) F_0s of Voice 1 and Voice 2 are given different modulations and achieve a maximum difference of N STs. (B) F_0s of Voice 1 and Voice 2 are given the same modulation with a constant difference of N STs. A role for CFM is established only if performance is better in (A) than (B).

With modulated targets, conditions (1) to (5) and (8) were analogous to the conditions involving static targets. Conditions (6) and (7) were different. Here, both masker and target were

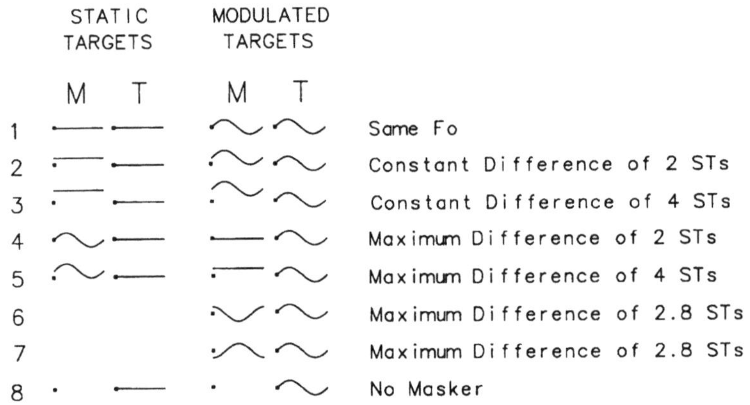

Fig. 4 F_0 contours of maskers (M) and targets (T) in the conditions of the experiment. The small squares mark a fixed frequency/time point for reference.

modulated. In (6), the phase of the masker modulation led that of the target by 90°. In (7), it lagged by 90°. The maximum difference in F_0 occurring over the course of these stimuli is 2.8 STs. In accordance with Fig. 3, a control condition is needed in which maskers and targets are modulated coherently with a constant difference of 2.8 STs. However, effects of F_0-differences on vowel segregation are constant for differences between 2 and 4 STs (Scheffers, 1983; Summerfield and Assmann, 1991). Thus, conditions (2) and (3) provide controls for (6) and (7).

4. "Harmonic" and "Random" Stimuli

Maskers and targets were synthesised digitally. The input to the cascade synthesiser was a set of formant frequencies and bandwidths, along with the frequencies of a set of "components". The synthesiser computed an appropriate amplitude and phase for each component in relation to the frequency and phase spectra defined by the formant frequencies and bandwidths. In "harmonic" stimuli, the components were related harmonically, with F_0s in the range from 100 Hz to 141 Hz. To create a sound whose F_0 differed by N STs, the frequency of every component was changed by N STs. The "random" stimuli were created by displacing the frequency of each component from its harmonic frequency by a random number of Hz chosen from the range $+F_0/2$ to $-F_0/2$. Then, to create a sound with a nominal difference in "F_0" of N STs, the frequency of each component was changed by N STs. In modulated stimuli, components "traced out" the spectral envelope as they changed in frequency.

5. Listeners

Three well-practised listeners were tested. They had audiometrically normal hearing in both ears. Stimuli were presented monaurally to their left ears through one ear-piece of a Sennheiser HD414 head-set. The average peak level of maskers was 60 dB(A). Each listener provided two thresholds in each condition.

6. Results and Discussion

Fig. 5 shows thresholds averaged over the three listeners for each of conditions (1) to (7). Thresholds measured in the absence of the masker (condition 8) were 15-20 dB below the lowest masked threshold. Thus absolute sensitivity did not constrain masked thresholds. The variability of repeated thresholds was similar for the three listeners and was such that differences greater than 3.2 dB between thresholds in any pair of conditions are significant ($p<0.01$).

Interpretation of Fig. 5 is helped by considering the following arguments. To identify a target, a listener must locate the frequencies of its formants despite the presence of an unpredictable pattern of formants contributed by the masker. When there are no cues to distinguish the components of the target from those of the masker, the formants of the target must be sufficiently intense to create identifiable *peaks* in the envelope of the combined spectrum. The complete set of peaks, from maskers and targets, can then be examined to establish the best match to stored templates representing the five targets (Assmann and Summerfield, 1989). Thresholds are lower when there are cues that listeners can use to distinguish the two sets of components. To be located, the formants of the targets need only

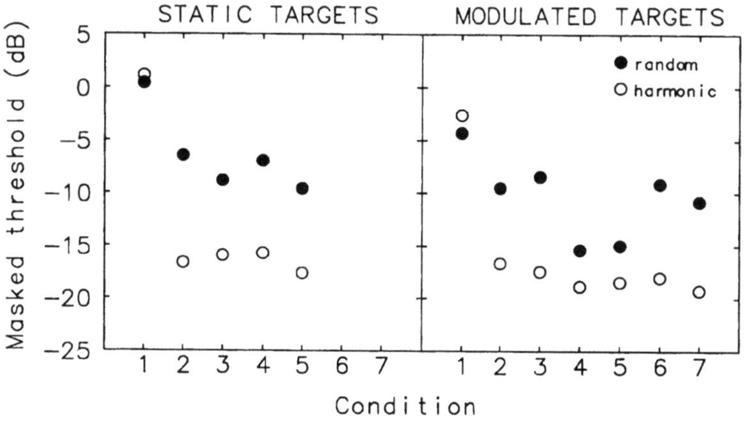

Fig. 5 Mean thresholds for random stimuli (filled circles) and harmonic stimuli (open circles), averaged over the three listeners. See Figure 4 for descriptions of the seven conditions.

to be locally more intense than the components of the maskers. They need not form peaks as such. Fig. 6 illustrates this distinction. It shows excitation patterns (Moore and Glasberg, 1987) of a masker (thin lines) and the combination of that masker with the vowel /a/ at threshold (thick lines) in two conditions. In (A), both masker and /a/ have F_0s of 100 Hz. At threshold (0 dB), the first two formants of /a/ create peaks in the excitation pattern of the combined stimulus. In (b), the F_0 of /a/ is 112 Hz. At threshold (-17 dB), the first two formants of the /a/ are merely the locally most intense features in the combined stimulus.

The major results, and their possible interpretations, are these:

(a) *A difference in F_0 lowers thresholds for harmonic stimuli by up to 17 dB.* [Compare condition (1) in Fig. 5 with all other conditions involving harmonic stimuli.]

(b) *A difference in "F_0" lowers thresholds for random stimuli by up to 8 dB.* [Compare condition (1), where corresponding components in random maskers and targets had the same frequencies, with (2) and (3) where they differed by 2 or 4 STs.] In (1), the same number of components was presented in both observation intervals, making it difficult to locate the interval containing the target. Moreover, the components of targets and maskers had different amplitudes and phases. Therefore, summation distorted the evidence of the formants of the targets, unless targets were relatively intense compared to maskers. Hence thresholds were high. In (2) and (3), different numbers of components were presented in the two intervals, making it easier to locate the interval containing the target. In addition, the difference of 2 or 4 STs between corresponding components in maskers and targets reduced distorting interactions (c.f. Culling, 1990). Thus, thresholds were lower. These factors are likely to have been beneficial with harmonic stimuli, too. If so, harmonicity would have contributed only 9 dB of the total fall in thresholds produced by introducing a difference in F_0 between harmonic maskers and targets. [Compare random and harmonic thresholds in conditions (2) and (3).]

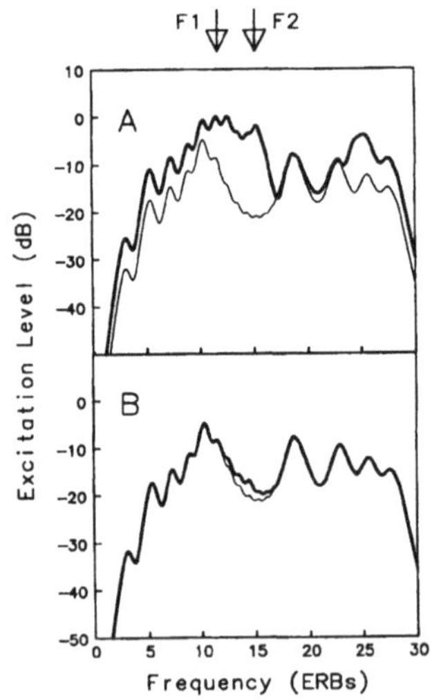

Fig. 6 Excitation patterns of a masker (F_0=100 Hz) (thin lines), and the combination of that masker with two versions of /a/ at threshold (thick lines). Panel (A): F_0 of /a/ = 100 Hz, relative level = 0dB. Panel (B): F_0 of /a/ = 112 Hz, relative level = -17 dB.

(c) *Listeners cannot use incoherent modulation between maskers and targets to hear out targets.* [Compare conditions (6) and (7) with (2) and (3) for random modulated targets.] This is the major issue which the experiments sought to address. The heights of the bars in Fig. 7 show the size of the effect of CFM with random stimuli (filled bars) and harmonic stimuli (open bars) for individual subjects and the mean. Although all effects are positive, none is significant.

(d) *With random modulated targets, segregation is easier against a static masker giving a maximum difference of N STs than against a modulated masker giving a constant difference of N STs.* [Compare conditions (2) and (3) with (4) and (5) for random modulated targets.] At threshold, the static masker dominates the combined spectrum. It is easy to estimate the formant frequencies of the targets because they generate local regions of the spectrum where frequencies and amplitudes are changing.

(e) *With random static targets, segregation is no easier against a modulated masker giving a maximum difference of N STs than against a static masker giving a constant difference of N STs.* [Compare conditions (2) and (3) with (4) and (5) for random static targets.] At threshold, the modulated masker dominates the combined spectrum. To be detectable, the formants of the target must be sufficiently intense either to generate locally static regions of the spectrum, or to generate spectral peaks. Hence, thresholds are high.

7. General Discussion

From previous results, it was possible that listeners *could* use CFM, but appeared not to when tested with harmonic stimuli because harmonicity allows all the segregation that can be achieved. The results obtained here with random stimuli rule out that possibility. Thresholds were moderately high when random stimuli were modulated coherently. Thus, there was room for thresholds to fall when they were modulated incoherently. However, thresholds did not fall, confirming Carlyon's (1991) demonstration (Fig. 1) that listeners cannot use CFM for grouping. Why not? One possibility was offered by Gardner et al. (1989). They speculated that the ear and brain have omitted CFM from their repertoire of grouping principles because reverberation degrades evidence of FM, making it an unreliable cue.

This idea provides the basis for a further explanation. There is logical and empirical evidence that the auditory system cannot detect FM as such, but can only infer its presence from the patterns of AM that it generates (Moore et al., 1991). Fig. 8 illustrates the type of evidence available. It shows the waveforms emerging from three simulated auditory filters (Assmann and Summerfield, 1991) when the F_0 of the /3/ vowel in the present stimulus set was modulated around a mean F_0 of 112 Hz. The F1 of the /3/ is at 506 Hz. Thus, the AM in the 450-Hz channel is created as the 4th harmonic (448 Hz) sweeps *up* and

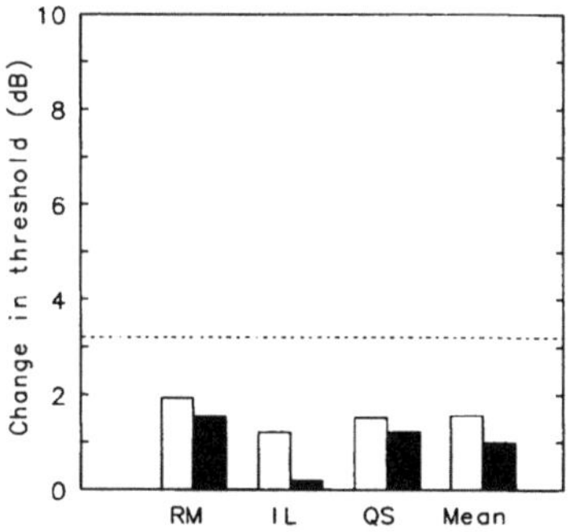

Fig. 7 Absence of effects of CFM. Changes in threshold for individual subjects (initials) and the mean, obtained with harmonic stimuli (open bars) and random stimuli (filled bars) comparing the average of conditions (6) and (7) with the average of conditions (2) and (3). The dotted line marks the criterial difference of 3.2 dB.

down the low-frequency skirt of the formant. The AM in the 550-Hz channel is created as the 5th harmonic (560 Hz) sweeps *down* and up the high-frequency skirt of the formant. Hence, the AM in these two channels is 180° out of phase. The AM in the 500-Hz channel is generated as the 4th and 5th harmonics alternately sweep into its filter. Thus, the three channels display different patterns of AM with different phases. Nonetheless, they must be interpreted together, because they convey evidence of the same source. One implication, therefore, is that the auditory system should not *segregate* channels on the basis of differences in AM phase. Carlyon's (1991) demonstration (Fig. 1) illustrates one instance in which the auditory system clearly does not segregate channels on the basis of differences in AM phase. Brian Moore's key paper provides further examples.

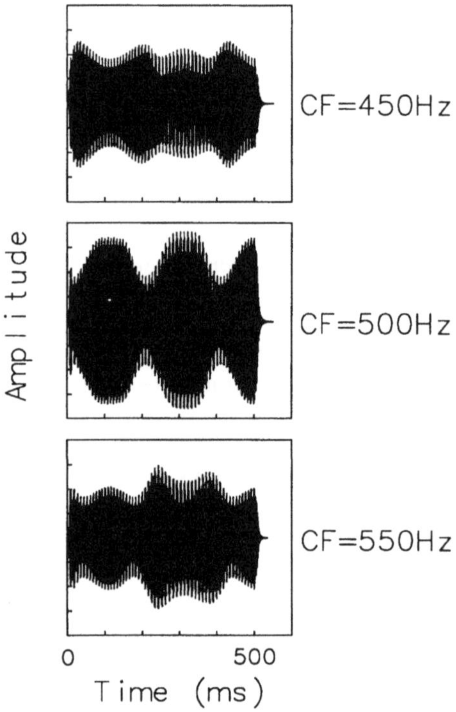

Fig. 8 Outputs of three simulated auditory filters excited by /3/ (F1 = 506 Hz; F_0 = 112 Hz, modulation rate = 2.5Hz, modulation amplitude = 2 STs).

Finally, consider the problem of inferring the pattern of CFM that gave rise to the three patterns of AM shown in Figure 8. The problem may be tractable in the example shown here where one source was present with static resonances, in a quiet communication channel, with a flat frequency response. The problem would certainly be more complex, and might be intractable, when reverberation makes the frequency response uneven, when resonances are changing in frequency, and when a second harmonic source is present. Possibly, the computational cost of deducing the pattern of CFM outweighs the benefits. Accordingly, as the present experiments have shown, auditory analysis relies on harmonicity for segregating competing harmonic sources, and ignores CFM.

Acknowledgments

I thank Alan Palmer for constructive comments on a draft of this paper.

References

Assmann, P.F. and Summerfield, Q. (1989). Modeling the perception of concurrent vowels: Vowels with the same fundamental frequency, *J. Acoust. Soc. Am.*, 85, 327-338.

Assmann, P.F. and Summerfield, Q. (1990). Modeling the perception of concurrent vowels: Vowels with different fundamental frequencies, *J. Acoust. Soc. Am.*, 88, 680-697.

Bregman (1990). *Auditory Scene Analysis*, MIT Press, Cambridge, Mass.

Broadbent, D.E. and Ladefoged, P. (1957). On the fusion of sounds reaching different sense organs, *J. Acoust. Soc. Am.*, 29, 708-710.

Carlyon, R.P. (1991). Discriminating between coherent and incoherent frequency modulation of complex tones, *J. Acoust. Soc. Am.*, 89, 329-340.

Chalikia, M.H. and Bregman, A.S. (1985). The perceptual segregation of simultaneous auditory signals: pulse train segregation and vowel segregation, *Percept. Psychophys.*, 46, 487-496.

Culling, J.F. (1990). Exploring the conditions for the perceptual separation of concurrent voices using F_0 differences, *Proceedings of the Institute of Acoustics*, 12, 559-566.

Darwin, C.J. (1990). Environmental influences on speech perception, *Advances in Speech, Hearing, and Language Processing, Volume 1*, JAI Press, 219-241.

Demany, L. and Semal, C. (1990). The effect of vibrato on the recognition of masked vowels, *Percept. Psychophys.*, 48, 436-444.

Gardner, R.G. and Darwin, C.J. (1986). Grouping of vowel harmonics by frequency modulation: Absence of effects on phonemic categorization, *Percept. Psychophys.*, 40, 183-187.

Gardner, R.G, Gaskill, S., and Darwin, C.J. (1989). Perceptual grouping of formants with static and dynamic differences in fundamental frequency, *J. Acoust. Soc. Am.*, 85, 1329-1337.

Marin, C.M.H. and McAdams, S. (1991). Segregation of concurrent sounds. II: Effects of spectral-envelope tracing, frequency modulation coherence, and frequency modulation width, *J. Acoust. Soc. Am.*, 89, 341-351.

McAdams, S. (1989). Concurrent sound segregation. I: Effects of frequency modulation coherence, *J. Acoust. Soc. Am.*, 86, 2148-2159.

Moore, B.C.J. and Glasberg, B.R. (1987). Formulae describing frequency selectivity as a function of frequency and level, and their use in calculating excitation patterns, *Hear. Res.*, 28, 209-225.

Moore, B.C.J., Glasberg, B.R., Gaunt, T., and Child, T. (1991). Across-channel masking of changes in modulation depth for amplitude- and frequency-modulated signals. *Quart. J, Exp. Psychol.* (in press).

Scheffers, M.T.M. (1983), *Sifting Vowels: Auditory Pitch Analysis and Sound Segregation*, Ph.D. Thesis, Rijkuniversiteit Groningen, The Netherlands.

Summerfield, Q. and Assmann, P.F. (1991). Perception of concurrent vowels: Effects of harmonic misalignment and pitch-period asynchrony, *J. Acoust. Soc. Am.*, 89, 1364-1377.

Terhardt, E. (1987). Psychophysics of audio signal processing and the role of pitch in speech, In M.E.H. Schouten (Ed.), *The Psychophysics of Speech Perception*, Martinus Nijhoff, Dordrecht, 271-283.

Comodulation Masking Release and Modulation Discrimination Interference

Brian C.J. Moore
Department of Experimental Psychology
University of Cambridge
Downing Street
Cambridge CB2 3EB
U.K.

1. INTRODUCTION

It is widely assumed that the peripheral auditory system contains a bank of overlapping bandpass filters (the auditory filters) which are approximately linear (Fletcher, 1940). The shape of the auditory filter at a given centre frequency can be thought of as a weighting function which is applied to the power spectrum of a sound to determine the effective magnitude of the output of the filter. The auditory filters seem to play an important role in many aspects of auditory perception and discrimination, including masking, loudness perception, timbre perception and pitch perception (for reviews, see Plomp, 1976, and Moore, 1989).

To those who work on speech perception, it may seem obvious that we are able to compare the outputs of different auditory filters. Speech perception depends at least partly on the recognition of spectral shapes, and changes in those shapes over time, and this requires the comparison of filter outputs. However, the masking of one sound by another has traditionally been explained by considering just one filter at a time. For example, when an observer is trying to detect a sinusoidal signal of a given frequency in the presence of a masking sound, it is usually assumed that performance is based on the output of the single auditory filter which gives the highest signal-to-masker ratio, and threshold is assumed to correspond to a constant signal-to-masker ratio.

Although this model works well in many situations (Patterson and Moore, 1986) it clearly fails in others. In some cases, the outputs of auditory filters tuned away from the signal frequency can be used to *enhance* signal detection, as in profile analysis (for a review see Green, 1988) or comodulation masking release (CMR) (Hall et al., 1984a; see below for details). In other cases, the outputs of auditory filters tuned away from the signal frequency *degrade* signal detection. This degradation seems to happen mainly when the masker and signal are modulated in some way and the task of the subject is to detect a change in the modulation of the signal (Yost and Sheft, 1989; Moore, Glasberg and Schooneveldt, 1990a). Hence, this phenomenon has been called modulation detection interference (Yost and Sheft, 1989) or modulation discrimination interference (Moore and Jorasz, 1992). Fortunately, the same acronym (MDI) can be used for both.

In this paper, each of these situations is reviewed in turn. The implications of the phenomena for mechanisms of perceptual grouping are then discussed. Finally, the relevance of the phenomena to speech perception is considered.

2. COMODULATION MASKING RELEASE

2.1 Initial demonstrations of comodulation masking release

Hall et al. (1984a) provided one of the first demonstrations that across-filter comparisons could enhance the detection of a sinusoidal signal in a fluctuating noise masker. The crucial feature for achieving this enhancement was that the fluctuations should be correlated across different frequency bands. In one of their experiments, the threshold for a 1-kHz 400-ms signal was measured as a function of the bandwidth of a continuous noise masker, keeping the spectrum level constant. The masker was centred at 1 kHz. They used two types of masker. One was a random (Gaussian) noise; this has irregular fluctuations in amplitude, and the fluctuations are independent in different frequency regions. The other was a random noise which was modulated in amplitude at an irregular, low rate. The modulation resulted in fluctuations in the amplitude of the noise which were the same in different spectral regions. This across-frequency correlation was called 'comodulation' by Hall et al. (1984a). Fig. 1 shows the results of this experiment.

For the random noise (denoted by R), the signal threshold increased as the masker bandwidth increased up to about 100 - 200 Hz, and then remained constant. This is exactly as expected from the traditional model of masking (Fletcher, 1940; Patterson and Moore, 1986). The auditory filter at this centre frequency has a bandwidth of about 130 Hz (Moore and Glasberg, 1983). Hence, for noise bandwidths up to about 130 Hz, increasing the bandwidth results in more noise passing through the filter. However, increasing the bandwidth beyond 130 Hz does not increase the amount of noise passing through the filter, so threshold does not increase. The pattern for the modulated noise (denoted by M) is quite different. For noise bandwidths greater than 100 Hz, the signal threshold decreases as the bandwidth increases. This indicates that subjects can compare the outputs of different auditory filters to enhance signal detection. The fact that the decrease in threshold with increasing bandwidth only occurs with the modulated noise indicates that fluctuations in the masker are critical and that the fluctuations need to be correlated across frequency bands. Hence, this phenomenon has been called 'comodulation masking

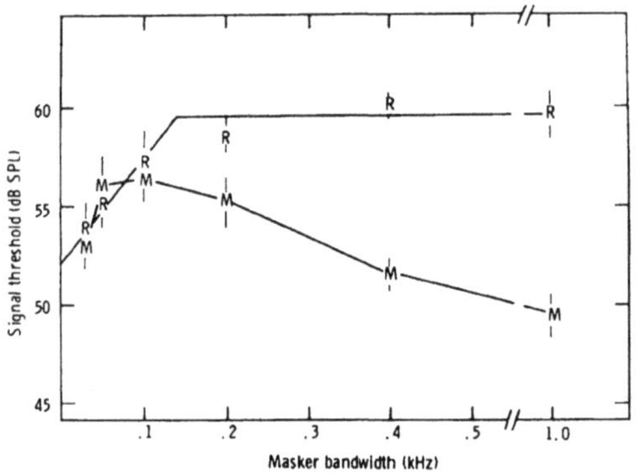

Fig. 1 Thresholds for a sinusoidal signal plotted as a function of the bandwidth of a noise masker centred at the signal frequency. The noise was either random (R) or modulated (M). From Hall et al. (1984a) by permission of the authors and publisher.

release' (CMR). The amount of CMR in this experiment, defined as the difference in thresholds for random noise and modulated noise, was maximally about 10 dB.

A second way in which CMR can be demonstrated is by using narrow bands of noise, which have inherent relatively slow amplitude fluctuations. One band, the on-frequency band, is centred at the signal frequency. One or more other bands, the flanking bands, are centred away from the signal frequency. If the flanking bands are uncorrelated with the on-frequency band, then when they are added to the on-frequency band they either have no effect on signal threshold, or they increase the signal threshold slightly. However, when the envelopes of the flanking bands are correlated with that of the on-frequency band (i.e. they have the same pattern of fluctuation over time), the flanking bands can produce a release from masking, a CMR (Hall et al., 1984a; McFadden, 1986; Cohen and Schubert, 1987; Schooneveldt and Moore, 1987). The release from masking can occur even if the signal and on-frequency band are presented to one ear and the flanking bands are presented to the other ear, although in this case the magnitude of the release is usually a little smaller (Hall et al., 1984b; Cohen and Schubert, 1987, Schooneveldt and Moore, 1987). The magnitude of the CMR is usually defined as the difference in signal threshold for the condition with the uncorrelated flanking bands and the condition with the correlated flanking bands. Sometimes it is defined as the difference in thresholds for the condition with the on-frequency band alone and the condition with the correlated flanking bands.

2.2 The role of within-channel cues

Schooneveldt and Moore (1987, 1989a) have shown that modulation of a masker can produce a release from masking even when the masker's bandwidth is less than the auditory-filter bandwidth (for example, when both on-frequency and flanking bands fall within the bandwidth of a single auditory filter). This release from masking cannot arise from comparisons of the outputs of different auditory filters, and hence it does not represent a CMR. Rather it results from a cue or cues available in the output of a single auditory filter. Schooneveldt and Moore called such cues 'within-channel cues.' One example of such a cue is a change in the pattern of envelope modulation which occurs when the signal is added to the masker; the envelope fluctuates less and the minima in the envelope tend to be less deep when the signal is present (Schooneveldt and Moore, 1989a). This cue appears to be used in band-widening experiments such as that illustrated in Fig. 1, but it can only be used when the signal duration is greater than about 100 ms (Schooneveldt and Moore, 1989a). Of course, this within-channel cue does not account for the decrease in thresholds with increasing bandwidth beyond 130 Hz. Its primary effect seems to be to reduce thresholds in modulated noise for all bandwidths.

A second possible within-channel cue is connected with the detailed temporal waveform at the output of auditory filters tuned close to the signal frequency. This waveform is reflected in the patterns of phase locking in neurones tuned to that frequency (Moore and Glasberg, 1987; Anderson, 1973); the nerve spikes tend to occur at a specific phase of the stimulating waveform. When the masker envelope is close to a maximum, the neurones are phase locked primarily to the masker. When the masker envelope is close to a minimum the neurones phase lock at least partly to the signal. This change in phase locking is a cue which may be used in experiments where an on-frequency band and a flanking band are used as maskers. When the two bands are close in frequency, they interact at the output of the auditory filter to give a waveform with regular envelope fluctuations, and with a centre frequency corresponding to the mean frequency of the two bands. Thus the pattern of phase locking fluctuates as the masker envelope fluctuates. Schooneveldt and Moore (1987) presented evidence that this cue was most effective for centre frequencies of 4000 Hz and below when the flanking band was close in frequency to the on-frequency band.

These within-channel cues make it easy to overestimate the magnitude of CMR. However, the cues do not appear to be important for brief signals in band-widening experiments, or when the on-frequency and flanking bands are widely separated in frequency. They also do not occur when the on-frequency and flanking bands are presented to opposite ears. Hence, results for these conditions can be used to estimate the magnitude of the 'true' CMR.

2.3 Factors influencing the magnitude of CMR

CMR measured in band-widening experiments (as in Fig. 1) occurs over a wide range of signal frequencies (500 to 4000 Hz), and does not vary greatly with signal frequency (Hall et al., 1984a; Haggard et al., 1990; Moore and Schooneveldt, 1989a). CMR is largest when the modulation of the masker is at a low rate, and when the masker covers a wide frequency range (Haggard et al., 1990; Schooneveldt and Moore, 1989a). For signal durations of 100 ms or less, for which within-channel cues probably have little effect, CMR can be as large as 11 dB (Schooneveldt and Moore, 1989a).

When CMR is measured using an on-frequency band and a flanking band, it generally falls in the range 1-6 dB when the flanking band is distant in frequency from the on-frequency band (Hall et al., 1984a; McFadden, 1986; Cohen and Schubert, 1987; Schooneveldt and Moore, 1987); this probably reflects a true CMR. The release from masking can be as large as 14 dB when the flanking band is close in frequency to the on-frequency band, but in this case within-channel cues probably influence the results (Schooneveldt and Moore, 1987). The 'true' CMR appears to vary little with centre frequency or with flanking-band frequency, although it may be somewhat greater for flanking band frequencies close to the signal frequency (Hall et al., 1990). CMR measured with a flanking band presented in the opposite ear to the signal-plus-masker also varies little with centre frequency or flanking-band frequency, and is typically 2-6 dB (Schooneveldt and Moore, 1987). Again, however, there is a trend for CMRs to be larger when the flanking bands are centred close to the signal frequency (Hall et al., 1990). Thus, across-filter comparisons can be made over a wide frequency range, but they are made most effectively for filters that are reasonably closely spaced in centre frequency.

CMR measured with an on-frequency band and a flanking band tends to increase as the width of the bands of noise is decreased. This is probably a consequence of the fact that the rate of envelope fluctuations decreases as the bandwidth decreases; slow fluctuations lead to large CMRs (Hall, 1987; Schooneveldt and Moore, 1987; 1989a; Carlyon et al., 1989). CMR also increases if more than one flanking band is used. Indeed, if a large number of bands is used, the CMR can be as large as 15 dB (Hall, 1987; Hall et al., 1988; Schooneveldt and Moore, 1989b; Moore and Shailer, 1991).

3. Modulation Discrimination Interference

I turn now to situations where the detection or discrimination of a target signal is *impaired* by the presence of frequency components remote from the target frequency. Usually, this happens when the task is either to detect modulation of the target sound, or to detect a change in depth of modulation of the target sound. Yost and Sheft (1989) showed that the threshold for detecting sinusoidal amplitude modulation (AM) of a sinusoidal carrier was increased in the presence of another carrier, amplitude modulated at the same rate, even when the second carrier was remote in frequency from the first. They called this modulation detection interference (MDI). They showed that MDI did not occur if the second carrier was unmodulated. Wilson, Hall and Grose (1990) have demonstrated a similar phenomenon for the detection of frequency modulation (FM). They showed that the threshold for detecting sinusoidal FM of a given carrier frequency could be elevated in the presence of a second carrier which was also frequency modulated. The effect showed some tuning for carrier frequency, being greater when the carrier frequencies of the target and interfering sounds were close, but it persisted even when the carriers were widely separated in frequency (by more than one octave). The effect also showed tuning for modulation rate, being greatest when the modulation rates of the target and interfering sounds were close.

Moore et al. (1990a) carried out a series of experiments measuring the threshold of a brief 700-Hz signal as a function of its temporal position relative to the modulation cycle of a 700-Hz masker 100% amplitude modulated at a 10-Hz rate. When extra components, also 100% amplitude modulated at 10 Hz, were added to the masker, signal detection was often impaired, even when all of the added components were remote in frequency from 700 Hz. The effect was usually greater when the added components were modulated in phase with the 700-Hz component than when they were modulated with a different phase. Moore et al. called this effect across-channel masking (ACM), since it did not seem to be explicable in terms of the output of the single auditory filter centred at the signal frequency.

It seems likely that the across-channel masking found by Moore et al. (1990a) is related to the MDI described by Yost and Sheft (1989). For the signal and maskers used by Moore et al., the main cue for signal detection was probably the change in the pattern of envelope modulation produced by adding the signal to the masker. The flanking modulated components appear to interfere with the ability to detect the change in modulation pattern (an effect opposite to CMR).

Moore et al. (1991) determined how thresholds for detecting an increase in modulation depth (sinusoidal AM or FM) of a 1000-Hz carrier frequency (the target) were affected by modulation of carriers (interference) with frequencies of 230 Hz and 3300 Hz. The target sound was presented twice for a duration of 1000 ms, with 300-ms inter-stimulus interval, and the subject was required to indicate the interval in which the sound was more modulated. The interference was gated with the target sound. The target sound was always modulated at a 10-Hz rate; the modulation index of the standard sound was 0.25 for AM and 2 for FM. An example of their results is shown in Fig. 2. They found that modulation increment thresholds

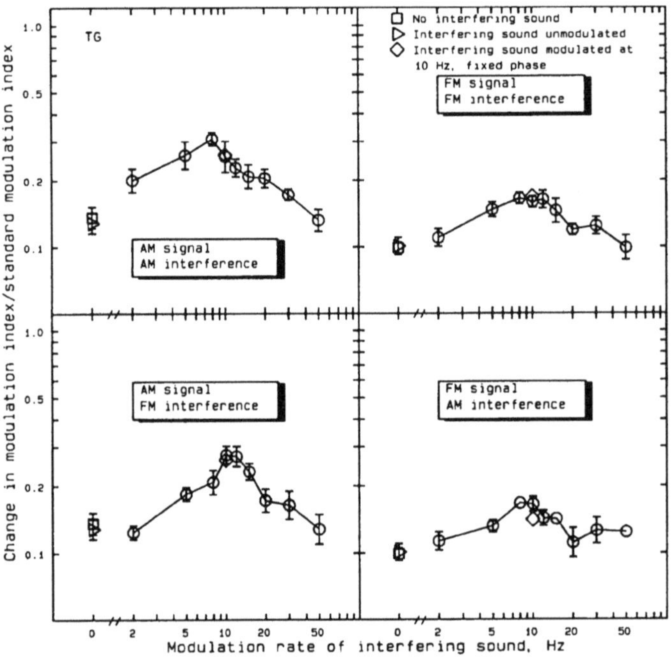

Fig. 2 Results for one subject from Moore et al. (1991). Thresholds for detecting a change in modulation depth are plotted as a function of the modulation rate of the interfering sound (log scale). The box in each panel indicates the signal type and interference type. Squares show thresholds in the absence of any interfering sound and triangles show thresholds with the interfering sound unmodulated. Diamonds show thresholds for interference modulated at a 10-Hz rate, the same as the target, averaged across the four values of modulator phase. Error bars show ± one standard error.

were increased (worsened) when the remote carriers were modulated. This MDI effect was greatest when the target and interference were modulated at similar rates, but the effect was broadly tuned for modulation rate. When the target and interfering sounds were both modulated at 10 Hz, there was no significant effect of the relative phase of modulation of the target and interfering sounds. Moore et al. also found cross-modal interference effects; the detection of an increment in AM depth was adversely affected by FM interference, and vice versa. Moore et al. suggested that this could be explained by the transformation of FM to AM in the peripheral auditory system.

In summary, the detection of modulation (either AM or FM) or the detection of changes in modulation depth in a target sound can be impaired by modulated sounds remote from the target frequency. The effects are greatest when the target and interference are modulated at the same rate, but they persist for quite large differences in modulation rate between the target and the interference.

4. The Role of Perceptual Grouping in CMR and MDI

In everyday life we often listen to several sound sources simultaneously. The auditory system is faced with the task of deciding which 'elements' of the complex mixture arise from one source, and which from another. The process of doing this is often described as 'perceptual grouping' or 'stream formation'; the elements of the sound are grouped across frequency and across time to form percepts of coherent streams each with its own loudness, pitch, timbre and location (Moore, 1989; Bregman, 1990). One principle that operates in perceptual grouping is 'common fate'; elements of a sound that change in the same way tend to be grouped and heard as a single stream. Two applications of this principle are relevant here: elements that start and stop together tend to be perceived as a single sound; and elements that are modulated in a similar way tend to be perceived as a single sound.

Consider first CMR. When the masker is a single narrow band of noise centred at the signal frequency, a sinusoidal signal added to the masker is not usually heard as a separate auditory 'object' or stream. Instead, the signal is detected as a slight change in loudness, or a subtle change in the pattern of fluctuation of the stimulus (Schooneveldt and Moore, 1989a; Moore et al., 1990b). However, when comodulated flanking bands are added to the masker, they tend to be grouped with the on-frequency band to form a coherent percept. When the signal is added it appears to 'pop out'; a pure tone is heard at the signal frequency. Moore and Shailer (1991) reported that this can even happen when the on-frequency band is presented to one ear, and multiple flanking bands are presented to the other. If the spectrum level of the flanking bands is close to or above that of the on-frequency band, then the entire masker may appear to come from the ear receiving the flanking bands. When a sinusoidal signal is added to the on-frequency band, it appears as a separate auditory event in the ear opposite to the ear receiving the flanking bands. In both these examples, the crucial feature seems to be that comodulation of the on-frequency band and flanking bands causes all bands to form a coherent perceptual stream. The signal causes a change in the modulation pattern in a local frequency region (i.e. at the output of the auditory filter centred at the signal frequency), and this disruption of the across-frequency comodulation causes the signal to 'pop out'.

Perhaps the most direct evidence for a role of perceptual grouping processes in CMR comes from some experiments of Hall and Grose (1990). They measured CMR in conditions where some flanking bands were comodulated with the on-frequency band, but other bands (called 'deviant' bands) were not. These deviant bands tended to reduce the magnitude of CMR, especially when they were centred close to the on-frequency band. In one condition of their experiment, CMR was measured for a 1000-Hz signal and a masker composed of seven comodulated 20-Hz wide bands, spaced from 400 to 1600 Hz (with one at 1000 Hz). The CMR for this condition, relative to the threshold for the on-frequency band alone, was about 15 dB. In a second condition, two deviant bands were added at 900 and 1100 Hz. These bands reduced the CMR to only 3-4 dB. They then investigated the effect of adding more deviant bands, interleaved in frequency with the comodulated bands. When the deviant bands shared a common envelope (codeviant bands) the extra bands resulted in increased CMR; the codeviant bands distant from the signal frequency reduced the disruptive effect of the codeviant bands close to the signal frequency. However, when the extra deviant bands all had independent envelopes (multideviant bands), no such beneficial effect was observed. The benefit of adding extra codeviant bands was also found when they were added in the opposite ear to the remainder of the stimulus. These results suggest a strong role for perceptual grouping. The added codeviant bands presumably formed a perceptual group with the codeviant bands close to the signal frequency, making all of the codeviant bands sound like a single stream. This helped to reduce their effect in disrupting CMR.

I turn now to the possible role of perceptual grouping in MDI. Yost and Sheft (1989) suggested that the MDI found by them might be a consequence of perceptual grouping; the common AM of the target and interfering sounds might make them fuse perceptually (McAdams, 1984; Bregman, Levitan and Liao, 1990), making it difficult to 'hear out' the modulation of the target sound. A similar explanation might apply to the other experiments demonstrating MDI, as described earlier. Certainly, the impression of subjects in these experiments is that the target sound is difficult to 'hear out' in the presence of the modulated interfering sounds. However, certain aspects of the results on MDI are difficult to reconcile with an explanation in terms of perceptual grouping. One would expect that widely spaced frequency components would only be grouped perceptually if their modulation pattern was very similar. Grouping would not be expected, for example, if the components were modulated out of phase or at different rates. While some experiments on MDI have found effects of modulator phase (Moore et al., 1990a; Wilson et al., 1990), others have not (Yost and Sheft, 1989; Yost et al., 1989; Moore et al., 1991). Thus, it is possible to obtain large amounts of MDI under conditions where the target and the interference are modulated out of phase.

Although these results do not appear to support an explanation of MDI in terms of perceptual grouping, it may be premature to reject such an explanation at this stage. The evidence that the phase of the modulators plays a critical role in perceptual grouping is not very strong, particularly in the case of frequency-modulated sounds (McAdams, 1989; Carlyon, 1991). Bregman et al. (1985) have presented evidence that modulator phase can be important for the perceptual grouping of amplitude-modulated signals. However, they used modulation rates much higher than those used in typical MDI experiments. Thus, it remains unclear whether perceptual grouping depends on modulator phase at low modulation rates. Until this is known, it is difficult to evaluate the significance of the finding that MDI can occur when the target and interfering sounds are modulated out of phase.

The broad tuning of MDI in the modulation domain does create clear difficulties for an explanation based on perceptual grouping. Bregman et al. (1990) have studied the effects of differences in AM rate on the perceptual fusion of two sinusoidal carriers. They found that fusion was strongest when the carriers were amplitude modulated at the same rate (114 Hz or 125 Hz), and fell off sharply when the carriers were modulated at rates differing by 7% (smaller differences were not tested). The tuning in the modulation domain found by them appears to be much sharper than that found by Moore et al. (1991). Of course, the overall difference in modulation rate makes the two sets of results difficult to compare. Nevertheless, their results lend support to the argument that the MDI found by Moore et al. was too broadly tuned in the modulation domain to be explained entirely in terms of perceptual grouping mechanisms.

Recently, we have been investigating the effects on MDI of gating the target sound on after the interfering sounds (Moore and Shailer, 1992). Onset asynchrony is known to be a powerful factor in perceptual grouping; when a new sound is introduced after another sound has been on for some time, the new sound seems to 'pop out' and to be perceived as a separate sound (for reviews, see Moore, 1989 and Bregman, 1990). Thus, if MDI depends on perceptual grouping of the target and interference, delaying the target sound relative to the interfering sounds should result in a marked decrease in MDI. The task of the subjects was to detect an increase in depth of 10-Hz AM of a 1000-Hz carrier, relative to a baseline modulation index of 0.25. The target sound was presented twice for a duration of 400 ms, with 300-ms inter-stimulus interval, and the subject was required to indicate the interval in which the sound was more modulated. An example of the results for one subject is shown in Fig. 3.

There were four conditions. In one, the target sound was presented alone. The modulation increment threshold in this case is indicated by the dashed line in Fig. 3. In the other conditions, interfering sounds were added at centre frequencies of 230 Hz and 3300 Hz. The interfering sounds were either gated synchronously with the target (0-ms asynchrony), or were gated on 25, 50 or 100 ms before the target. In one of these condition (circles), the interfering sounds were unmodulated. In another (up-pointing triangles) they were modulated in phase with the target with modulation index 0.5. In the last condition (down-pointing triangles), they were modulated in antiphase with the target.

Even when the interference was unmodulated, it produced some MDI; the amount of MDI declined as the onset asynchrony increased. The MDI in this case presumably occurred because gating the target and interference together tended to promote their perceptual fusion. MDI was markedly greater when the interference was modulated. Again, the MDI declined with increasing onset asynchrony, but, even at the largest asynchrony (100 ms) a substantial amount of MDI remained. It is noteworthy that there is some evidence for an effect of modulator phase at the largest onset asynchrony. In other experiments we have also sometimes found effects of modulator phase, but the effects are not usually large, and they vary across subjects.

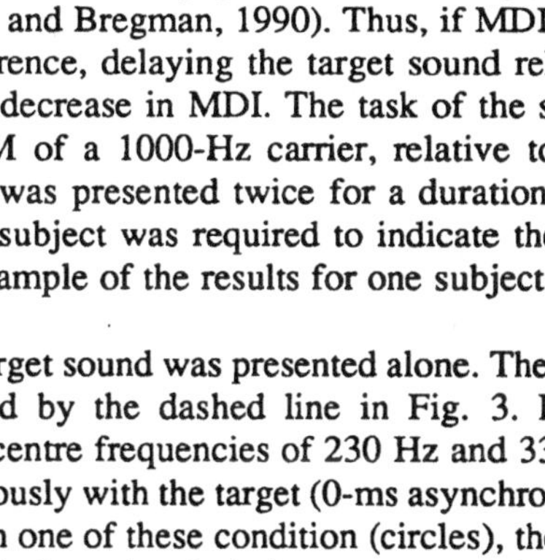

Fig. 3 Thresholds for detecting an increase in modulation index from a standard value of 0.25 for a 1000-Hz carrier modulated at a 10-Hz rate. The threshold without any interfering sound is indicated by the dashed horizontal line. The interfering sounds were centred at 230 and 3300 Hz. Symbols show thresholds plotted as a function of the onset asynchrony between the interference and the target sound.

Overall, these results suggest that perceptual grouping does play a role in MDI. The MDI for both modulated and unmodulated interference declined with increasing onset asynchrony. Similar results have been reported by Moore and Jorasz (1992) for AM modulation depth discrimination and by Hall and Grose (1991b) for the detection of AM and FM. Hall and Grose also found that they could reduce or even abolish MDI by presenting the interference continuously, rather than gated with the target. However, in our experiments, significant MDI remained even at large onset asynchronies, suggesting that some factor other than perceptual grouping plays a role.

Finally, it is worth noting that, if we were to intrepret both CMR and MDI as arising from perceptual grouping processes, we would come to quite different conclusions about the precision with which grouping mechanisms operate. Results from CMR experiments suggest that the auditory system is very sensitive to disparities in modulation pattern across bands; even a small disparity appears sufficient to cause the signal to 'pop out' and to enhance signal detection. In contrast, to explain MDI in terms of grouping, we would have to say that sounds with quite different modulation patterns tend to be fused and heard as a single sound.

5. Similarities and Differences between CMR and MDI

In many ways, the situations where CMR occurs and where MDI occurs are very similar. Both CMR and MDI involve modulated stimuli. In the case of CMR, the signal is added to a modulated sound (the on-frequency band), and results in a change in the modulation pattern of that sound. The flanking bands make it easier to detect the change in modulation pattern. In the case of MDI, the signal is also a change in modulation of a target sound. However, the flanking (remote) components make it harder rather than easier to detect the change. What then, determines whether CMR occurs or MDI occurs?

One difference between CMR and MDI concerns the relative modulation depths of the on-frequency and flanking bands. In the great majority of experiments demonstrating CMR, the flanking bands have been modulated in the same way, and with the same modulation depth, as the on-frequency band. Thus, the addition of the signal to the masker has resulted in a *disparity* in modulation depth across bands, providing a potential detection cue. In contrast, in experiments demonstrating MDI, the flanking bands have usually had a greater modulation depth than the on-frequency band. Thus, even in the non-signal interval there was a disparity in modulation depth across bands. However, this difference between CMR and MDI does not appear to be critical. Grose and Hall (1989) showed that when the on-frequency band was a sinusoid modulated with a modulation index of 0.63, substantial CMRs could be obtained when the flanking bands were modulated with a modulation index of 1.0. Thus, CMR *can* be obtained when the flanking bands are modulated more than the on-frequency band. Also, Moore and Jorasz (1992) have shown that MDI for AM increment detection can occur when the on-frequency band and the flanking bands are modulated at the same depth. Thus, the relative modulation depths of the on-frequency band and flanking bands do not seem to be critical in determining whether CMR or MDI will occur.

A second difference between CMR and MDI is related to the difficulty of signal detection in the condition with the on-frequency band alone (the reference condition). Usually, large CMRs occur when there is a high degree of stimulus uncertainty in the reference condition, or when thresholds are high for some other reason. For example, when the masker is a Gaussian noise with a very narrow bandwidth, the main cue for signal detection appears to be the change in level produced by adding the signal to the masker (Schooneveldt and Moore, 1989a; Moore et al., 1990b). However, this is a poor cue, because narrowband noise fluctuates markedly in level from moment to moment. Under these conditions, the signal level required for threshold has to be roughly equal to the masker level; the change in overall level at threshold is then about 3 dB. Comodulated flanking bands provide an indication of the inherent fluctuations in the masker, thus reducing uncertainty, and giving lower thresholds. Hence, a large CMR occurs.

In contrast, in experiments demonstrating MDI, thresholds in the reference condition tend to be quite low. For example, in Fig. 3, a change in modulation index from 0.25 to 0.286 was detectable. This corresponds to a change in level in the 'valleys' of the target of only 0.42 dB and a change in peak-to-valley ratio from 4.44 dB to 5.51 dB. In general then, one might argue that when performance in the reference condition is poor, possibly because of stimulus uncertainty, adding comodulated flanking bands tends to give a CMR. When performance in the reference condition is good, adding flanking bands either has no effect or produces MDI.

A third difference between CMR and MDI concerns the nature of the signal to be detected. In experiments demonstrating CMR, the addition of the signal to the masker usually results in an effective decrease in the modulation depth of the on-frequency band. If the signal is a relatively long duration sinusoid then it partially 'fills in' the valleys in a fluctuating noise masker (Schooneveldt and Moore, 1989a). Sometimes the signal consists of one or more brief tone pips presented in the valleys of an AM masker (Grose and Hall, 1989; Moore et al.,1990a). In either case, the result is that the level in the valleys increases. Several researchers have suggested that CMR may depend strongly on the detection of changes in the valleys ('dip listening'; see Buus, 1985; Grose and Hall, 1989; Moore et al., 1990a; Hall and Grose, 1991a). In contrast, experiments demonstrating MDI have usually required subjects to detect an *increase* in modulation depth, resulting in a decrease in level in the valleys. Moore et al. (1990a) showed that stimuli that were otherwise very similar could give CMR when the task was to detect an increase in level in the valleys, and MDI when the task was to detect a decrease. Moore and Jorasz (1992) studied the ability to detect changes in modulation depth of a target sound in the presence of added sounds modulated at the same rate. They found that MDI could occur when the task of the subject was either to detect an increase in modulation depth or a decrease in modulation depth. However, they were only able to demonstrate CMR when the task was to detect a decrease in modulation depth.

Finally, it may be the case that CMR depends on there being a difference in modulation *pattern* across bands, rather than simply a difference in modulation depth (Moore et al., 1990a). In experiments where large CMRs are observed, the addition of the signal usually changes the modulation pattern of the on-frequency band, for example transforming a local minimum to a local maximum or plateau. Most experiments on MDI have involved only a change in modulation depth, not a change in modulation pattern. Moore and Jorasz (1992) showed that it was possible to obtain CMR when the only cue was an across-band disparity in modulation depth, but the effect was small, and it only occurred for large modulation depths of the target sound.

In summary, large CMRs tend to occur when the signal threshold is high in the reference condition (on-frequency band alone), when the signal produces an increase in level in the valleys of the on-frequency band, and when the addition of the signal to the on-frequency band results in a change in modulation *pattern*. When all these conditions are satisfied, the addition of comodulated flanking bands to the on-frequency band results in a large masking release. When only one of these conditions is satisfied, a small CMR may occur. When none of these conditions is satisfied, the addition of flanking bands either produces no effect or produces MDI.

6. Implications of CMR and MDI for the Perception of Speech

It seems likely that across-filter comparisons of temporal envelopes are a general feature of auditory pattern analysis, which may play an important role in extracting signals from noisy backgrounds, or separating competing sources of sound. As pointed out by Hall et al. (1984a): "Many real-life auditory stimuli have intensity peaks and valleys as a function of time in which intensity trajectories are highly correlated across frequency. This is true of speech, of interfering noise such as 'cafeteria' noise, and of many other kinds of environmental stimuli". This suggests that the phenomena of CMR and MDI may have some relevance to the understanding of speech, particularly in situations where there are competing sounds.

6.1 CMR and speech perception

It is difficult to assess the role of CMR in speech perception since there are several major differences between speech and the types of stimuli typically studied in experiments on CMR. One difference is that the signal in CMR experiments has typically been either a single sinusoid or a narrow band of noise, while speech is a wideband signal whose spectral pattern is of major importance. A second difference is that speech itself is comodulated, whereas in most CMR experiments only the background noise was comodulated. There have been only a few CMR experiments using multi-component signals. Hall et al. (1988) measured CMR for signals consisting of either one, two or three sinusoidal components. In the three-component case, the sinusoids had frequencies of 400, 500 and 600 Hz, and they were presented in three narrowbands of noise centred at the same three frequencies. Thresholds for the complex signal were about 6 dB lower when the three masker bands were comodulated than when they were uncorrelated. Grose and Hall (1992) have extended this experiment and shown that masking release for a three-tone complex signal is greater in a 15-band background noise than in a three-band background noise. Thus CMR can be obtained for complex multi-component signals as well as for narrowband signals. However, the signals in this experiment still differed from speech in several important ways: they covered a relatively small frequency range compared to speech; all components were of equal amplitude; and the components were static rather than dynamically varying.

Grose and Hall (1992) have tried to examine more directly whether CMR plays a role in the identification of speech in noise. They filtered speech into a number of very narrow bands (typically 40 Hz wide). They then measured the threshold for identifying the speech in comodulated bands of noise centred on the passbands of the speech (reference condition). Finally, they measured the threshold for identifying the speech when additional comodulated noise bands were added to the masker at centre frequencies between the passbands of the speech. They argued that a CMR would be revealed as a reduction in threshold in this last condition in comparison to the reference condition. In one experiment, where the task was to identify which of six filtered vowels was present, a CMR was observed. However, in another experiment, where the task was a forced-choice rhyming test, no CMR was found. In a third experiment, using a somewhat modified procedure but with sentence materials, again no CMR was found.

Overall, these results do not support the idea that a CMR-like process can enhance the identification of speech in noise. However, caution is needed in reaching this conclusion. As Grose and Hall pointed out, the filtered speech stimuli used by them were highly degraded and unnatural. Thus, the results may not reflect normal speech perception mechanisms. One consequence of filtering speech into narrow bands is to introduce 'spurious' amplitude fluctuations; this would occur, for example, as a harmonic with changing frequency swept through one of the passbands. Furthermore, these spurious amplitude fluctuations would be relatively independent in the different passbands. CMR-like mechanisms might help the auditory system to separate the fluctuations inherent in the speech from fluctuations due to the background noise, but this would not improve speech intelligibility if the fluctuations in the speech were 'spurious', and it would not help to tie the speech together as a coherent perceptual whole. It is possible that, with more natural stimuli, a CMR would be obtained.

6.2 MDI and speech perception

One explanation of MDI, not mentioned so far, is that it reflects the operation of 'channels' specialised for detecting and analysing modulation. There is both physiological evidence (Kay, 1982; Rees and Moller, 1983; Schreiner and Urbas, 1986) and psychophysical evidence (Kay and Mathews, 1972; Tansley and Suffield, 1983; see, however, Wakefield and Viemeister, 1984) for such channels. Yost et al. (1989) suggested that MDI might arise in the following way. The stimulus is first processed by an array of auditory filters. The envelope at the output of each filter is extracted. When modulation is present, channels are excited that are tuned for modulation rate. All filters responding with the same modulation rate excite the same channel, regardless of the filter centre frequency. Thus, modulation at one centre frequency can adversely affect the detection and discrimination of modulation at other centre frequencies.

Recently, Hall and Grose (1991b) have described some results consistent with the idea that modulation is detected in channels responsive to a range of centre frequencies. Subjects were presented with 1- and 2-kHz tones, gated synchronously. On each trial, one of the tones, selected at random, was amplitude modulated and the other was unmodulated. The task of the subjects was to identify which tone was modulated. Remarkably, most subjects performed rather poorly at this task. Even when the modulation was clearly audible, it was hard to say whether the higher or lower tone was modulated. A very different experiment, conducted by Moore and Shailer (1992), also suggests that subjects can have difficulty assigning modulation to particular components. Subjects were presented with a 1-kHz tone modulated at a 10-Hz rate, followed by that same tone together with some interfering sounds. They were asked to listen to the modulation of the 1-kHz tone alone, and to rate how clearly they could hear the modulation of that tone in the complex mixture. When the interfering sounds were modulated at a 10-Hz rate (a condition giving maximum MDI), clarity ratings were higher than when the interfering sounds were modulated at 4 Hz or 25 Hz (conditions giving less MDI). Thus there was a discrepancy between the MDI results and the clarity ratings. It appears that subjects could make an overall judgement of how clearly they could hear 10-Hz modulation, but it was hard to judge the modulation of the 1-kHz component alone.

The purpose of the hypothetical modulation channels remains unclear. Since the physiological evidence for such channels comes from studies of animals, we can assume that they did not evolve for the purpose of speech perception. Nevertheless, it is possible, even likely, that speech analysis makes use of the modulation channels.

There is considerable evidence that amplitude modulation patterns in speech are important for speech recognition (Steeneken and Houtgast, 1980). Thus, anything that adversely affects the detection and discrimination of the modulation patterns would be expected to impair intelligibility. One way of describing MDI is: modulation in one frequency region may make it more difficult to detect and discriminate modulation in another frequency region. Thus, it may be the case that MDI makes speech recognition more difficult in situations where there is a background sound that is modulated, such as another person talking. For normally hearing persons, speech reception thresholds in noise are lower (better) for a fluctuating background noise (a single competing talker) than for a continuous speech-shaped noise (Duquesnoy, 1983). This has been explained by assuming that people can listen in the 'dips' of a fluctuating noise (a CMR-like process?). However, the advantage to dip listening may be partly offset by MDI. In other words, the advantages of dip listening might be even larger if it were not for the effects of MDI.

All of this is highly speculative. Clearly, more data are needed to assess the possible role of MDI in affecting speech intelligibility in fluctuating background noise.

Acknowledgements

This work was supported by the Medical Research Council (U.K.). I thank Michael Stone and Joe Hall for helpful comments on an earlier version of this paper.

References

Anderson, D.J. (1973). Quantitative model for the effects of stimulus frequency upon synchronization of auditory discharges, *J. Acoust. Soc. Am.*, 54, 361-364.

Bregman, A.S. (1990). *Auditory Scene Analysis*, MIT Press, Cambridge, MA.

Bregman, A.S., Abramson, J., Doehring, P., and Darwin, C.J. (1985). Spectral integration based on common amplitude modulation, *Percept. Psychophys.*, 37, 483-493.

Bregman, A.S., Levitan, R., and Liao, C. (1990). Fusion of auditory components: Effects of the frequency of amplitude modulation, *Percept. Psychophys.*, 47, 68-73.

Buus, S. (1985). Release from masking caused by envelope fluctuations, *J. Acoust. Soc. Am.*, 78, 1958-1965.

Carlyon, R.P. (1991). Discriminating between coherent and incoherent frequency modulation of complex tones, *J. Acoust. Soc. Am.*, 89, 329-340.

Carlyon, R.P., Buus, S., and Florentine, M. (1989). Comodulation masking release for three types of modulator as a function of modulator rate, *Hearing Research*, 42, 37-46.

Cohen, M.F. and Schubert, E.D. (1987). Influence of place synchrony on detection of a sinusoid, *J. Acoust. Soc. Am.*, 81, 452-458.

Duquesnoy, A.J. (1983). Effect of a single interfering noise or speech source upon the binaural sentence intelligibility of aged persons, *J. Acoust. Soc. Am.*, 74, 739-743.

Fletcher, H. (1940). Auditory patterns, *Reviews of Modern Physics*, 12, 47-65.

Green, D.M. (1988). *Profile Analysis*. Oxford University Press, New York, 1-138.

Grose, J.H. and Hall, J.W. (1989). Comodulation masking release using SAM tonal complex maskers: Effects of modulation depth and signal position, *J. Acoust. Soc. Am.*, 85, 1276-1284.

Grose, J.H. and Hall, J.W. (1992). Comodulation masking release for speech stimuli. Submitted to *J. Acoust. Soc. Am.*

Haggard, M.P., Hall, J.W., and Grose, J.H. (1990). Comodulation masking release as a function of bandwidth and test frequency, *J. Acoust. Soc. Am.*, 88, 113-118.

Hall, J.W. (1987). Experiments on comodulation masking release, in: Yost, W.A. and Watson, C.S. (Eds.), *Auditory Processing of Complex Sounds*, Erlbaum, New Jersey, 57-66.

Hall, J.W. and Grose, J.H. (1988). Comodulation masking release: Evidence for multiple cues, *J. Acoust. Soc. Am.*, 84, 1669-1675.

Hall, J.W. and Grose, J.H. (1990). Comodulation masking release and auditory grouping, *J. Acoust. Soc. Am.*, 88, 119-125.

Hall, J.W. and Grose, J.H. (1991a). Relative contributions of envelope maxima and minima to comodulation masking release, *Quarterly Journal of Experimental Psychology*, 43a, 349-372.

Hall, J.W. and Grose, J.H. (1991b). Some effects of auditory grouping factors on modulation detection interference (MDI), *J. Acoust. Soc. Am.*, 90, 3028-3035.

Hall, J.W., Grose, J.H., and Haggard, M.P. (1988). Comodulation masking release for multi-component signals, *J. Acoust. Soc. Am.*, 83, 677-686.

Hall, J.W., Grose, J.H., and Haggard, M.P. (1990). Effects of flanking band proximity, number, and modulation pattern on comodulation masking release, *J. Acoust. Soc. Am.*, 87, 269-283.

Hall, J.W., Haggard, M.P., and Fernandes, M.A. (1984a). Detection in noise by spectro-temporal pattern analysis, *J. Acoust. Soc. Am.*, 76, 50-56.

Hall, J.W., Haggard, M.P., and Harvey, A.D.G. (1984b). Release from masking through ipsilateral and contralateral comodulation of a flanking band, *J. Acoust. Soc. Am.*, 76, Suppl. 1, S76.

Kay, R.H. (1982). Hearing of modulation in sounds, *Physiological Reviews*, 62, 894-975.

Kay, R.H. and Mathews, D.R. (1972). On the existence in human auditory pathways of channels selectively tuned to the modulation present in frequency modulated tones, *Journal of Physiology*, 225, 657-667.

McAdams, S. (1984), *Spectral fusion, spectral parsing, and the formation of auditory images.* Doctoral dissertation, Stanford University, Stanford, CA.

McAdams, S. (1989). Segregation of concurrent sounds. I. Effects of frequency modulation coherence, *J. Acoust. Soc. Am.*, 86, 2148-2159.

McFadden, D. (1986). Comodulation masking release: Effects of varying the level, duration and time delay of the cue band, *J. Acoust. Soc. Am.*, 80, 1658-1667.

Moore, B.C.J. (1989). *An Introduction to the Psychology of Hearing*, Third Edition, Academic Press, London.

Moore, B.C.J. and Glasberg, B.R. (1983). Suggested formulae for calculating auditory filter bandwidths and excitation patterns, *J. Acoust. Soc. Am.*, 74, 750-753.

Moore, B.C.J. and Glasberg, B.R. (1987). Factors affecting thresholds for sinusoidal signals in maskers with fluctuating envelopes, *J. Acoust. Soc. Am.*, 82, 69-79.

Moore, B.C.J. and Jorasz, U. (1992). Detection of changes in modulation depth of a target sound in the presence of other modulated sounds, *J. Acoust. Soc. Am.*, (in press).

Moore, B.C.J. and Shailer, M.J. (1991). Comodulation masking release as a function of level, *J. Acoust. Soc. Am.*, 90, 829-835.

Moore, B.C.J. and Shailer, M.J. (1992). Modulation discrimination interference and auditory grouping, *Philosophical Transactions of the Royal Society*, B (in press).

Moore, B.C.J., Glasberg, B.R., and Schooneveldt, G.P. (1990a). Across-channel masking and comodulation masking release, *J. Acoust. Soc. Am.*, 87, 1683-1694.

Moore, B.C.J., Glasberg, B.R., Gaunt, T., and Child, T. (1991). Across-channel masking of changes in modulation depth for amplitude- and frequency-modulated signals. Quarterly *Journal of Experimental Psychology*, 43a, 327-347.

Moore, B.C.J., Hall, J.W., Grose, J.H., and Schooneveldt, G.P. (1990b). Some factors affecting the magnitude of CMR, *J. Acoust. Soc. Am.*, 88, 1694-1702.

Patterson, R.D. and Moore, B.C.J. (1986). Auditory filters and excitation patterns as representations of frequency resolution, in: B.C.J. Moore (Ed.) *Frequency Selectivity in Hearing*, Academic Press, London, 123-177.

Plomp, R. (1976). *Aspects of Tone Sensation*, Academic Press, London.

Rees, A. and Moller, A.R. (1983). Responses of neurons in the inferior colliculus of the rat to AM and FM tones, *Hearing Research*, 10, 301-310.

Schooneveldt, G.P. and Moore, B.C.J. (1987). Comodulation masking release (CMR): Effects of signal frequency, flanking-band frequency, masker bandwidth, flanking-band level, and monotic versus dichotic presentation of the flanking band, *J. Acoust. Soc. Am.*, 82, 1944-1956.

Schooneveldt, G.P. and Moore, B.C.J. (1989a). Comodulation masking release as a function of masker bandwidth, modulator bandwidth and signal duration, *J. Acoust. Soc. Am.*, 85, 273-281.

Schooneveldt, G.P. and Moore, B.C.J. (1989b). Comodulation masking release for various monaural and binaural combinations of the signal, on-frequency and flanking bands, *J. Acoust. Soc. Am.*, 85, 262-272.

Schreiner, C.E. and Urbas, J.V. (1986). Representation of amplitude modulation in the auditory cortex of the cat. I. The anterior auditory field (AAF), *Hearing Research*, 21, 227-241.

Steeneken, H.J.M. and Houtgast, T. (1980). A physical method for measuring speech-transmission quality, *J. Acoust. Soc. Am.*, 67, 318-326.

Tansley, B.W. and Suffield, J.B. (1983). Time course of adaptation and recovery of channels selectively sensitive to frequency and amplitude modulation, *J. Acoust. Soc. Am.*, 74, 765-775.

Wakefield, G.H. and Viemeister, N.F. (1984). Selective adaptation to linear frequency-modulated sweeps: Evidence for direction-specific channels? *J. Acoust. Soc. Am.*, 75, 1588-1592.

Wilson, A.S., Hall, J.W., and Grose, J.H. (1990). Detection of frequency modulation (FM) in the presence of a second FM tone, *J. Acoust. Soc. Am.*, 88, 1333-1338.

Yost, W.A. and Sheft, S. (1989). Across-critical-band processing of amplitude-modulated tones, *J. Acoust. Soc. Am.*, 85, 848-857.

Yost, W.A., Sheft, S., and Opie, J. (1989). Modulation interference in detection and discrimination of amplitude modulation, *J. Acoust. Soc. Am.*, 86, 2138-2147.

Across-band Processing of Dynamically Varying Stimuli

Deborah A. Fantini
MRC Institute of Hearing Research
University of Nottingham
Nottingham NG7 2RD
England

Brian C.J. Moore
Department of Experimental Psychology
University of Cambridge
Cambridge CB2 3EB
England

1. INTRODUCTION

When a subject is trying to detect a change in level of one component of a complex sound, then the level may be monitored simply in a single critical band around that component, or the subject may compare the level across critical bands. If the overall level of the stimuli is randomised, this forces the subjects to adopt the second strategy: tasks of this type have been given the name Profile Analysis (Green, 1988). Typically, the stimuli used in this task are complex signals constructed by summing together sine waves, equally spaced in log-frequency. The subject is instructed to discriminate the stimulus in which all sine waves are equal in amplitude from the stimulus in which one of these sinusoids, typically the centre one, is incremented in level. In order to prevent subjects from basing their discrimination on a level change within a single auditory filter or critical band, the entire stimulus is randomly varied in level from presentation to presentation, thus making level an unreliable cue. Subjects must make use of the presence of the additional sine waves for relative level information to make their discrimination. The main point which comes out of studies on Profile Analysis is that subjects are very good at detecting the change in level in the target sinusoid when flanking sinusoids of equal amplitude are also present. Furthermore, subjects can integrate the relative level information across frequency in order to perform well on this task; performance improves, within limits, when more flanking components are added.

Another masking situation which is directly relevant to the present paper is Comodulation Masking Release or CMR. In this task, subjects are better at detecting a signal masked by a narrowband noise when a second noise, with the same amplitude envelope (amplitude fluctuations over time) as the original masker band, is added. It has become rather widely accepted that CMR depends on across-channel comparisons of the amplitude envelopes of the noise bands present, where the signal interval is marked by a disparity among the envelopes across frequency channels. Recently, however, Hall and Grose (1988) presented data which indicate that a masking release can occur even when the signal produces no across-channel envelope disparity. In their task, the signal was a noise band added back to itself in phase, resulting in an increment in level of the band but causing no change to the envelope pattern or modulation depth. Subjects were better at detecting this increment in level to the target band when a correlated noise band (one with the same amplitude envelope as the target) was present than when an uncorrelated noise band (one with a different amplitude envelope) was present. In a separate experiment, Hall and Grose demonstrated that a CMR could also occur when there were no across-band differences in level. They cite the improvement in performance with a correlated flanking band (or FB) as evidence for multiple cues available in a CMR task. However, for the case where only across-band level cues were available, one might interpret the improvement as due to a discrimination in spectral shape, i.e., Profile Analysis.

The present experiment examines this possibility by studying Profile Analysis for complex stimuli composed of bands of noise. Consider first the situation where the task is to detect an increment in level in the centre band of a complex composed of several bands, and all bands have the same envelope (i.e., the same pattern of fluctuation over time). In this case, the overall level of the stimulus will vary over time, but the spectral shape will be static. Thus, this task resembles the normal Profile Analysis task, except for the variation in overall amplitude across time. This type of stimulus situation also resembles that occurring for some speech sounds, e.g., vowels. The question addressed here is: how do the dynamic fluctuations in overall amplitude affect the ability to compare spectral shapes?

Consider now the situation where all of the noise bands are independent. Now there are fluctuations both in overall amplitude and in spectral shape during the presentation time of each stimulus. If subjects base their judgements on the moment-by-moment spectral shape, then the random fluctuations in spectral shape should markedly impair the ability to compare the spectral shapes of different stimuli. If, on the other hand, there is a temporal integration or smoothing process prior to the stage where Profile Analysis takes place, then good Profile Analysis may still be possible; essentially the spectral shape could be extracted from the long-term average spectrum, rather than from the time-varying short-term spectrum.

Presumably, when the amplitude fluctuations are slow (for narrow noise bandwidths), subjects will be able to follow the moment-by-moment fluctuations of the noise bands. Thus we would expect efficient Profile Analysis for the case where all the noise bands are correlated, and poor Profile Analysis when the bands are independent. When the amplitude fluctuations are rapid (for wider noise bandwidths), subjects should not be able to follow the moment-by-moment fluctuations. In this case, performance will be based on the long-term spectrum, and efficient Profile Analysis should be possible both when the noise bands are correlated and when they are independent. Transitions in performance as the bandwidth of the noise bands increases, and the rapidity of the fluctuations in the noise bands increases correspondingly, thus give a measure of the time over which integration takes place for Profile Analysis.

2. METHOD

Subjects were asked to discriminate a change in level in a noise band which was centred in a complex of four FBs. Noise bands were digitally generated at each of five bandwidths from 4 Hz to 64 Hz. Examples of some of these noise stimuli are shown in Fig. 1.

Let us examine the top row of Fig. 1 first. The top panel in the left-hand column shows the waveform resulting from adding four uncorrelated FBs centred at 1.02 kHz, 1.43 kHz, 2.8 kHz, and 3.92 kHz; each noise band is 4-Hz wide. These noises were generated by summing nine sinusoids at 0.5-Hz spacing. Each of the nine components in one FB had an amplitude and a phase which was randomly chosen from a Rayleigh and a rectangular distribution (0° to 360°), respectively. The four uncorrelated bands were generated by allowing all of the sinusoids composing each of the four noise bands to have independent, randomly

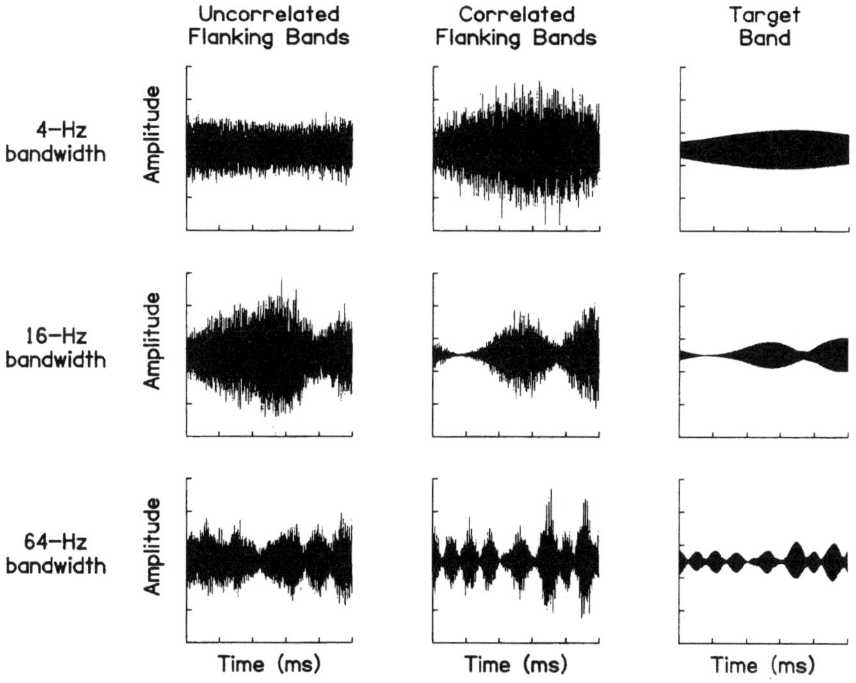

Fig. 1 Examples of the waveforms used. The total duration shown is 200 ms.

chosen phases and amplitudes. When four uncorrelated FBs are summed, the resulting waveform is relatively smooth, as the peaks and valleys of the four waveforms tend to average out.

The top panel of the middle column shows the sum of four correlated FBs. The correlation was achieved by specifying that the first sinusoid in each of the four noise bands had the same amplitude and phase; the same applied to the second sinusoid, the third, and so forth. Only the actual frequencies were different, and depended on the desired centre frequency of the noise band.

The top panel of the right-hand column shows the central target noise band. To get a target band which was correlated with a set of FBs, the nine sinusoids composing the target band all had the same amplitudes and phases as those in the correlated FBs. Only the frequencies were different to generate a noise band whose centre frequency was 2.0 kHz. Note that the amplitude fluctuations are very slow; the time scale shown here is 200 ms. At a 4-Hz bandwidth, the average or expected number of envelope maxima is 2.56 per second or about 0.5 within the 200-ms stimulus duration illustrated here (Rice, 1954). Ten pairs of correlated FBs and target bands, plus ten samples of uncorrelated FBs were generated for each bandwidth condition.

The second row shows three more samples of noise, this time at a 16-Hz bandwidth, with each noise band composed of 33 sinusoids. Note that the amplitude fluctuations are faster at this bandwidth; the expected number of envelope maxima increases to about 10 per second.

Finally, the bottom row illustrates FBs and target bands which are 64-Hz wide, with each band composed of 129 sinusoids. Here again the amplitude fluctuations are faster than in the top two rows; the expected number of envelope maxima increases to about 41 per second.

In the experiment, four conditions were run at each bandwidth. In the Reference (REF) condition, the target band was presented alone, and the subject had to detect an increment in level of this band. In the Correlated condition (COR), all five noise bands were correlated, and both the overall level, and the moment-by-moment level provided relative level or profile information. The third condition was the All-Uncorrelated (A-U) condition, in which a target band was presented with FBs which were uncorrelated with each other and with the target band. In this case, all five bands had independent amplitude fluctuations over time. The final condition was the Co-Uncorrelated (C-U) condition, in which the four FBs were all correlated with each other, but were not correlated with the target band.

Thresholds were estimated using a 3I3AFC adaptive procedure tracking 70.7% correct performance (Levitt, 1971). Visual feedback was provided via LEDs. Signal increments were varied in equal steps of 10 log(ΔI/I). Three experienced subjects ran in blocks of 20 reversals, the last 16 of which were averaged to achieve an estimate of threshold. Subjects continued to run in each condition until their thresholds had reached a clear asymptote. Then three final blocks of data were collected in each condition, and the thresholds were averaged over these three blocks for each subject. For all conditions, the median overall level of each noise band was 60 dB SPL, with a 20-dB range of random variation about this value. All stimuli were 200 ms in duration with a 50-ms rise/fall time. Stimuli were digitally generated at a 10 kHz sampling rate and stored in waveform files on a Masscomp 6600 computer. When played, the digital waveforms were converted using a pair of CED 1401 12-bit D/As, and anti-alias filtered at 4300 Hz, before being gated, mixed, and played to subjects in a sound-attenuating room via Sennheiser HD414 headphones.

3. Results

Fig. 2 illustrates the results for each subject in the REF, COR, and A-U conditions. Each panel shows thresholds, in units of 10 log(ΔI/I), as a function of bandwidth for the three subjects. The fourth panel shows the average results; error bars indicate one standard error about the mean. In the REF condition, the signal was merely an increment in level to the target band. All of the REF thresholds (circles) were about 6-9 dB, with the 4-Hz REF threshold being the highest, presumably due to the inherent random fluctuation in level of noises with very narrow bandwidths which occurred over and above the imposed random variation in level. The addition of COR FBs provided both instantaneous relative amplitude information, and average relative amplitude information. For each bandwidth, the presentation of the COR FBs (upward-pointing triangles) aided performance. The benefit to performance was roughly the same magnitude across the range of bandwidths tested (except at 4 Hz where it was a bit bigger), thresholds being lowered to about 0 dB.

Consider now the results for the A-U condition (inverted triangles in Fig. 2). If subjects are using the average level of the noise bands for their source of relative level information, then additional FBs which are uncorrelated with the target band (i.e. have different amplitude fluctuations over time) should still result in good performance. If, however, subjects are sensitive to the moment-by-moment relative level cues, then the addition of uncorrelated FBs should not aid performance until the envelope fluctuations become too fast for the auditory system to follow. Thresholds in the A-U condition decreased with increasing bandwidth, indicating that, as the rapidity of the fluctuation increased, the four uncorrelated FBs became more useful for providing relative level information. It appears that subjects were able to use the average spectral shape information provided by the FBs for bandwidths of 16 Hz and above. However, even at the 64-Hz bandwidth, performance in the A-U condition was not quite as good as in the COR condition. The short-term amplitude fluctuations did disrupt performance to some extent, even at the widest bandwidth.

In the C-U condition, the four FBs were present, and were correlated with each other, but not with the target band. The results of this condition may have implications for the role of perceptual grouping in the present experiment. That is, if grouping were to play a part in the present stimulus situation, the coherent modulation of the four FBs might cause them to be grouped as a separate auditory object from the target band. This separation might interfere with performance on a task which requires integration of information across the frequency range of a stimulus. The results of this condition are shown in Fig. 3.

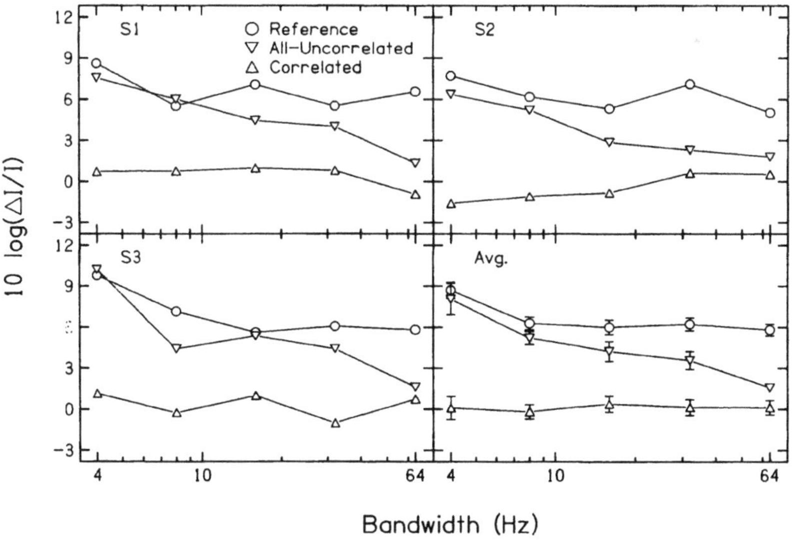

Fig. 2 Thresholds, in units of 10 log(ΔI/I) as a function of the bandwidth of the noise bands, for each of the three subjects. The lower right-hand panel gives the mean results, and one standard error about the mean. Circles are results from the REF condition, inverted triangles from the A-U condition, and triangles from the COR condition.

In Fig. 3 we have replotted the REF and the COR thresholds from Fig. 2 for comparison. We see almost the same pattern of results in the C-U condition as in the A-U condition. Thresholds in the C-U condition (squares) decreased with increasing bandwidth, and the advantage to having the target band also correlated with the four FBs decreased as the bandwidth increased. There was no tendency for a greater impairment to performance in the C-U condition relative to the A-U condition. Thresholds in the two conditions were almost identical as a function of bandwidth. Thus subjects can use the long-term average spectral shape information equally well for FBs that are correlated with each other or are independent. Differences in perceptual grouping caused by the correlation of the bands appear to play little role.

The results of the various conditions are summarised in Fig. 4, which shows the average benefit to performance resulting from having correlated FBs, compared to the other three conditions. To obtain the masking release values, each of the thresholds in units of 10 log(ΔI/I) was first converted to a ΔI value. This allowed us to compare the change in level in dB required for the signal to be detected in each of the conditions. To assess the benefit to performance gained by having correlated FBs, thresholds, in ΔI, for the COR condition were subtracted from those for each other condition for each subject. These difference values, or masking release values, were then averaged across subjects, and the means and one standard error presented as a function of bandwidth.

The top left-hand panel shows the relative benefit to performance when the target band alone (REF) was flanked by correlated FBs (COR). At the narrowest bandwidth there was about 6 dB of benefit, which decreased and reached an asymptote of about 4 dB by the 8-Hz bandwidth. The benefit to performance in the COR condition relative to the A-U and the C-U conditions was about 6 dB at the narrowest bandwidth, decreasing monotonically to about 0 dB by the 64-Hz bandwidth.

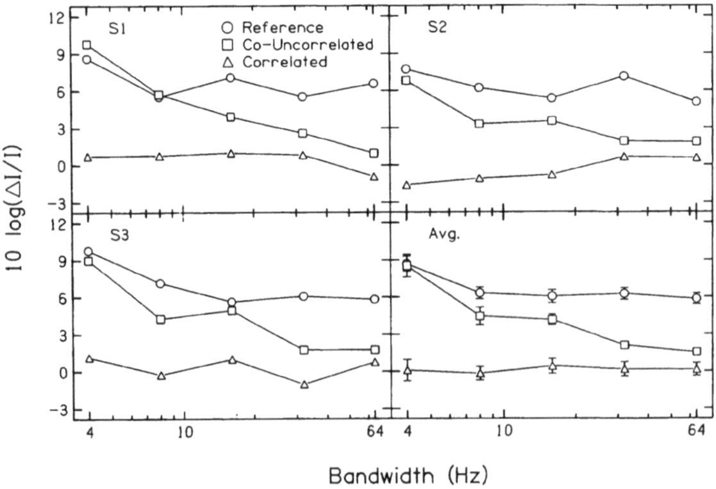

Fig. 3 As Fig. 2, but squares indicate thresholds for the C-U condition.

4. Summary and Conclusions

In summary, it is clear that subjects were able to perform well on a Profile Analysis task in which the components composing the profile were dynamically varying. At narrow bandwidths, less than about 32 Hz, subjects could follow the slow amplitude fluctuations and perform a dynamic spectral shape discrimination using the moment-by-moment levels of the FBs. At these bandwidths, the presence of uncorrelated FBs did not improve performance (thresholds in the A-U and C-U conditions were not different from those in the REF condition, see Figs. 2 and 3). However, when the amplitude fluctuations became faster, at 32 Hz and above, subjects were able to make use of the overall level of the FBs. At these wider bandwidths, subjects performed well regardless of whether the FBs were correlated with the target band or not. Thus there may be a temporal integration mechanism operating in Profile Analysis which smooths amplitude fluctuations. If so, then the smoothing which is operating for the present stimuli occurs for bandwidths between 16 and 32 Hz, corresponding to between 10 and 20 maxima per second. This suggests an integration time on the order of 100 ms.

Acknowledgements

We thank Tim Folkard and David Marshall for assistance with the signal-generation programming.

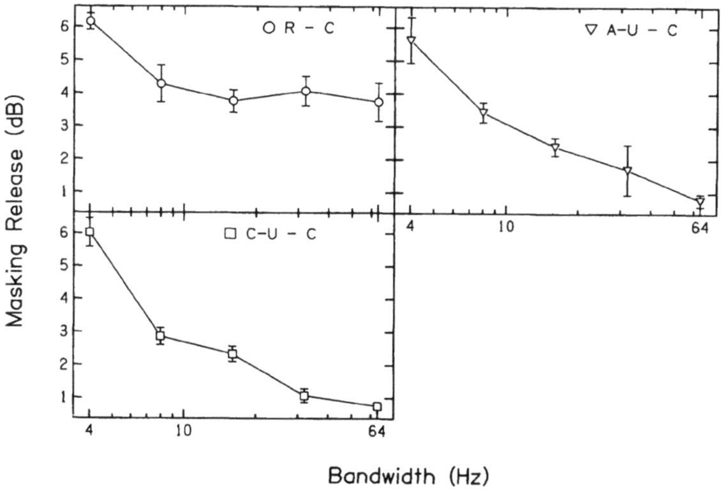

Fig. 4 Mean masking release values (see text). The top left-hand panel shows the advantage of having COR FBs relative to the REF condition (circles). The top right-hand panel shows the benefit of COR FBs relative to the A-U condition (inverted triangles). And the bottom left-hand panel shows the benefit of COR FBs relative to the C-U condition (squares).

References

Hall, J.W., III, and Grose, J.H. (1988). Comodulation masking release: Evidence for multiple cues, *J. Acoust. Soc. Am.*, 84, 1669-1675.

Green, D.M. (1988). *Profile Analysis*, Oxford University Press, New York.

Levitt, H. (1971). Transformed up-down methods in psychoacoustics, *J. Acoust. Soc. Am.*, 49, 467-471.

Rice, S.O. (1954). Mathematical analysis of random noise, in: N. Wax (ed.), *Selected Papers on Noise and Stochastic Processes*, Dover, New York.

Effectiveness of Comodulation Masking Release

Willem A.C. van den Brink,
Tammo Houtgast,
Guido F. Smoorenburg
TNO Institute for perception
P.O. Box 23
3769 ZG Soesterberg
The Netherlands

1. Introduction

A great number of recent experiments on signal detection in temporally modulated wide-band noise have revealed that the detection cue is not solely based on the information in the critical band centered at the signal but that information (about temporal modulation) in off-signal comodulated frequency bands also plays a part.

The phenomenon of comodulation masking release (CMR) was initially demonstrated by Hall et al. (1984). They found a release from masking for the detection of a tone pulse in a narrow band of noise if a second narrow band of noise was added remote in frequency. Release from masking occurred when the two bands of noise had similar temporal envelopes, and was thus called comodulation masking release.

The comodulated masker bands are usually obtained with the multiplication/filtering method as described by Hall et al. (1984). Thus, multiple narrow bands of noise with statistical comodulated envelope fluctuations are obtained. Amplitude, or intensity, modulation of the on-signal and off-signal masker bands provides another way of generating comodulated masker bands.

These two approaches yield different results with respect to the effect of CMR. For instance, in the multiplication/filtering approach a reduction in the amount of CMR was found with decreasing signal duration (Schooneveldt and Moore, 1989). The amplitude modulation approach yields a large CMR effect if the short-duration signal is placed in the dip of the masker envelope (e.g. Grose and Hall, 1989; Moore et al., 1990; van den Brink, 1991).

The results on CMR as found in the literature (e.g. Hall et al., 1988; Hall and Grose, 1990; Haggard et al., 1990; Schooneveldt and Moore, 1987; Moore and Schooneveldt, 1990) suggest that the CMR effect is observed especially when no obvious detection cues for retrieving the signal from the valleys in the masker are available within the signal band itself. In this paper we will present some experiments, using a deterministic (sinusoidal) amplitude modulation of a noise masker, eliminating as much as possible the within-signal-band detection cues. This will result in a number of stimulus configurations especially sensitive to a comodulation release from masking.

2. METHODS

2.1 Procedure

A two-interval forced choice procedure was used in all experiments. Each trial consisted of two 300-ms observation intervals, separated by 200 ms. The signal was presented with equal probability in the first or second interval. The masking noise was presented continuously, and the intervals were marked by a light on the listener's response box. Feedback was provided after each response. The signal level was varied adaptively with a stepsize of 2 or 1 dB. Initially, the signal level was set well above masked threshold, and the level was reduced by 2 dB after three successive correct responses; after the first incorrect response the level was increased by 2 dB and the stepsize was reduced to 1 dB. A three-down one-up procedure (Levitt, 1971) was applied in order to estimate the level that would produce a correct score of 79.4%. After three reversals the data collection started up to a total of thirteen reversals. Threshold was defined as the mean of the signal levels at the last ten reversals in either direction. Three threshold estimates were obtained for each stimulus condition.

2.2 Apparatus

The experiments were performed under control of an IBM-AT computer. Signals were generated, at 40-μs sample intervals, using a digital signal processor based on a TMS320-10. Broadband noise was generated, using a Wandel & Golterman RG-1 analog noise generator. The 100% SAM noise was created by leading the noise from the noise generator through an analog amplitude modulator (TNO, custom built) of which the modulation depth and modulation frequency could be programmed. The modulation frequency at the amplitude modulator was set to 20 Hz. The noise was bandpass filtered (filter slopes > 180 dB/oct) by programmable digital filters (TNO, custom built). It was verified that, for the bandwidth applied, the amplitude modulation of the noise remained 100% SAM. The stimuli were presented diotically (same stimulus to both ears) by means of Beyer DT-48 headphones. The first author served as a subject in this pilot study and was seated in a soundproof room.

2.3 Level Definition

The energy spectra of all stimuli were determined using a real-time frequency analyzer (Brüel & Kjær 2123). All maskers were derived from white noise. The noise level was defined by the noise spectral density N_0. Using a masker bandwidth of 13/3-octs, the level of the masking noise was set to approximately 50 dB SL, corresponding to a noise spectral density, in case of non-modulated noise, of about 20 dB/Hz. In this pilot study 1.6 kHz was used as a signal center frequency. In the experiments with a 1/3-oct bandwidth (about 390 Hz at 1.6 kHz), the noise spectral density was kept constant which implied lower sensation levels. The threshold levels of the signals were defined in terms of their total energy relative to the spectral density of the masking noise: E/N_0 (van den Brink, 1991).

The release from masking was always determined relative to the masking conditions with no comodulated flanking bands present. Results averaged across replications per condition are presented. The error bars in the figures represent the standard deviations.

3. EXPERIMENTS

3.1 Signal Duration

In this experiment signal duration was varied systematically in order to determine its effect on the masked threshold. The masker, which had a bandwidth of 390 Hz (approximately one critical band), was geometrically centered at the signal frequency and was presented continuously. The signal was a pure tone at 1.6 kHz having rise/fall times of 20 ms and steady state durations of 0, 2, 4, 8, 16, 32, 64, 128 and 256 ms. The temporal center of the signal was chosen to either coincide with a masker envelope dip (DIP) or a masker envelope peak (PEAK), in case of a 100% sinusoidal amplitude modulation applied to the white noise masker. Masked thresholds were also determined with non-modulated white noise having a bandwidth of 390 Hz geometrically centered at 1.6 kHz (REF).

The results are plotted in Fig. 1, showing the masked threshold as a function of signal duration for the three masking conditions. In case of non-modulated white noise the masked threshold in terms of E/N_0 is independent of signal duration. This is in line with classical experiments on temporal integration as performed by Plomp and Bouman (1959). However, in case of a dip or a peak placement the masked thresholds vary with signal duration. For very short signal durations the masked threshold for a dip and a peak placement are found to be essentially the same. It is surprising that the dip placement does not yield a lower masked threshold. Apparently, for the present 1/3-oct masker, the auditory system cannot benefit from a dip placement of a short-duration signal.

When signal duration is increased, the auditory system does benefit from the modulation of the masker; the masked threshold for both the peak and the dip placement decreases. For the larger signal durations there is actually no difference between the dip and the peak placement of the signal; the masked thresholds are equal. The masked threshold for this signal duration is about 10 dB below the masked thresholds of the short-duration signals. This indicates that for the long-duration signal, when compared to the short-duration signal, an additional

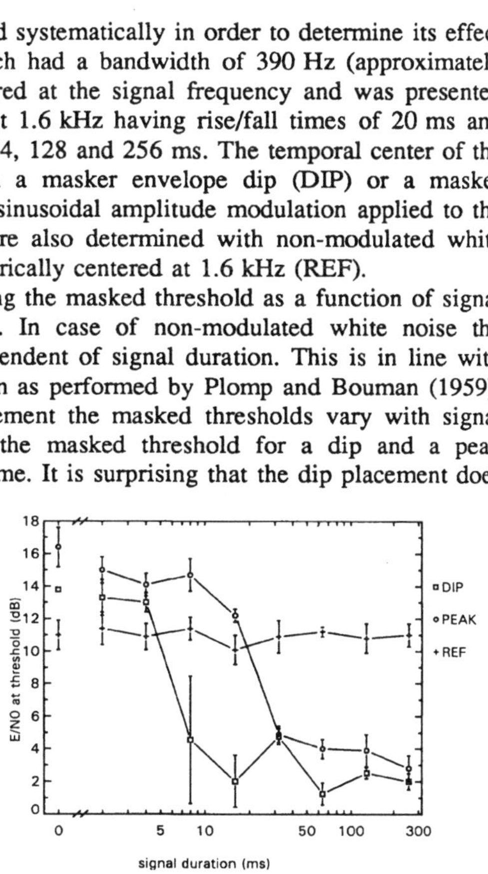

Fig. 1 Masked thresholds as a function of signal duration in non-modulated white noise (plus symbols) and in 100% SAM (F_{mod} = 20 Hz) white noise, with the temporal center of the signal either coinciding with a masker envelope peak (open circles) or a masker envelope dip (open squares). The masker bandwidth was set at 390 Hz.

detection cue is available. This detection cue will be eliminated in the following experiment.

3.2 Masker Bandwidth

With a 1.6 kHz pure tone of 256 ms duration (rise/fall times of 20 ms) as a signal, masked thresholds were determined. The masking noise was either non-modulated or 100% amplitude-modulated (F_{mod} = 20 Hz) bandpass-filtered white noise. The bandwidth of the noise was set to 390, 320, 260, 196, 130, 98, and 60 Hz. The masked thresholds in case of the 390 Hz masker bandwidth (=1/3-oct) has already been determined in the previous experiment.

The results are plotted in Fig. 2, showing the masked thresholds in terms of E/N_0 as a function of masker bandwidth for both masking conditions.

In case of non-modulated bandpass-filtered white noise the masked threshold, in terms of E/N_0, increases when the bandwidth is increased within the 1/3-oct. However, in case of the 100% SAM noise masker an increase in masker bandwidth up to 1/3-oct results in a decrease in masked threshold. Assuming the decrease of threshold with masker bandwidth to be due to CMR, the data indicate that for a long-duration signal the appropriate on-signal masker bandwidth for studying CMR would be about 100 Hz. For this condition there is essentially no difference between the modulated (SAM) and non-modulated (REF) masked thresholds.

3.3 Optimal CMR Conditions

The results of the two previous experiments have provided two stimulus configurations (short signal in 1/3-oct and long signal in noise with bandwidth ≤ 100 Hz) for which signal detection is poor, showing essentially no difference between non-modulated and modulated noise masked thresholds. These stimulus configurations seem especially suitable to determine the effect of CMR by adding flanking bands. The short-duration signal placed in 390 Hz 100% SAM masking noise and the long-duration signal placed in 100 Hz 100% SAM masking noise both have masked thresholds that do not differ from the masked threshold in the non-modulated white noise condition determined with identical masker bandwidths. The masked thresholds of these signal, were determined when two

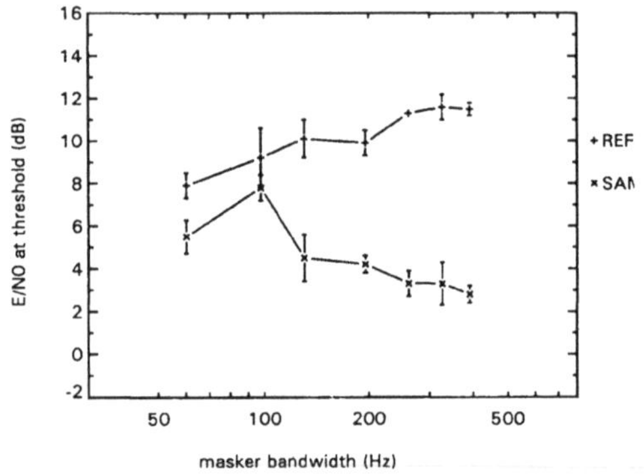

Fig. 2 Masked thresholds of a pure-tone signal with a duration of 256 ms as a function of masker bandwidth for the two masking conditions. The plus signs represent the masked thresholds in case of non-modulated bandlimited white noise, the cross symbols represent the masked thresholds in 100% SAM bandlimited white noise.

comodulated flanking bands, having a bandwidth of just within 1/3-oct, were added to the masker band centered at the signal frequency. The flanking bands were placed at frequencies of 1.0 kHz and 2.5 kHz.

In case of the short-duration signal the on-signal maskerband had a width of 390 Hz. For the long-duration signal the masked thresholds were determined for both a 100 Hz and a 390 Hz on-signal masker bandwidth.

The results are plotted in Fig. 3, showing the amount of CMR for the four stimulus configurations. Only two stimulus configurations exhibit a CMR effect: The short-duration signal placed in a masker dip and the long-duration signal for which the on-signal masker bandwidth is narrow (100 Hz). For the other two masking conditions no CMR is found. For a long-duration signal in a 390 Hz on-signal masker band adding the comodulated flanking bands causes an increase in the masked threshold indicating across-channel masking (Moore et al., 1990) or modulation detection interference (MDI; Yost and Sheft, 1989). It also seems that detection of a short-duration signal placed at a peak of the temporal envelope is governed by a within-channel cue, since no benefit from CMR is found. This indicates that for a peak placement of the signal all signal energy is effectively masked by the on-signal masker and that comodulated flanking bands cannot assist in retrieving the signal from the masker, as is the case when the signal is placed in a masker dip.

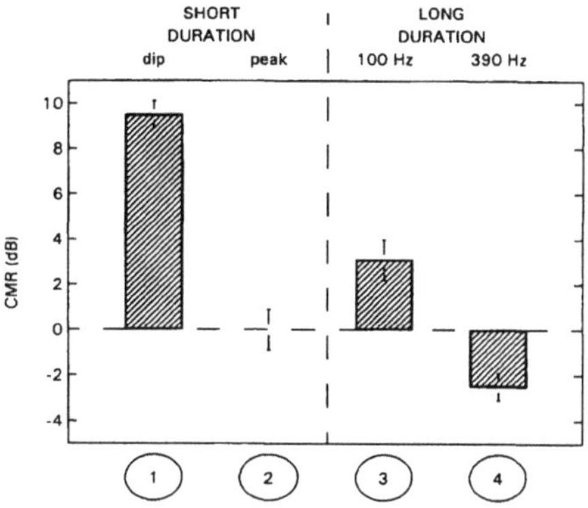

Fig. 3 The amount of CMR, i.e., the decrease in masked threshold when adding comodulated flanking bands, for four stimulus configurations. Configurations 1 and 3 are especially sensitive to comodulated flanking bands.

1 : *short-duration signal placed in the dip of 1/3-oct 100% SAM noise.*

2 : *short-duration signal placed in the peak of 1/3-oct 100% SAM noise.*

3 : *long-duration signal placed in a narrowband (100 Hz at a 20 Hz modulation frequency) of 100% SAM noise.*

4 : *long-duration signal placed in a narrowband (390 Hz at a 20 Hz modulation frequency) of 100% SAM noise.*

4. Conclusions

The experiments presented in this paper indicate that a facilitation of signal detection due to comodulation occurs for stimulus configurations for which detection is already poor: no clear within-channel detection cues are available for retrieving the signal from the valleys in the masker.

Two stimulus configurations that are especially sensitive to CMR, when a deterministic masker envelope is applied to a noise masker in order to achieve comodulation, are the following:

1. short-duration signal placed in a masker envelope valley of a 100% SAM 1/3-oct bandwidth masker.
2. long-duration signal in a narrow-band (100 Hz 100% SAM) masker.

References

Brink, W.A.C. van den (1991). *Aspects of spectro-temporal processing in auditory signal detection*, Ph. D. Dissertation, Utrecht, The Netherlands.

Grose, J.H. and Hall, J.W. III (1989). Comodulation masking release using SAM tonal complex maskers: Effects of modulation depth and signal position, *J. Acoust. Soc. Am.*, 85, 1276-1285.

Haggard, M.P., Hall, J.W. III, and Grose, J.H. (1990). Comodulation masking release as a function of bandwidth and test frequency, *J. Acoust. Soc. Am.*, 88, 113-119.

Hall, J.W. III, Haggard, M.P., and Fernandez, M.A. (1984). Detection in noise by spectro-temporal pattern analysis, *J. Acoust. Soc. Am.*, 76, 50-57.

Hall, J.W. III, Grose, J.H., and Haggard, M.P. (1988). Comodulation masking release for multi-component signals, *J. Acoust. Soc. Am.*, 83, 677-687.

Hall, J.W. III and Grose, J.H. (1990). Comodulation masking release and auditory grouping, *J. Acoust. Soc. Am.*, 88, 119-126.

Levitt, H. (1971). Transformed up-down methods in psychoacoustics, *J. Acoust. Soc. Am.*, 49, 467-477.

Moore, B.C.J., Glasberg, B.R., and Schooneveldt, G.P (1990). Across-channel masking and comodulation masking release, *J. Acoust. Soc. Am.*, 87, 1683-1695.

Moore, B.C.J and Schooneveldt, G.P. (1990). Comodulation masking release as a function of bandwidth and time delay between on-frequency and flanking-band masker, *J. Acoust. Soc. Am.*, 88, 725-732.

Plomp, R. and Bouman, M.A. (1959). Relation between hearing threshold and duration for tone pulses, *J. Acoust. Soc. Am.*, 31, 749-758.

Schooneveldt, G.P. and Moore, B.C.J. (1987). Comodulation masking release (CMR): Effects of signal frequency, flanking band frequency, masker bandwidth, flanking band level, and monotic versus dichotic presentation of the flanking band, *J. Acoust. Soc. Am.*, 82, 1944-1957.

Schooneveldt, G.P. and Moore, B.C.J. (1989). Comodulation masking release as a function of masker bandwidth, modulation bandwidth, and signal duration, *J. Acoust. Soc. Am.*, 85, 273-282.

Yost, W.A. and Sheft, S. (1989). Across-critical band processing of amplitude- modulated tones, *J. Acoust. Soc. Am.*, 85, 848-858.

The Masking of Modulations in Relation to Speech Perception

Joost M. Festen
Department of Otolaryngology
Free University Hospital
Amsterdam, The Netherlands

1. INTRODUCTION

Speech is a signal modulated both in frequency and in time. Usually, the carrier sound wave consists of an alternation of noise and a periodic signal, but it may also be noise only, as in whispered speech. To a large extent, the information in speech is conveyed by the modulations. Therefore, not only is a good transfer of these modulations essential for intelligibility, but ultimately the auditory system itself must be sensitive enough to process the modulations.

A way of studying the auditory processing of modulations is in masking experiments, where the characteristics of the system are evaluated in terms of the detection threshold for modulations in the presence of other modulations. Along this line of research Yost and Sheft (1989) showed that a 10-Hz modulation on a 1-kHz carrier is able to mask a 10-Hz modulation on a 4-kHz carrier. Also, modulation on the high-frequency tone can mask modulation on the low-frequency tone. Yost and Sheft interpreted their data in terms of theories suggesting that common modulations help the auditory system to group signals from different frequency regions into one auditory object.

Using noise as a carrier signal, both Houtgast (1989) and Bacon and Grantham (1989) found the detection mechanism for modulations to be frequency- or rate-selective. The greatest amount of masking occurs when probe and masker modulations have a comparable rate. In speculations on a physiological basis for this mechanism, Bacon and Grantham adhered to the existence of specialized modulation-processing channels. These channels were suggested earlier to explain results on adaptation experiments in AM and FM modulation (see Kay, 1982; Tansley and Suffield, 1983). However, the validity of these adaptation experiments has been seriously questioned by Moody et al. (1984), who showed, at least for FM modulation, that the effects of adaptation could be completely canceled with listener training.

Houtgast (1989) estimated the bandwidth of the modulation-rate analyzer by measuring the modulation threshold as a function of the bandwidth of masker modulations (the classic "band-widening experiment" modified to the domain of modulations). In this experiment the masking increased with masker bandwidth up to about ½ - 1 oct. and was constant for a further widening of masker bandwidth. Although the modulation-detection mechanism behaves as if it is rate-selective, it is not clear whether a real decomposition of modulation frequencies is performed on the envelope. The selective masking may just as well be a figure-background problem in which the detection of modulations is easier for rates that show a large contrast with the background.

The experiments presented here were initiated to solve this problem by investigating the masking of modulations at harmonics of a complex modulator. Appearance of the harmonics in the masking pattern supports an explanation in terms of frequency decomposition, while masking at harmonics would not occur if a modulation were only detected by its rate, and not by its Fourier components. The possibilities of this approach are, however, very limited, due to the shallow masking slopes in modulation detection. Even with a square wave modulation (containing only odd harmonics), detection of the third harmonic at -9.5 dB would be very difficult. For periodic modulations the phase relation between masker and probe modulation can be an additional complicating factor. Therefore, it was decided to use noise as masker modulation, and to study the masking pattern of two simultaneously presented modulation bands of equal amplitude and clearly separated in modulation rate. The presented data are from one listener only.

2. Detection of Modulation in a Masker Modulation

Modulations were presented on a pink noise carrier from 1 and 4 kHz, as shown in Fig. 1. Effects of modulation on the carrier skirts were masked by the addition of a complementary unmodulated band-rejected noise. Masker modulations were low-frequency bands of noise, and the probe modulation was a sinusoid with frequency ω_p. The two modulations were applied to one carrier by passing it through successive modulators. This led to the following signal equation:

$$s(t) = [\ 1 + m(t)\ ] \cdot [\ 1 + A_p \cos(\omega_p . t)\ ] \cdot n(t), \qquad (1)$$

where m(t) is the masker modulation, A_p and ω_p are amplitude and frequency of the probe modulation, respectively, and n(t) is the pink noise carrier.

Fig. 1 Modulated pink noise from 1 to 4 kHz with two unmodulated flanking bands.

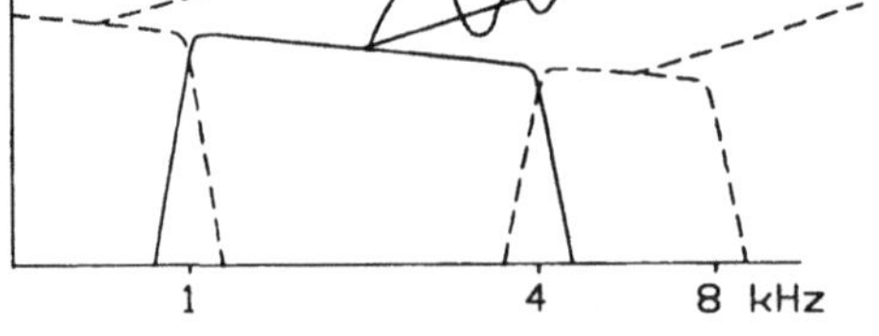

Thresholds were determined in a 2AFC procedure in which the masker modulation was presented continuously and the probe was added in one of two visually indicated observation intervals of two seconds each, with one second separation. The probe modulation was gated on and off in 200 ms. The level of the probe modulation was adjusted in 2-dB steps according to an adaptive procedure (two-down one-up) aiming at 71% correct. The probe level averaged over eight reversals in the adaptive procedure was taken as the threshold and is expressed in dB re 100% modulation depth [20log(A_p)]. Signals were presented diotically over Beyer DT48 earphones at a level of 55 dB SL.

In a first test the unmasked threshold for modulation detection was determined. Results from 1 to 64 Hz are given by the filled squares in Fig. 2. Next, masked modulation thresholds were measured for ½-oct wide masker modulations with 4 and 16 Hz center frequency, respectively. The results are shown in Fig. 2 (closed circles) and agree with those by Houtgast (1989) and Bacon and Grantham (1989). The masking pattern has a bandpass character; a high threshold is obtained when masker and probe modulation rates are about equal and the threshold decreases as masker and probe are separated in modulation rate. The shallow slopes of these masking curves limit the possibility of measuring a spectral decomposition of the masker in the modulation-detection mechanism. The threshold obtained for simultaneous modulation with the two masker noise bands (open circles) shows only a very small masking dip between the modulation noise bands.

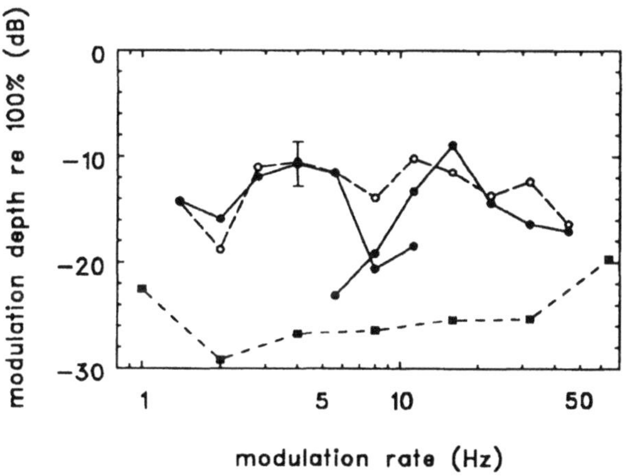

Fig. 2 Detection threshold for modulation as a function of modulation rate. Squares represent the unmasked threshold and filled circles the threshold masked by ½-oct wide modulation bands at 4 and 16 Hz, respectively. The open circles show the masked threshold for both masker modulation bands simultaneously present. The standard deviation averaged over all data is indicated at the peak of the lower masking curve.

In a final test, thresholds were determined for an 8-Hz probe modulation masked by a band of modulations (2 - 32 Hz) with a notch centered at 8 Hz. Results, as a function of the notch width, are shown in Fig. 3 for two levels of the modulation depth. Once again the data show some rate selectivity, but with a rather poor resolution. The main difference between these results for modulation rate and the comparable results for audio frequencies is that with a widening of the notch there seems to be at first a plateau in the modulation data before the notch becomes effective. Such a plateau is not found in the audio-frequency domain, not even in listeners with broadened auditory filters (see Glasberg and Moore, 1986).

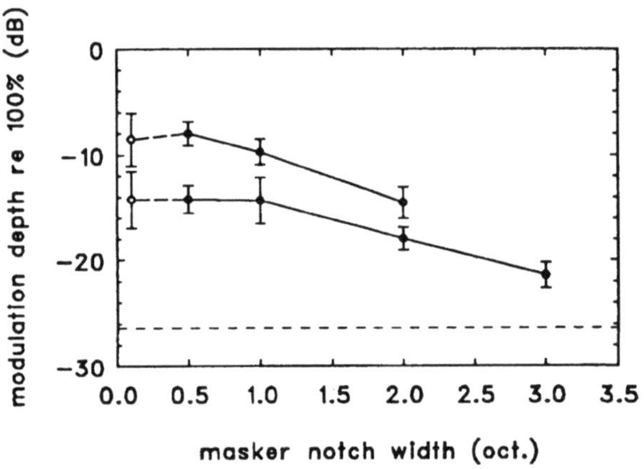

Fig. 3 Detection threshold for 8-Hz modulations masked by a notched-noise modulator as a function of the notch width. Two levels of the masker modulation were used with 6-dB difference. Thresholds obtained for a noise modulator without a notch are represented by open symbols.

In conclusion, the frequency selectivity in modulation detection is so poor that the auditory system is not able to resolve the harmonics of a complex modulation. Therefore, it seems inappropriate to describe this selectivity in terms of a Fourier analysis on the modulation waveform; hence the existence of modulation-rate filters in the auditory system is unlikely.

3. Significance for Speech Perception

The data presented above show that modulations can be masked by other modulations. This occurs even when test and masker modulations have carriers with very wide frequency separation (see Yost and Sheft, 1989). At the same time however, it is shown that masking is limited when test and masker modulations have a different rate. Although modulations are very important for speech intelligibility, this selective masking may be the reason that two simultaneous voices, each with their own pattern of modulations, do not strongly interact. The large width of the modulation spectrum of speech (more than 5 octaves from 0.5 to 20 Hz) sees to it that two different speech patterns meet only occasionally. Apart from this, the introduction of modulations in a masking noise creates intervals with a high signal-to-noise ratio and, due to the redundancy of speech, listeners are very well capable of reconstructing the intervals with low S/N-ratio. Consequently, the speech-reception threshold for sentences in a modulated masker is considerably lower than in a steady-state masker of the same intensity [see for sinusoidal modulations (Festen, 1987) and for an interfering voice (Festen and Plomp, 1990)].

Because the fluctuations in the sound-pressure level of speech mainly contain modulations below about 20 Hz, the envelope can be represented by 40 samples per second. Assuming that a 5-bit quantisation of level variation is sufficient, we can estimate the rate of information in the speech envelope to be about 200 bits/s. As the information transmitted in speech is largely conveyed by the modulations, data on the processing of modulations in the auditory system can augment our knowledge on the information-transmission capacity of the ear. In normal-hearing listeners this capacity is of course well matched with the rate of changes that occur in speech, but for hearing-impaired listeners, and in particular for those with severe impairment, this need not be so. If we want to recode speech for this group of listeners, in order to present amplitude information in an alternative way, the transmission capacity of the alternative receiver should be at least comparable to the capacity of the modulation detector in the ear.

References

Bacon, S.P. and Grantham, D.W. (1989). Modulation masking: Effects of modulation frequency, depth, and phase, *J. Acoust. Soc. Am.*, 85, 2575-2580.

Festen, J.M. (1987). Speech-reception threshold in a fluctuating background sound and its possible relation to temporal auditory resolution, in M.E.H. Schouten (ed.), *The Psychophysics of Speech Perception*, Nijhoff, The Netherlands (NATO ASI Series D).

Festen, J.M. and Plomp, R. (1990). Effects of fluctuating noise and interfering speech on the speech-reception threshold for impaired and normal hearing. *J. Acoust. Soc. Am.*, 88, 1725-1736.

Glasberg, B.R. and Moore, B.C.J. (1986). Auditory filter shapes in subjects with unilateral and bilateral cochlear impairment, *J. Acoust. Soc. Am.*, 79, 1020-1033.

Houtgast, T. (1989). Frequency selectivity in amplitude-modulation detection, *J. Acoust. Soc. Am.*, 85, 1676-1680.

Kay, R.H. (1982). Hearing of modulation in sound, *Physiol. Rev.*, 62, 894-975.

Moody, D.B., Cole, D., Davidson, L.M., and Stebbins, W.C. (1984). Evidence for a reappraisal of the psychophysical selective adaptation paradigm, *J. Acoust. Soc. Am.*, 76, 1076-1079.

Tansley, B.W. and Suffield, J.B. (1983). Time course of adaptation and recovery of channels selectively sensitive to frequency and amplitude modulation, *J. Acoust. Soc. Am.*, 74, 765-775.

Yost, W.A. and Sheft, S. (1989). Across-critical-band processing of amplitude-modulated tones, *J. Acoust. Soc. Am.*, 85, 848-857.

Chapter 3
Perception of Spectral Change and Timbre

What Do We Know about Perception of Dynamic and Complex Signals, and how Relevant Is It to Speech Perception?

A.J.M. Houtsma
Institute for Perception Research
Eindhoven
The Netherlands

1. Introduction

A noticeable shift in interest has taken place in psychoacoustics during the past twenty years, away from simple and static sounds towards more complex and dynamic sounds. Studies of detection, discrimination, identification, loudness scaling or pitch matching with simple steady-state sinusoidal tones have to a large extent made place for an interest in modulation, masking release, profile analysis and scene analysis. The main moving forces behind this shift of interest may have been, on the one hand, the growing awareness that the auditory system as a whole is so nonlinear and time-variant that its total behavior will never be completely understood in terms of its behavior for simple steady-state sinusoidal tones, while, on the other hand, there has been mounting pressure on the discipline of psychoacoustics to become and remain relevant with respect to modern sound-technology developments such as telephone communication, speech coding, hearing aids and high-fidelity sound reproduction.

A comprehensive description of modern studies on complex and dynamic auditory behavior would go far beyond the limits and scope of a single review paper. On profile analysis and on auditory scene analysis alone two books were published during the last few years (Green, 1988; Bregman, 1990). This paper will focus on those aspects of auditory behavior that appear directly relevant for the topic of speech perception. One aspect concerns the dynamic sensation of voice pitch, which is probably the main carrier of prosodic information in spoken sentences. This aspect is discussed in the first part of the paper. The second aspect concerns the ability of our auditory system to discriminate and identify sounds by details of their spectral shape in a dynamic context. Spectral shape is the principal carrier of phonetic information in speech, and will be discussed in the second part of the paper.

2. Pitch and Pitch Tracking

In the literature on speech perception the term "pitch" is used almost synonymously with a vowel's fundamental frequency f_0. Strictly speaking this is incorrect because pitch denotes a perceptual, subjective attribute of a sound (ANSI, 1963), whereas f_0 is clearly a physical attribute. Within the context of speech sounds, however, this well-rooted but incorrect terminology is not likely to lead to serious misconceptions. Speech vowels and voiced consonants represent nearly perfect harmonic sounds with discrete frequency components that are integral multiples of the fundamental vocal-chord vibration rate f_0. Independent of the relative intensities of the various harmonics, which characterize each particular vowel or voiced consonant, the perceived voice pitch always corresponds to the fundamental frequency f_0, even if this fundamental as a spectral component has little or no acoustical power.

Experiments by Plomp (1967), Ritsma (1967), and Houtsma and Goldstein (1972) on the relationships between the perceived Gestalt pitch of a harmonic complex tone and the frequencies of its partials have shown that the central part of the brain primarily uses information derived from aurally resolved partials to find f_0. Aural resolution implies that harmonics are of an order below the tenth. Other experiments (Hoekstra, 1979; Cullen and Long, 1986; Houtsma and Smurzynski, 1990) have shown that harmonics well above the tenth can also contribute to the f_0 percept. Such a percept is not very salient, however, and occurs only if there are many high-order harmonics. In natural speech, particularly in a male voice with low f_0, there are indeed many of such high-order harmonics, but even in that case there are enough low-order harmonics to dominate the f_0 percept. Only in filtered speech can we encounter a situation where voice pitch would be conveyed only by high-order, aurally unresolved harmonics.

The percept of pitch in speech as well as in music is a dynamic and not a static one. It is not so much the pitch of a sound itself, but rather a pitch change or pitch contrast that catches our attention. In music we usually deal with discrete pitch changes according to steps along well-established tone scales. Numerous experiments on the perception of musical tones, intervals and scales (see Deutsch, 1982) have shown that perceptual musical relationships are best described in terms of log-frequency units. Musical intervals, triads, and other chords appear to have a strong perceptual similarity if the constituent frequencies have the same ratios. Already Pythagoras seems to have been aware of this when he tried to express the consonance or dissonance of harmonic intervals (diads) in terms of string-length ratios measured on a monochord. Most professional and quite a few amateur musicians possess the ability to recognize melodic and harmonic musical intervals within a span of a couple of octaves. This is a skill that can be learned through standard solfeggio training, taught at every music school. (Only very few musicians have the special skill of "absolute" or "perfect" pitch, i.e. the ability to name tones by their proper name without any external reference.) This shows that the subjective categories used to store musical interval information in short-term memory (Wickelgren, 1966, 1969; Durlach and Braida, 1969) correspond with log-frequency units in the physical world.

Pitch of natural or synthetic speech is also a dynamic percept. In a spoken sentence it is not so much the instantaneous pitch, but rather an entire pitch contour that is being perceived. The main difference with musical pitch seems to be that music tends to treat fundamental frequencies f_0 mostly in a discrete, step-wise manner, whereas in speech f_0 changes in a continuous fashion. One might wonder whether continuous pitch variations in speech give rise to a different perceptual organization of pitch in comparison with music.
There is evidence that this is indeed the case.

Hermes and van Gestel (1991) performed an experiment in which subjects were given two versions of the utterance / mamáma/, spoken by a male speaker in two different f_0 registers. One was a fixed reference stimulus, the other a comparison stimulus in which subjects had to adjust the f_0 excursion until it subjectively matched the reference in prominence of the pitch accent. Both stimuli had f_0 contours that were piece-wise linear on either a linear frequency scale, a log-frequency scale or an equivalent rectangular bandwidth (ERB) scale. Reference stimuli were presented in a low and comparison stimuli in a high register for half the trials, and vice versa for the other half.

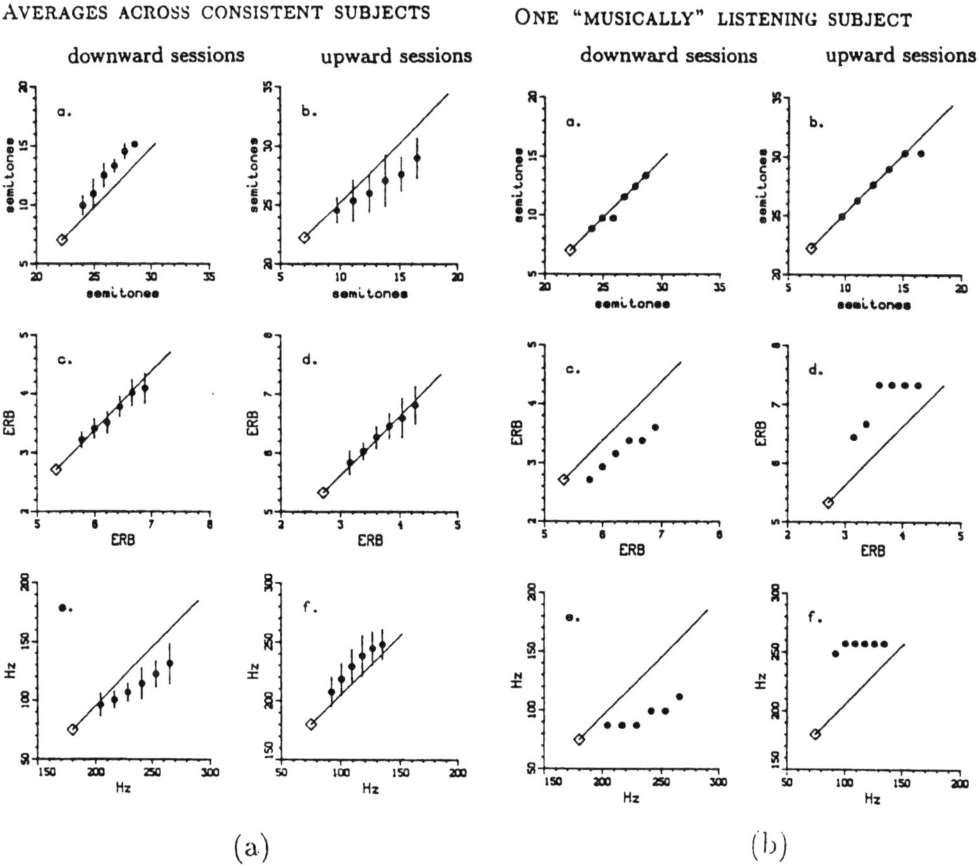

Fig. 1 Average results of matching comparison stimuli (ordinate) to test stimuli (abscissa) by five consistent subjects operating in the "speech mode" (a), and by one of those subjects operating in the "musical mode" (b). The diamond represents the end point of the (lower) declination line of the test and comparison stimulus. (From Hermes and Van Gestel, 1991).

Averaged results of five consistent subjects (out of a total of nine) are shown in Fig. 1a. The abscissa shows the f_0 excursion of the reference stimulus, expressed in either semitones, ERBs or Hz. The diamond in each panel represents the final f_0 value of the lower declination line of the utterance, so excursion size should be taken from this reference point. In a similar manner the ordinate shows the matched f_0 excursions of the comparison stimulus. One can clearly see that matches fall along a line of unit slope only if expressed in ERB units. This implies that two accented speech utterances, spoken in different f_0 registers, sound equally prominent if they sweep through the same number of critical-band filters expressed in ERBs (Patterson, 1976; Glasberg and Moore, 1990; Greenwood, 1961, 1990)

This is very different from typical musical behavior where one would expect two frequency excursions to be subjectively matched if they are equal on a log-frequency (e.g. semitone) scale. In fact, one of the subjects in Hermes and van Gestel's study volunteered to repeat the mamáma matching experiment under exactly the same experimental conditions as before, but subjectively using a musical interval matching criterion. The subject produced a set of matches that perfectly fit the semitone scale, and did not fit a line of unit slope at all if stimuli were measured and plotted on an ERB or Hz scale, as is shown in Fig. 1b. Apparently the use of a prosodic or a musical pitch criterion can lead to consistent but very different experimental results, even for physically identical stimuli. Although it has not been shown experimentally, it seems likely that prosodic or musical perception behavior can be enhanced by the choice of the f_0 modulation function. A smooth, continuous rise-fall function, as one typically finds at pitch accents in natural speech, may enhance prosodic perception, whereas a discrete step-wise modulation function may induce musical behavior. Future research will have to show whether this is true or not.

Despite all the differences between speech and musical modes of perception, most psychoacoustical studies on pitch perception should be considered relevant for understanding speech perception, especially those that deal with complex and dynamic stimuli. One area in which that has become quite evident is the development of techniques to measure pitch in running speech. From a purely mathematical or technical point of view there are several ways to approach the problem (see Hess, 1983). The most stable, robust and noise-resistant algorithms, however, have turned out to be the ones based on knowledge of auditory pitch perception (Duifhuis et al., 1982; Allik et al., 1984; Hermes, 1988), i.e. those algorithms that apply bandpass filtering and use frequency information of all resolved stimulus partials to compute the underlying, best-fitting fundamental frequency.

3. Timbre and Spectral Shape

Another essential attribute of a speech signal which allows us to grasp the phonetic and semantic content of a spoken message is the timbre or sound color of its segments. Expressed in physical terms, this attribute depends primarily on the quasi-instantaneous spectral shape of a signal or, in phonetic terms, on its formant structure. A spectral shape or formant structure refers to the spectral envelope of a short segment of a speech signal, typically 40 ms. Such an envelope can be a really continuous function, for instance for sounds with continuous spectra such as fricatives, but is also often an artificial function determined by only a finite number of spectral values, for instance for vowels and voiced consonants.

Spectral shapes of sounds normally change with time in speech and in music, and our perception of timbre is very sensitive to this transient behavior. If one listens, for instance, to a piano piece in which all the tones have been turned backwards in time, one will not recognize the sounds as coming from a piano. This is despite the fact that tone spectra, computed over the duration of each tone, are exactly the same for forward and backward notes. Also a speech message, recorded in a room with some reverberation, has a very different timbre due to the fact that echoes precede rather than follow each speech sound. Both effects have been demonstrated on a CD "Auditory Demonstrations" (Houtsma et al., 1987). The point of these demonstrations is to show that our auditory system computes spectral images over a short time window in the immediate past, typically a few milliseconds, and is very sensitive to the manner in which these computed images change with time. The rather complex relationships of the subjective attribute of timbre with both spectral and temporal properties of complex and dynamic sound is probably the main reason why the American National Standards Institute in essence defined timbre as those subjective attributes that are neither loudness nor pitch (see ANSI, 1973).

Many attempts have been made to study the perception of timbre in a systematic manner and to come up with a set of functional relationships with the many physical attributes it potentially depends on. Plomp (1970) proposed representing the steady-state condition of a complex tone by means of an n-dimensional vector with components equal to the sound power measured in n critical bands (actually 1/3-octave bands). He found that for a set of musical instrument sounds the total differences between these vectors, computed either in Euclidean or in city-block metrics, showed a high degree of correlation with subjective timbre differences measured in a triadic comparison experiment. Pols (1970) found something similar for the perceptual similarity of 11 Dutch vowels and a six-dimensional vector formed by the first three formant frequencies and corresponding sound pressure levels. More recently Pollard and Jansson (1982), inspired by earlier work of von Bismarck (1974) and Grey (1977), proposed modeling both transient and steady-state properties of musical instrument sounds by the time course of a three-dimensional vector, the components being the respective loudnesses (in sones) of (1) the fundamental, (2) harmonics 2, 3, and 4, and (3) harmonics 5 and higher, all normalized with respect to total loudness. Because the sum of these vector components is always unity, a two-dimensional representation in the form of a triangle suffices. Fig. 2a shows such a triangle, with the x-axis representing the fractional loudness of the high and the y-axis the fractional loudness of the 2nd, 3rd and 4th harmonics. A pure tone will by construction always be located at the origin. Fig. 2b shows traces in this plane made by viola, clarinet and trumpet tones, beginning at the onset of the sound and ending where the steady state is reached.

It is interesting to see that steady-state positions for these three instruments are rather close, but that the paths they follow to get there are very different. This is consistent with experimental evidence that sounds of some musical instruments are easily confused if attack transients are removed or exchanged (Berger, 1964; Clark et al., 1964). Pollard and Jansson's sound triangle, however, appears too crude to adequately describe speech sounds because their perceptually important formant structure is insufficiently represented.

An entirely different research strategy is represented by the work of Green and co-workers on Profile Analysis (see Green, 1988, for a comprehensive review). In that work the auditory system's sensitivity to intensity changes in one or more spectral components is measured in the presence of other spectral components. The experiments in this work are mostly of the forced-choice type and the experimental tasks are therefore defined in an

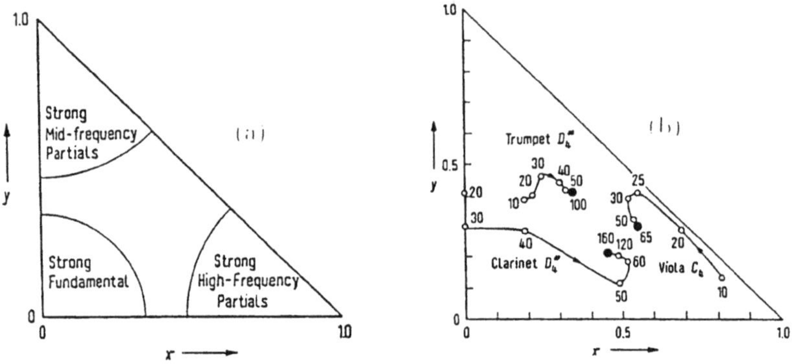

Fig. 2 Tristimulus diagrams representing timbre of musical instruments. (a) Regions of tones with strong fundamental, strong midfrequency partials, and strong high partials; (b) Course of attack transients for various instruments. (From Pollard and Jansson, 1982)

objective sense, with right and wrong responses. The concepts of timbre, pitch or loudness and their exact meaning do not play an important role in this research, because the experimenter does not care, in principle, what subjective clues subjects use to arrive at their responses.

A characteristic feature of the profile analysis research methods is the rando-mization of overall intensity of each sound, the so-called roving intensity. This prevents subjects from using cues related to simple intensity changes, and forces them to use the entire spectral profile in order to detect a small increase or decrease of some target component. An example of a between-trial and a within-trial roving-level discrimination paradigm, taken from a study by Green et al. (1983), is shown in Fig. 3. The work of Green's group has yielded a wealth of experimental data that show under what conditions and to what extent the auditory system can make within-channel and across-channel comparisons to obtain a measure of a spectral profile.

A potentially very useful model of profile analysis behavior is the channel model illustrated in Fig. 4 (Durlach et al., 1986). This model is a stochastic formulation of Plomp's vector model in which at various levels noise is added to variables derived from aurally resolved stimulus components. For instance, independent noise processes are injected into each channel immediately after the filtering operation, representing the stochastic nature of the physiological filtering processes in the peripheral part of the auditory system (Fig. 4a). A common noise signal may be added to all channels, representing, for instance, the uncertainty introduced by the use of a roving-intensity paradigm (Fig. 4b). After all channel outputs have been reduced to some optimal decision variable, for instance a log likelihood ratio, another random variable may be added to represent the stochastic nature of the decision process itself (Fig. 4c). The model accounts for effects of inter-channel correlation and central noise on discrimination sensitivity. It explains some of the behavior observed in profile analysis experiments, for instance the fact that subjects' performance with multiple targets is well below predictions by the optimum combination rule in which the sensitivity d' for the

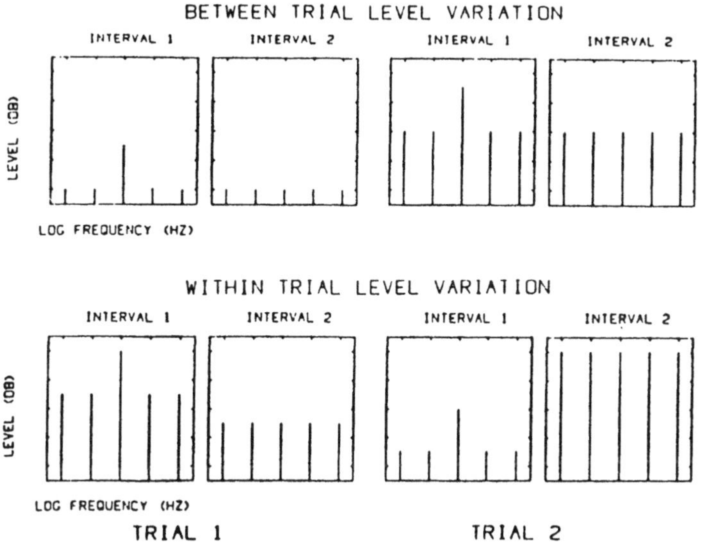

Fig. 3 Example of roving-level stimuli used in roving-level profile analysis experiments. The task is to detect the interval with the incremented component. Top: between-trial roving; bottom: within-trial roving. (From Green et al., 1983)

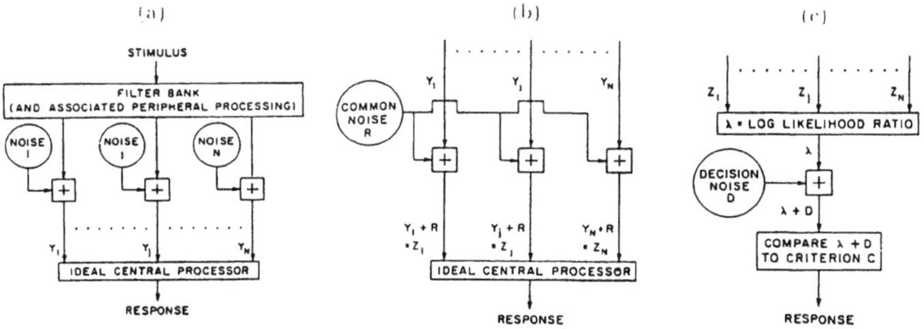

Fig. 4 Illustration of three stages of the channel model, according to Durlach et al., 1986.

complex target equals the square root of the sum of d's squared for the individual targets (Green and Swets, 1966; Green et al., 1987).

An entirely different model mentioned by Green (1988) as a possible explanation of profile analysis behavior is the EWAIF (Envelope Weighted Average Instantaneous Frequency) model (Feth, 1974; Feth and O'Malley, 1977; Stover and Feth, 1983). The model is based on the fact that for any complex sound s(t) the waveform can be expressed as the product of an instantaneous envelope function e(t) and the cosine of an instantaneous phase angle p(t):

$$s(t)=e(t) \cos p(t). \tag{1}$$

The instantaneous frequency f(t) is given by the time derivative of p(t) divided by 2π. We can then define the EWAIF as the envelope-weighted average of this instantaneous frequency over a period T:

$$EWAIF=\frac{\int_0^T f(t)e(t)dt}{\int_0^T e(t)dt} \tag{2}$$

The integration time T may be taken equal to the stimulus duration if it is small (in the order of 10 ms), or equal to the repetition period for periodic sounds. For other sounds the choice of T becomes somewhat arbitrary, which is unfortunate because EWAIF can be quite sensitive to T.

Despite the potential power of the EWAIF model, there are some conceptual and empirical facts which limit its applicability to auditory profile analysis behavior. Perhaps the most important one is that the model applies only to within-channel comparisons, since the EWAIF is formed through the interaction of signal components with one another. If one applied the formulas blindly to broadband stimuli, one would ignore the fact that the stimulus is bandpass filtered by the ear at a very early stage. The model therefore cannot account for the very apparent across-channel comparisons which are so characteristic of profile analysis behavior. An empirical problem with the EWAIF model as a description of within-channel discrimination concerns the frequency dependence of discrimination thresholds for two-tone complexes that differ in the relative amplitude of their components (Feth and O'Malley, 1977; Versfeld and Houtsma, 1991a). In one such experiment the frequency difference between components was kept at 60 Hz, and in another experiment at one semitone. If EWAIF were the sole discrimination statistic, one might expect that differential EWAIF values computed from experimental threshold conditions would be the same in both experiments. This was found to be the case for frequencies of 1000 Hz and higher, but for lower frequencies the EWAIF difference limen for the 60-Hz inter-tone spacing could be as much as ten times larger than the EWAIF difference limen obtained with the one-semitone spacing (Versfeld and Houtsma, 1991b).

Another auditory phenomenon which is thought to be closely related to profile analysis is comodulation masking release (CMR), first described by Hall (Hall et al.,1984; Hall, 1986). It means that the amount of masking of a pure-tone signal presented in narrow-band modulated noise (masker band) decreases when other co-modulated noise bands (flanking bands) away from the masker band are added. The most common interpretation of this phenomenon is that the central auditory system makes an across-channel comparison and attempts to detect an envelope disparity in one of the channels which would be caused by a signal in that channel. In a recently completed study, van den Brink (1991) was able to show that about 12 dB of CMR is obtained when a brief signal (the impulse response of a 1/3-octave filter) is spectrally centered in a 4-octave, 100 % amplitude modulated noise band with a modulation frequency of 32 Hz, and temporally placed in a valley of the masker. When the signal bandwidth was increased to 4 octaves (impulse response of 4-octave filter), however, the amount of masking release remained virtually unchanged. Under that condition there are no flanking noise bands without signal power, so that the observed CMR cannot be explained as the detection of across-channel disparity. It thus appears that much more work needs to be done before we can claim to understand the exact relationship between profile analysis and broadband masking behavior of the auditory system.

Finally an example is presented that illustrates differential sensitivity to real musical instrument tones. The experiment was meant as a test of the often heard claim that a good pianist can change the tone color of a piano tone merely by the "touch" of the key. A well-known piano teacher who strongly supported this claim was asked to produce isolated tones, played on the same key and at as much as possible the same intensity, but with two clearly different "touches". Analysis of the tones showed that there were differences in overall intensity of between 1 and 6 dB for the tones to be compared. Due to the nonlinear nature of the collision between hammer and string, a more forceful stroke not only produces a tone of greater intensity but also one with slightly stronger high harmonics. This can be seen in Fig. 5 which shows the spectra, measured for the first 50 ms, of two piano tones played with a different touch. The absolute total intensity of the tone shown in Fig. 5b was 1.2 dB above that of the tone shown in Fig. 5a. The plots have been normalized with respect to their strongest component. The inserts in each Fig. give the precise levels of the harmonics. One can see that, except for partials 2 and 7, all harmonics of (b) are somewhat stronger relative to the fundamental than the harmonics of (a). In order to see whether these spectral differences are also audible, a two-interval two-alternative forced choice discrimination experiment was done, with three subjects, using 1-s tone fragments. In order to eliminate

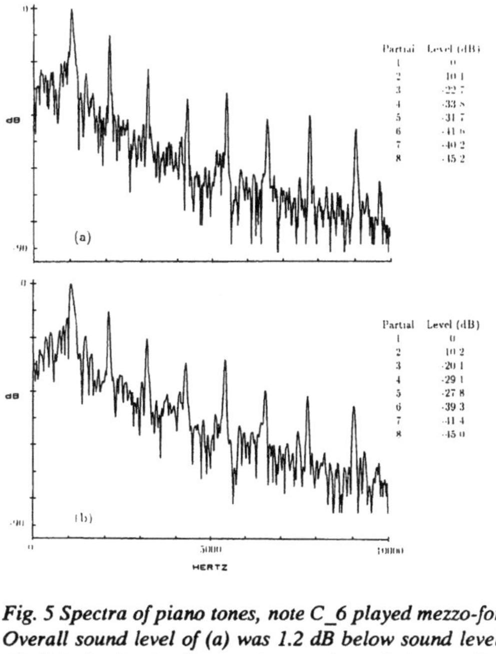

***Fig. 5** Spectra of piano tones, note C_6 played mezzo-forte. Overall sound level of (a) was 1.2 dB below sound level of (b). Relative levels of harmonics are shown in inserts. Tones were aurally barely discriminable with within-trial roving intensity.*

possible intensity cues, stimuli were equalized with respect to their peak value and presentation intensity was randomized over a range of 4 dB. The results showed that the pair shown in Fig. 5, which was about the most difficult pair in the entire test, yielded 55 % correct responses for one subject, and 75 % correct for the other two. This shows that complex and dynamic tones can still be discriminated at about threshold level despite only very small differences in details of their spectra.

References

Allik, J., Mihkla, M. and Ross, J. (1984). Comment on measurement of pitch in speech: An implementation of Goldstein's theory of pitch perception, *J. Acoust. Soc. Am.*, 75, 1855-1857.

American National Standard Institute (1973), *American national psychoacoustical terminology*, S3.20, New York.

Berger, K.W. (1964). Some factors in the recognition of timbre, *J. Acoust. Soc. Am.*, 36, 1888-1891.

Bismarck, G. von (1974). Timbre of steady sounds: a factorial investigation of its verbal attributes, *Acustica*, 30, 146-159.

Bregman, A. (1990), *Auditory Scene Analysis*, MIT Press, Cambridge.

Brink, W.A.C. van den (1991), *Aspects of spectro-temporal processing in auditory signal detection,* Ph. D. Thesis, Utrecht.

Clark, M., Luce, D., Abrams, R., Schlossberg, H., and Rome, J. (1964). Preliminary experiments on the aural significance of parts of tones of orchestral instruments and on choral tones, *J. Audio Engr. Soc.*, 12, 28-31.

Cullen, J.K., Jr. and Long, G. (1986). Rate discrimination of high-pass filtered pulse trains, *J. Acoust. Soc. Am.*, 79, 114-119.

Deutsch, D. (1982), *The psychology of music*, Academic Press, New York.

Duifhuis, H., Willems, L.F., and Sluyter, R.J. (1982). Measurement of pitch in speech: An implementation of Goldstein's theory of pitch perception, *J. Acoust. Soc. Am.*, 71, 1568-1580.

Durlach, N.I. and Braida, L.D. (1969). Intensity perception I. Preliminary theory of intensity resolution, *J. Acoust. Soc. Am.*, 46, 372-383.

Durlach, N.I., Braida, L.D., and Ito, Y. (1986). Towards a model for discrimination of broadband signals, *J. Acoust. Soc. Am.*, 80, 63-72.

Feth, L.L. (1974). Frequency discrimination of complex periodic tones, *Perc. and Psychophys.*, 15, 375-378.

Feth, L.L. and O'Malley, H. (1977). Two-tone auditory spectral resolution, *J. Acoust. Soc. Am.*, 62, 940-947.

Glasberg, B.R. and Moore, B.C.J. (1990). Derivation of auditory filter shapes from notched-noise data, *Hearing Res.*, 47, 103-138.

Green, D.M. (1988), *Profile Analysis*. Oxford Univ. Press, New York.

Green D.M. and Swets, J.A. (1966). *Signal detection theory and psychophysics*. J. Wiley, New York.

Green, D.M., Kidd, G., and Picardi, M.C. (1983). Successive versus simultaneous comparison of auditory intensity discrimination, *J. Acoust. Soc. Am.*, 73, 634-643.

Green, D.M., Onsan, Z.A. and Forrest, T.G. (1987). Frequency effects in profile analysis and detecting complex spectral changes, *J. Acoust. Soc. Am.*, 81, 692-699.

Greenwood, D.D. (1961). Critical bandwidth and the frequency coordinates of the basilar membrane, *J. Acoust. Soc. Am.*, 33, 1344-1356.

Greenwood, D.D. (1990). A cochlear frequency-position function for several species --- 29 years later, *J. Acoust. Soc. Am.* 87, 2592-2605.

Grey, J.M. (1977). Multidimensional perceptual scaling of musical timbres, *J. Acoust. Soc. Am.*, 61, 1270-1277.

Hall, J.W., Haggard, M.P. and Fernandes, M.A. (1984). Detection in noise by spectro-temporal pattern analysis, *J. Acoust. Soc. Am.*, 76, 50-56.

Hall, J.W. (1986). The effect of across-frequency differences in masking level on spectro-temporal pattern analysis, *J. Acoust. Soc. Am.*, 79, 781-787.

Hermes, D.J. (1988). Measurement of pitch by subharmonic summation, *J. Acoust. Soc. Am.*, 83, 257-264.

Hermes, D.J. and van Gestel, J.C. (1991). The frequency scale of speech intonation, *J. Acoust. Soc. Am.*, 90, 97-102.

Hess, W. (1983), *Pitch determination of speech signals*. Springer Verlag, New York.

Hoekstra, A. (1979), *Frequency discrimination and frequency analysis in hearing*. Ph. D. Thesis, Groningen.

Houtsma, A.J.M. and Goldstein, J.G. (1972). The central origin of the pitch of complex tones: Evidence from musical interval recognition, *J. Acoust. Soc. Am.*, 51, 520-529.

Houtsma, A.J.M. and Smurzynski, J. (1990). Pitch identification and discrimination for complex tones with many harmonics, *J. Acoust. Soc. Am.*, 87, 304-310.

Houtsma, A.J.M., Rossing, T.D., and Wagenaars, W.M. (1987). Auditory Demonstrations. Philips CD No. 1126-06, Acoust. Soc. Am., Woodbury, N.Y.

Patterson, R.D. (1976). Auditory filter shapes derived with noise stimuli, *J. Acoust. Soc. Am.*, 59, 640-654.

Plomp, R. (1967). Pitch of complex tones, *J. Acoust. Soc. Am.*, 41, 1526-1533.

Plomp, R. (1970). Timbre as a multidimensional attribute of complex tones, in: *Frequency Analysis and Periodicity Detection in Hearing*, R. Plomp and G.F. Smoorenburg, eds., Sijthoff, Leiden.

Pollard, H.F. and Jansson, E.V. (1982). A tristimulus method for the specification of musical timbre, *Acustica*, 51, 162-171.

Pols, L.C.W. (1970). Perceptual space of vowel-like sounds and its correlation with frequency spectrum, in: *Frequency Analysis and Periodicity Detection in Hearing*, R. Plomp and G.F. Smoorenburg, eds., Sijthoff, Leiden.

Ritsma, R.J. (1967). Frequencies dominant in the perception of the pitch of complex sounds, *J. Acoust. Soc. Am.*, 42, 191-198.

Stover, L.J. and Feth, L.L. (1983). Pitch of narrow-band signals, *J. Acoust. Soc. Am.*, 73, 1701-1707.

Versfeld, N.J. and Houtsma, A.J.M. (1991a). Perception of spectral changes in multi-tone complexes, *Q. J. Exp. Psychol.*, 43A, 459-479.

Versfeld, N.J. and Houtsma, A.J.M. (1991b). Spectral shape discrimination of two-tone complexes, in: *Auditory Physiology and Perception*, Y. Cazals, ed., Pergamon Press, Oxford, in press.

Wickelgren, W.A. (1966). Consolidation and retroactive interference in short-term recognition memory for pitch, *J. Exp. Psychol.*, 72, 250-259.

Wickelgren, W.A. (1969). Associative strength theory of recognition memory for pitch, *J. Math. Psychol.*, 6, 13-61.

On the Perception of Spectral Changes in Noise Bands

Niek J. Versfeld
Institute for Perception Research
P.O. Box 513
5600 MB Eindhoven
The Netherlands

1. Introduction

In the last two decades a growing number of psychoacoustic studies has been reported, dealing with the detectability of a change in the amplitude of a single component in a multi-tonal masker (profile analysis; Green, 1988), or of a sinusoid in amplitude-modulated noise bands flanked by other modulated noise bands (co-modulation masking release). The detectability of broadband spectral changes in a multi-tone spectrum has received less attention. Green, Onsan and Forrest (1987) studied the detectability of the change from a flat to a rippled spectrum; Bernstein and Green (1987) studied the detectability of several types of complex broadband changes. In general, they found that thresholds obtained with complex changes were much higher than would be expected from extrapolation of thresholds obtained with simple-sinusoid changes.

Only few papers deal with the detectability of broadband spectral changes in noise (Farrar, Reed, Ito, Durlach, Delhorne, Zurek and Braida, 1987; Moore, Oldfield and Dooley, 1989; Versfeld, 1990). The present paper is an attempt to relate the perception of spectral changes in discrete spectra to spectral changes in dense (hence more noise-like) spectra. Firstly, results obtained with noise bands are presented and compared to earlier results of experiments with two- and multi-tone complexes (Versfeld and Houtsma, 1991, 1992) in order to gain some insight into how changes in a spectrum are perceived and what features in the spectral shape are important in the discrimination process. Secondly, a simple model is proposed which may account for these results, and more evidence for this model is given by comparison of the present results with data reported in the literature.

2. Experiment

In the present experiment the ability of the auditory system to discriminate between noise bands that differ only with respect to their spectral slope was investigated. In an adaptive, three-interval, three-alternative, forced-choice procedure, the subject's task was to discriminate between a noise band having a positive spectral slope and one having a negative spectral slope (see Fig. 1). The idea of using these sounds was derived from earlier experiments with two-tone complexes (Houtsma, this volume). The spectral shape was chosen such that changes in the shape were very simple and symmetric, while the overall intensity remained constant.

Thresholds for changes in the spectral slope were measured:

(1) as a function of the bandwidth of the noise, while the centre frequency was kept fixed at 1000 Hz;
(2) as a function of the centre frequency, while the bandwidth was kept fixed at 58 Hz;
(3) as a function of the centre frequency, while the bandwidth was kept fixed at 1 semitone (ST).

In condition (1), the bandwidth was varied between 0.5 and 24 ST. In conditions (2) and (3), the centre frequency was varied between 125 and 4000 Hz. In order to force subjects to listen purely to changes in the spectral shape of the noise band, the intensity of each and every presentation within a trial was roved randomly between 30 and 50 dB above the subject's empirically established absolute threshold for the investigated sound.

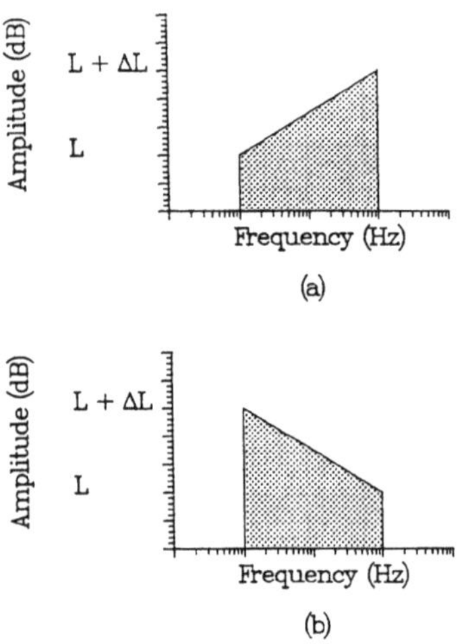

Fig. 1 Frequency spectrum of stimuli used in the experiment. (a) Noise band with a positive spectral slope. (b) Noise band with a negative spectral slope.

2.1 Stimuli

Stimuli were generated digitally by summation of sinusoids of the appropriate amplitude and random phase. The separation between sinusoids was 1 Hz. In each particular condition the phase relation was preserved, which means in fact that the signal should not be considered as true noise in a statistical sense, but rather as frozen noise, or simply as a signal with a very dense spectrum. The spectral slope was linear on a log-frequency, log-amplitude scale, and was expressed as the difference in amplitude ΔL between the spectral edges (see Fig. 1). One stimulus consisted of three stimulus intervals, each with a duration of 400 ms (20-ms onset and offset ramps included). Intervals were separated by a 100-ms silent period. A stimulus interval comprised a noise band with either a positive or a negative spectral slope. A stimulus contained two identical and one different interval, and the subject's task was to indicate the odd interval. Response time was unlimited and feedback was provided immediately after each response. The difference in spectral slope, ΔL, was varied adaptively, and the threshold was defined as that point of the psychometric function at which d' equalled one. Under condition (1), at least 750 trials per subject and per bandwidth were conducted; under conditions (2) and (3), at least 600 trials per subject and centre frequency were conducted.

2.2 Subjects

In condition (1) six subjects participated. In conditions (2) and (3), two subjects participated. The latter two subjects had also participated in condition (1).

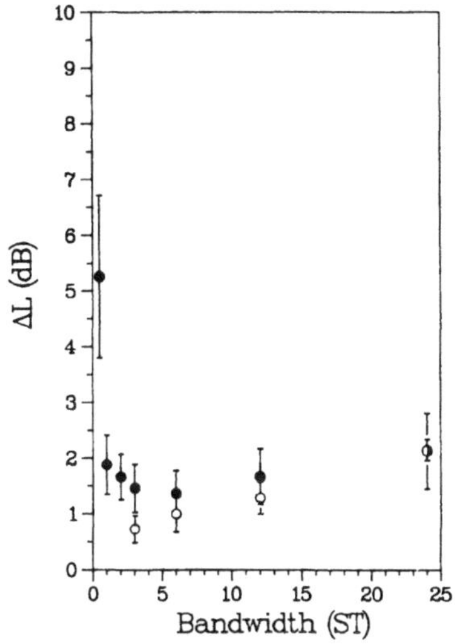

Fig. 2 Thresholds for changes in the spectral slope of noise bands (•) and two-tone complexes (∘) as a function of bandwidth. Bars indicate the standard deviation between subjects.

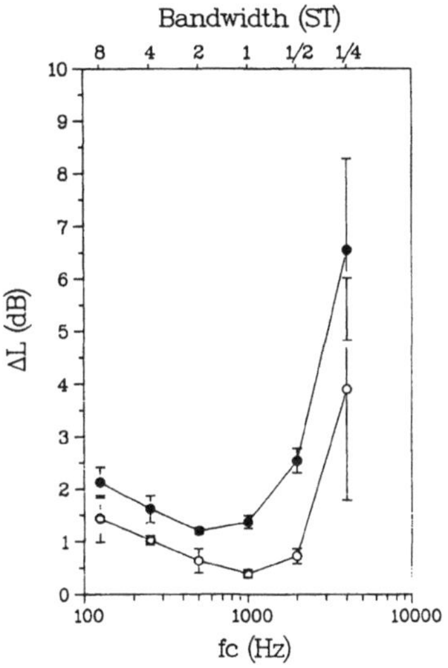

Fig. 3 Thresholds for changes in the spectral slope of noise bands (•) and two-tone complexes (∘) with a bandwidth of 58 Hz, as a function of the centre frequency. Bars indicate the standard deviation between subjects.

2.3 Results

Fig. 2 displays the results as filled circles for condition (1), where thresholds ΔL are plotted as a function of bandwidth. Since all subjects behaved similarly, only the averaged results are plotted. Individual results can be found in Versfeld (1990). One symbol corresponds to about 4500 trials. Also indicated is the between-subject standard deviation.

The results show that performance is best if the bandwidth of the noise is 3-6 ST. For smaller bandwidths the threshold rapidly increases. The subjective cue here is a change in pitch. For bandwidths larger than 6 ST, the threshold increases slowly. Now the perceptual cue is more timbre-like: noise bands with a positive spectral slope are perceived as sharper than those with a negative slope. Even for large bandwidths, the auditory system is apparently still able to discriminate between the two noise bands, which indicates that - since the overall intensity was roved - the output of different critical bands or frequency channels are compared in a relative fashion (profile analysis; Green, 1988). The open symbols represent thresholds obtained with two-tone complexes, and will be discussed below.

Fig. 3 displays the thresholds ΔL as filled circles for condition (2), as a function of centre frequency f_c. The behaviour of the two subjects was very similar, so that again only averaged results are plotted. One symbol represents on average 1200 trials. Before going into detail, it should be noted that a fixed bandwidth in Hz corresponds to a decreasing bandwidth in ST if the centre frequency is increased. Therefore, the corresponding bandwidth of the noise band in ST is given by the upper axis in Fig. 3. A minimum in threshold is observed near f_c = 500 Hz (2 ST). Furthermore, the threshold increases rapidly for higher centre frequencies (smaller bandwidths, if expressed in semitones), and increases slowly when the centre frequency decreases. This trend is similar to the one displayed in Fig. 2, with the difference that now the centre frequency has been varied too.

The results of the third condition are displayed in Fig. 4. For a bandwidth of 1 ST, averaged thresholds (filled circles) are plotted as a function of the centre frequency. For convenience, the bandwidth in Hertz is given by the upper axis. Thresholds are hardly dependent on centre frequency, except for perhaps a slight decrease in threshold at increasing centre frequencies. Note that for f_c = 1000 Hz, a bandwidth of 1 ST corresponds to a bandwidth of 58 Hz. Comparison of Figs. 2, 3, and 4 shows excellent agreement between these points (ΔL = 1.3 dB).

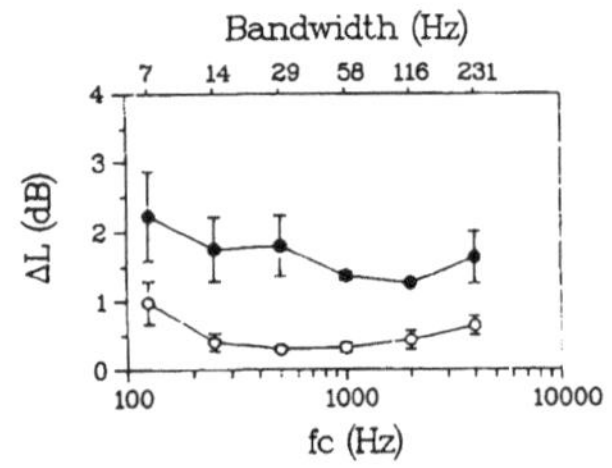

Fig. 4 Thresholds for changes in the spectral slope of noise bands (•) and two-tone complexes (∘) with a bandwidth of 1 ST, as a function of the centre frequency. Bars indicate the standard deviation between subjects.

3. Comparison with Two-Tone Complexes

In a previous study, Versfeld and Houtsma (1991) measured thresholds ΔL for two-tone complexes as a function of the bandwidth at a centre frequency of 1000 Hz. They did not rove the overall intensity, except for a control experiment. Their main finding was that threshold reached an extremely low minimum (of about 0.25 dB) near 1 ST. Because in this paper interest is focused on thresholds obtained with large bandwidths, and because the present experimental paradigm differs from the one used by Versfeld and Houtsma (1991), thresholds for large-bandwidth two-tone complexes have been measured again. The experimental set-up was identical to the one described above. Fig. 5 displays the two complexes between which the subject had to discriminate. The two-tone complexes had a bandwidth of 3, 6, 12 or 24 ST. Four subjects participated, and about 600 trials per subject and per bandwidth were conducted. The (averaged) thresholds (corresponding to d' = 1) are plotted as open circles in Fig. 2. The results show that the threshold decreases with decreasing bandwidth. Furthermore, previous research has shown that the threshold reaches a minimum near a bandwidth of 1 ST, whereafter it rapidly increases. Another study (Versfeld and Houtsma, 1992) investigated the discriminability of amplitude changes in two-tone complexes as a function of frequency separation (bandwidth) and centre frequency. The results are displayed in Figs. 3 and 4 as open circles.

In all three figures, the threshold behaviour of two-tone complexes shows a remarkable similarity to that of noise bands: Only absolute values are different. In all cases thresholds of noise bands are larger. The slope of the noise band, as depicted in Fig. 1, is valid only if the signal is integrated over an infinitely long time period. The successive short-term spectra, however, differ from each other, and these temporal fluctuations in the spectrum cause thresholds to be elevated in comparison with those of the two-tone complexes.

The independence of the threshold from centre frequency in Fig. 4 suggests an invariance of the U-shaped curve in Fig. 2 under transformation of centre frequency. The results in Fig. 3 are in line with this idea.

4. MODELS

The results in Fig. 2 (for both noise bands and two-tone complexes) can be separated into two subgroups, namely those obtained with narrow-band signals and results obtained with broadband signals. The minimum in Fig. 2 reflects the transition from narrowband to broadband signals. Narrowband signals fall entirely into one frequency channel, hence they are processed as a whole (within-channel processing). Broadband signals excite more than one channel, and between-channel processing will take place as well.

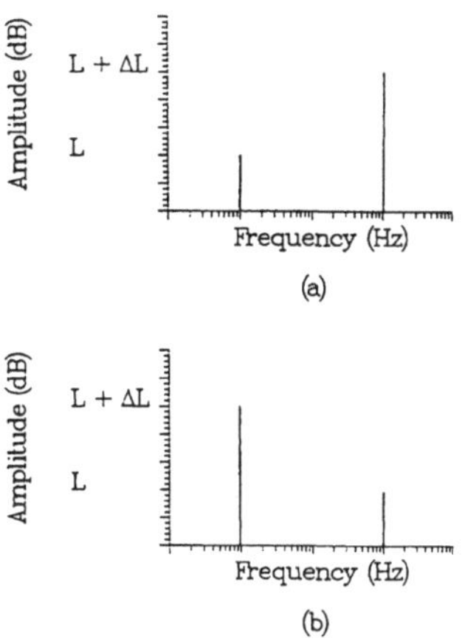

Fig. 5 Frequency spectrum of two-tone stimuli. (a) Two-tone complex with a positive spectral slope. (b) Two-tone complex with a negative spectral slope.

4.1 Narrowband signals

The results of Fig. 2 (for bandwidths smaller than 3 ST), Fig. 3 and Fig. 4 (except for the two points with centre frequencies of 125 and 250 Hz in Fig. 4) are obtained with noise bands or two-tone complexes having bandwidths that fall into a single critical band (according to conventional estimates). However, only if the signal's bandwidth is smaller than 1 ST, can these results can be accounted for with the EWAIF model of Feth (1974). This model assumes that a change in spectral shape is perceived as a change in pitch — which is in agreement with the reported perceptual cue. This model is applicable only if the signal is processed as a whole; hence, at bandwidths larger than 1 ST, the signal obviously excites more than one band, and between-channel processing will also take place.

4.2 Broadband signals

If the signal's bandwidth is larger than 1 ST, more frequency channels are excited. One may then try to describe the results with multi-channel models. Filter-bank models of e.g. Plomp (1976) or Durlach, Braida and Ito (1986) state that the sensitivities in the individual channels add in a vector-like manner. Hence, every spectral change occurring in a stimulated channel generally improves detectability. If the auditory system were to use all information regarding changes in the spectrum of a signal — as is assumed in these filter-bank models — one would expect (if ΔL is kept fixed) a greater sensitivity for noise bands as the bandwidth increases, since more frequency channels become available, and, at the same time, the changes in the outermost bands remain constant. Hence, if the bandwidth increases, the threshold should decrease. Fig. 2, however, does not display this trend for bandwidths beyond the critical bandwidth. This suggests that either the auditory system does not use all information with equal weight (i.e. the variance of the internal noise differs between the individual bands), or that the information of the different critical bands is not combined optimally, probably in the sense that remote bands are less comparable. Even both suggestions may be valid. With two-tone complexes, a threshold independent from bandwidth would indicate that comparison between the outputs of near-by frequency channels goes equally well as comparison between remote channels. Hence, the amount of increase in threshold with the two-tone complexes is a direct measure of the ability of the auditory system to compare the output of different frequency channels. Results plotted in Fig. 2 show that such an increase indeed exists. The threshold increase with noise bands is almost identical to that of two-tone complexes, which makes it plausible that, while processing the noise bands, *changes in only two regions of the spectrum are used in the discrimination process* ("two-region" model). Obviously, the auditory system uses those two regions that give the most reliable information. In this case they are situated most probably at the spectral edges. In that sense the auditory system treats the noise bands in the same way as two-tone complexes. However, since the increase in threshold is slightly less for noise bands, compared to that for two-tone complexes, it is possible that the auditory system uses more than only the spectral edges.

5. DISCUSSION

In other experiments by Versfeld and Houtsma (1991), thresholds of changes in the spectral slope of multi-tone complexes were measured as a function of the number of components, where the distance between two adjacent components remained 1 ST (as illustrated in Fig. 6). They did not use a roving intensity level. Results are plotted in Fig. 7 as filled circles. Results obtained with two-tone complexes, (also measured without a roving level) are included in Fig. 7 as open circles. It was found that for bandwidths beyond the critical band an increase in the number of components did not produce a decrease in threshold, as would be expected from a multi-channel model, but that threshold instead remained constant. Moreover, results resemble the ones obtained with two-tone complexes, suggesting that only the outermost components play a role. Only at the largest bandwidths, thresholds of multi-tone complexes are smaller than those of the two-tone complexes, suggesting influence (*viz.* information) of components lying inside the complex.

Bernstein and Green (1987) reported a series of experiments where the detection of complex, broadband changes in a flat 21-component spectrum was studied. They found that these results could be accounted for by a model stating that "detection of a change in spectral shape occurs when the addition of the signal to the flat multicomponent background produces a reliable and sufficient difference in level between only two regions of the spectrum".

A typical profile-analysis experiment is the measurement of the detectability of an increment of the amplitude in one component of an otherwise flat multicomponent spectrum. The model of Bernstein and Green (1987) — which is essentially the same as the present "two-region" model — cannot account for these results, but the so-called COSS analysis by Berg (1990) can. This analysis derives a spectral weight for each component in the spectrum. The weights indicate the degree to which individual components aid the detection of a change in one component of an otherwise flat spectrum. The COSS analysis has only been performed for single-component changes. Therefore, it is very interesting to note what spectral weights

Berg's model would predict with complex, broadband spectral changes. It might well be that the results of this analysis show, too, that only two regions have large weights.

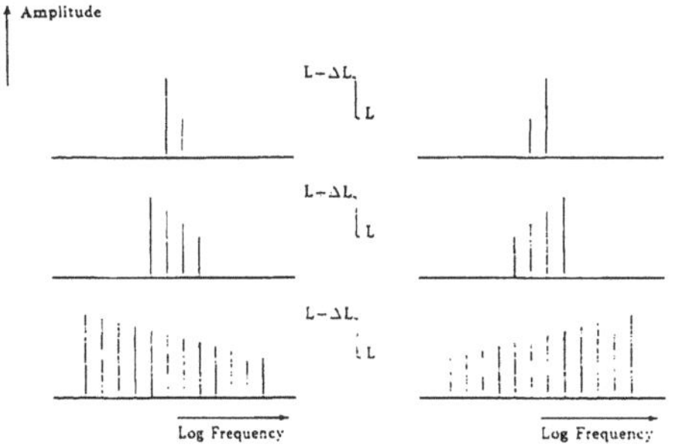

Fig. 6 Frequency spectrum of multi-tone stimuli. Stimuli with 2, 4, and 12 components are plotted. Inter-tone spacing was always 1 ST.

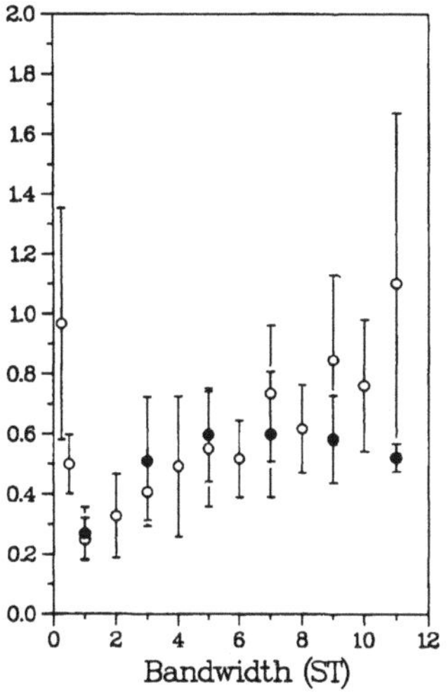

Fig. 7 Thresholds for changes in the spectral slope of multi-tone complexes (•) and two-tone complexes (∘) as a function of bandwidth. Bars indicate the standard deviation between subjects.

Moore *et al.* (1989) performed experiments in which the detectability of a peak in an otherwise flat broadband noise band was measured. They found that threshold (i.e. the difference in spectrum level between the peak and the noise band) hardly depended on the peak's bandwidth. Though Moore *et al.* could predict these results with an energy-detector model having a very low efficiency, they can also be explained easily with the present "two-region" model. Here, one region is situated at the peak, the other at the noise band.

Farrar *et al.* (1987) studied the discriminability of two speech-like noise spectra, embedded in long-term averaged speech noise. They tried to match their results with the filter-bank model of Durlach *et al.* (1986), but found very large values for the internal-noise variance. Inspection of their Fig. 6 shows that, if presented at threshold, the two speech-like sounds differ from each other only with respect to two regions in the spectrum. The "two-region" model can probably account for these data, at least in a qualitative manner.

In general, results reported in the literature indicate that the discriminability of complex broadband changes is much less efficient than would be expected on the basis of thresholds obtained with narrowband changes. This suggests that not all regions of a broadband spectrum are used with equal weight in the discrimination process. In terms of a filter-bank model, one can view this as a set of frequency channels, of which the variance of the internal noise for each channel is different. The larger the channel variance, the smaller the weight in the decision process. In the extreme case, only two channels have a small variance, with the consequence that only two regions are used.

Though the idea that only two regions of a changing complex spectrum are used in the discrimination process is supported by several experiments reported in the literature, one should keep in mind that the idea might hold only for a limited set of stimuli.

Another result is that experiments with broadband two-tone complexes convincingly show that comparison of remote channels is more difficult than comparison of adjacent channels. This might be used to gain more insight into interchannel correlation (Durlach et al., 1986).

6. Summary and Conclusions

This paper reports experiments on the discriminability of changes in the spectral shape of noise bands and two-tone complexes. Results show that threshold behaviour for noise bands is very similar to that for two-tone complexes. Changes in the spectral shape of signals with a bandwidth of 1 ST or less are processed as a whole, and thresholds can be accounted for by Feth's EWAIF model (1974). For bandwidths beyond 1 ST, signals are processed in more than one channel. From the similarity in threshold behaviour it was concluded that the processing of broadband noise bands is analogous to that of two-tone complexes, in the sense that discrimination cues were derived from only two regions of the spectrum, *viz.* the spectral edges. Results also show that the ability to compare the outputs of different critical bands decreases when the bands are more remote.

Acknowledgements

This research was supported by the Netherlands Organization for the Advancement of Pure Research (N.W.O.) through the psychon Foundation, Grant No. 560-262-034. The author is grateful to Jack Cullen, Dik Hermes, Aad Houtsma, Armin Kohlrausch and Tino Trahiotis for their comments on the manuscript and their helpful discussions.

References

Berg, B.G. (1990). Spectral weights in profile listening. *Journal of the Acoustical Society of America*, 88, 758-766.

Bernstein, L.R. and D.M. Green (1987). Detection of simple and complex changes of spectral shape. *Journal of the Acoustical Society of America*, 82, 1587-1592.

Durlach, N.I., L.D. Braida and Y. Ito (1986). Towards a model for discrimination of broadband signals. *Journal of the Acoustical Society of America*, 80, 63-72.

Farrar, C.L., C.M. Reed, Y. Ito, N.I. Durlach, L.A. Delhorne, P.M. Zurek and L.D. Braida (1987). Spectral-shape discrimination. I. Results from normal-hearing listeners for stationary broadband noises. *Journal of the Acoustical Society of America*, 81, 1085-1092.

Feth, L.L. (1974). Frequency discrimination of complex periodic tones. *Perception & Psychophysics*, 15, 375-378.

Green, D.M. (1988). *Profile Analysis*. Oxford University Press, New York.

Green, D.M., Z.A. Onsan and T.G. Forrest (1987). Frequency effects in profile analysis and detecting complex spectral changes. *Journal of the Acoustical Society of America*, 81, 692-699.

Houtsma, A.J.M. (this volume). What do we know about perception of dynamic and complex signals, and how relevant is it to speech perception? This issue.

Moore, B.C.J., S.R. Oldfield and G.J. Dooley (1989). Detection and discrimination of spectral peaks and notches at 1 and 8 kHz. *Journal of the Acoustical Society of America*, 85, 820-836.

Plomp, R. (1976). *Aspects of Tone Sensation*. Academic Press, London.

Versfeld, N.J. (1990). Perception of spectral changes in noise bands with varying bandwidth. *IPO Annual Progress Report*, 25, 23-31.

Versfeld, N.J. and A.J.M. Houtsma (1991). Perception of spectral changes in multi-tone complexes. *The Quarterly Journal of Experimental Psychology*, 43A, 459-479.

Versfeld, N.J. and A.J.M. Houtsma (this volume). Spectral-shape discrimination of two-tone complexes, *Auditory Physiology and Perception*. Y Cazals, L. Demany, K. Horner, eds. (Pergamon Press, Oxford).

Young Infants' Discrimination of Confusable Speech Signals

Francisco Lacerda
Institute of Linguistics
Stockholm University
S - 106 91 Stockholm
Sweden

1. Introduction

Some years ago infant speech perception studies seemed to suggest a "universal discrimination power" allowing infants to handle most of the sound contrasts used both in their ambient languages and even in foreign languages (Jusczyk, 1985a; Studdert-Kennedy, 1986). Given that the infant's ambient language will only use a subset of the universal sound contrasts, the infant, in order to evolve towards adult speech perception, must learn to focus on those meaningful contrasts while ignoring acoustic differences that are non-functional in its mother-tongue. This has been in fact supported by a growing body of empirical data indicating that the infant's perceptual system tunes to the ambient language by the end of its first year of life (e.g. Werker and Tees, 1984; Aslin, Pisoni, Hennessy and Perey, 1981; Eilers, Gavin and Wilson, 1979) or even as early as by six months of age (Kuhl, Williams, Lacerda, Stevens and Lindblom, 1992). Besides, evidence has been found that infants can distinguish the phonotatic patterns of their native languages (Jusczyk, Friederici, Wessels and Svenkerud, 1992). Thus infants are able to attend selectively to their mother-tongues and even focus on relevant contrasts that may be signaled by motherese (Fernald and Kuhl, 1987; Kelmer Nelson, Hirsh-Pasek, Jusczyk, and Wright Cassidy, 1989).

This, along with the infant's ability to discriminate among speech-like sounds, has often been interpreted as granting the infant a general proclivity for speech perception and even a competence similar to that of the adult. Generally, little notice has been taken of the possibility that young infants and adults might be treating the speech signal in distinct ways but nevertheless produce similar discrimination results. In fact, because the goal has been to investigate the infants' discrimination of speech sounds, the stimuli used in most studies have been realistic synthetic replicas of natural utterances, therefore usually contrasting in several acoustic cues (for instance burst, VOT, and formant transitions). Thus, while demonstrating that infants discriminate among various types of speech utterances (e.g. Bertoncini, Bijeljac-Babic, Blumstein and Mehler, 1987), these experiments cannot answer the more stringent issue of whether infants treat the stimuli as speech (in an adult sense) or rather evidence discrimination because they attend to general acoustic differences among the stimuli (Jusczyk, Pisoni, Walley and Murray, 1980; Jusczyk, Rosner, Reed and Kennedy, 1989).

The present study attempted to tap into the possible basis for infant discrimination of speech-like stimuli by directly equating infant and adult discrimination of sounds that contrast along single acoustic dimensions. The rationale was that contrasts along a single phonetic dimension, which suffice for adult categorical judgement and discrimination, may not be salient enough to enable discrimination by the young infant (Eilers, Morse, Gavin and Oller, 1981; Jusczyk et al., 1989). Hence, if adults can perceive speech contrasts conveyed by single acoustic cues but infants cannot, that may indicate that infants will have to establish functional categories of speech sounds prior to being able to recognize isolated acoustic cues that constitute the natural contrasts.

The focus of this study was therefore the infant's discrimination of complex speech-like stimuli which differed along a single acoustic cue. Specifically, it addressed the question of how discrimination based on a single formant distinction (F_2) was affected when the acoustic cue was presented both as a time-varying formant transition and as a shift in a static formant. In addition, the study was designed to assess possible ontogenetic changes in the infant's discrimination of this type of stimuli and to compare infant and adult performance for the same stimuli.

2. METHOD

2.1 Stimuli

Pairs of stimuli were generated by introducing a fixed F_2 difference between the stimuli in each of the pairs. Across pairs, the F_2 shift was applied to either a static F_2 formant (producing a contrast between two vowels) or to the onset (or offset) of F_2 formant transitions (producing a CV (or VC) contrast). Thus, while keeping, in a sense, a constant acoustic difference, the dynamic characteristics of its occurrence were systematically varied[1].

Two additional pairs of vowels were created - an [ae]/[ae] and a [i]/[u] pair - to assess the limits of infant discrimination performance. The first one was a control pair providing a reference for the statistical analysis. The second assures that infants display the expected behavior when the contrast is large enough.

The stimuli were generated on-line by a hardware serial speech synthesizer (VOX-PC, research version, INFOVOX) and included neither bursts nor aspiration noises. The stimuli in each pair were loudness-equalized with reference to a schwa vowel. The level of this reference vowel was 65 dB(A) at the subject's location.

Vowel stimuli

The formant frequencies and durations of the vowel stimuli are shown in Table I.

CV and VC stimuli

The CV syllables were obtained by introduction of formant transitions through adequate control of the temporal evolution of F_1 and F_2. The transitions were 50 ms long (for 90% sweep) exponential

Table I

Vowel	F_1	F_2	F_3	F_4	DR
[i]	282	2262	3108	3489	200
[u]	308	634	2397	3489	200
[æ]	565	1744	2467	3200	200
V4_4	733	1099	2467	3200	80
V4_6	733	1467	2467	3200	80

F1, F2, F3, F4 expressed in Hz
DR expressed in ms

trajectories in the frequency *vs* time domain. The total duration of these stimuli was 100 ms. Their maximum slopes were at CV or VC boundaries and the minimum was at the target vowels.

The initial and final formant frequencies are illustrated in Fig. 1 for the CV-stimuli. F_3 and F_4 have no formant transitions (F_3=2467Hz and F_4=3200Hz). Note that the stimuli differ only in F_2. The VC-stimuli are the reverse of of the CV-stimuli.

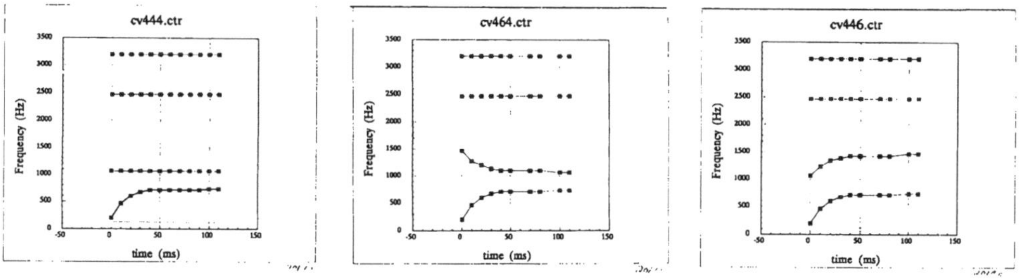

Fig. 1 Stylized spectrograms of the CV stimuli. The stimuli can only be distinguished by their F2 trajectories. The F2 frequency at CV464 onset is equal to the vowel's F2 of CV446.

2.2 Subjects

Adults

A labeling test was carried out with a reference group of eight adult normal hearing native Swedes. Four other adult subjects participated in a discrimination test.

Infants

The subjects for this experiment were recruited by advertising at the Barnavårdcentraler (BVC, Child Health Centers) in the Stockholm area. A total of 87 infants, whose ages varied from 16 to 230 days on the day of their first visit, participated in the study. A pragmatic five-month-old limit was imposed due to the characteristics of the experimental procedure.

2.3 Procedure

Adults

Adult identification

The stimuli were presented in random order, via headphones, and transcribed orthographically. The subjects used a computer keyboard to assign open-class labels to the stimuli.

Adult discrimination

The test was carried out under conditions that were assumed to be similar to those experienced by the infant. However, instead of using a habituation task, the adult stimuli were presented in pairs that included both target and control stimuli. To divert the adult subjects' attention during the test, subjects were requested to play a labyrinth game (BRIO, No. 35310) while performing the task. Subjects were instructed to look up to the video camera when they heard a pair of different stimuli. An experimenter, outside the booth, monitored the video screen and registered the subject's responses. The pairs of stimuli were presented with a 2 second ISI and a total of 40 stimuli pairs (three repetitions per pair) were used.

Infants

Environment

The experiments were carried out in a dimly lit studio. The infants sat on an AKTA/RÖMER "Baby Safe" chair and faced a colorful and highlighted doll, intended to keep the infant's concentration during the test session. Above the doll a loudspeaker (JBL pro III) and a video camera (HITACHI, VM-S83 E) were mounted.

One parent sat in the studio with the infant to keep it calm and make sure that the pacifier was held in place. The parent listened to classical music[2] presented through circumaural headphones and sat quietly on the infant's right side, slightly behind the infant's chair and outside the infant's visual field. If the infant became fussy, the experimenter instructed the parent to establish passive physical contact with the infant by laying a hand on the infant's stomach. This procedure usually calmed the infant, but when it did not help the experiment was interrupted.

The High-Amplitude Sucking procedure

The experiments were carried out using a traditional habituation/deshabituation paradigm in an operant conditioning high-amplitude sucking (HAS) technique (Siqueland and DeLucia, 1969; Eimas, Siqueland, Jusczyk and Vigorito, 1971; Jusczyk, 1985b). The HAS procedure used in this study was completely implemented by a computer program and the stimuli generated on-line by a hardware speech synthesis board (PC-VOX, INFOVOX, Sweden).

To make sure that the infants had sufficient opportunity to listen to the pre-shift stimuli, computations for the shift criterion were not started until a minimum of 20 HAS/minute was achieved. The shift criterion was a 75% decrease of the HAS frequency during two consecutive minutes, relative to the previously observed maximum. The pre-shift sucking frequency was, however, restricted to a minimum of 10 HAS. Data from subjects whose sucking frequency was below this value was not taken into consideration. The dependent variable used in this study was the change in sucking frequency between the first post-shift minute and the last pre-shift minute. Most of the studies referred to here use instead a two-minute interval, since infants often take a while to initiate their post-shift response[3].

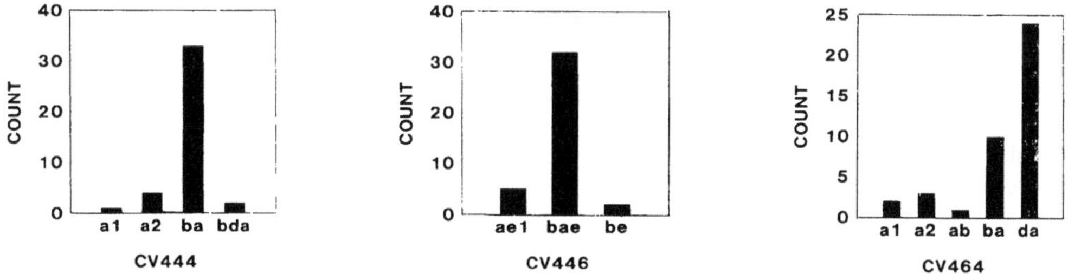

Fig. 2 Adult labeling. Each graph shows the actual labels attributed to a given stimulus. The long vowels that were indicated by two repeated vowels (e.g. aa) were replaced by a single vowel followed by : (e.g. a:).

Experiment design

The experiment was carried out in a repeated measures design, attempting to use each subject as his own control. To control for possible learning and developmental effects, the series of four experimental conditions were counterbalanced into 24 different sequences (test programs), corresponding to all the permutations of the four pairs of target stimuli. The "no-change" control condition was inserted in the beginning, middle or end of each individual program. The [i]/[u] contrast was always tested in the first session. To balance for possible effects of within pair presentation order, two infants were assigned to each of the programs. One of the infants was exposed to *stimulus 1* during the pre-shift period and to *stimulus 2* during the post-shift period whereas the other listened to *stimulus 2* during pre-shift and to *stimulus 1* during the post-shift period.

To run the 203 successful experiments reported here, it was necessary to carry out 328 experimental sessions (10% refused or cried, 11% fell asleep during the experiment, 10% did not wake up to begin the session, had bowel movements or vomited, 7% experimental errors).

3. Results

3.1 Adults

Identification test

Adult labeling indicates that the subjects' judgements were mainly guided by vowel quality differences (Fig. 2). Note the confusion between the /b/ and /d/ judgments ocurring for cv444 and cv464 which differed in their F_2 transitions. Henceforth the stimuli will be referred to by their most frequent adult labels, as shown in Table II.

Table II

v4_4	-> [A]	v4_6	-> [a]	
cv444	-> [bA]	cv464	-> [dA]	cv446 -> [ba]
vc444	-> [Ab]	vc464	-> [Ad]	

Discrimination tests

The bars in Fig. 3 indicate the average number of "different" judgements for each of the stimulus pairs. The maximum average score for any pair was 3, indicating unanimous "different" judgment.

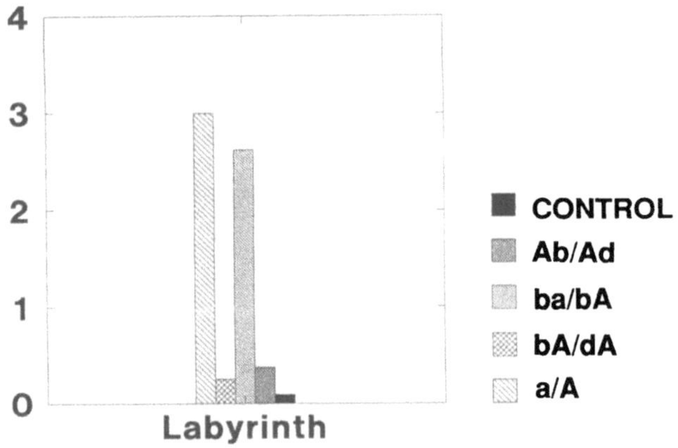

Fig. 3 Adult discrimination results.

3.2 Infants

Age ranges

Table III displays the distribution of ages vs experimental conditions, on which the present results are based.

Pairwise discrimination results

The average sucking differences between the first post-shift minute and the last pre-shift minute are displayed in Fig. 4.

Effect of design variables

The major consequence of the exposure to repeated measures was a progressive reduction in the number of completed experiments. A constant factor of 0.77 roughly accounts for the drop in the number of completed experiments between two consecutive sessions. The primary reasons for the drop-off were the parent's difficulty in allocating time for all the sessions, sickness of siblings, parents or subjects, and infants who became too mature for the HAS-technique. No significant differences were observed when the results were analysed in terms of matched pairs of subjects, nor between the groups reported as "pacifier" vs "non-pacifier" users. Furthermore, no systematic variation could be observed within subjects as the result of the exposure to the repeated measures. Hence, given that the differences observed in the post- to pre-

Table III Age is expressed in months. Columns A to X show conditions:

***A** = [A]/[a]; **B** = [bA]/[dA]; **C** = [bA]/[ba];*
***D** = [Ab]/[Ad]; **K** = [i]/[u]; **X** = [ae]/[ae];*

The table shows the number of experiments carried out for each of the conditions, with infants grouped by age groups.

Age	A	B	C	D	K	X	Total
Below 3	6	6	10	7	39	7	75
Age 3	10	12	8	12	12	10	64
Above 3	11	7	9	11	17	9	64
Total	27	25	27	30	68	26	203

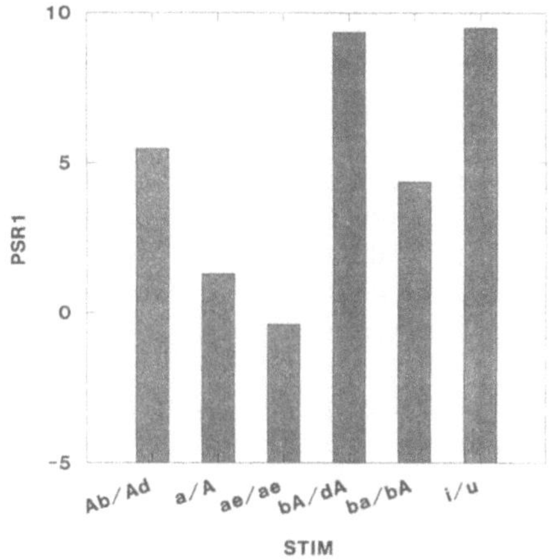

Fig. 4 Recovery from sucking under different conditions.

shift sucking frequencies could not be attributed to the repeated measures assessment and that missing cases impaired the full repeated measures analysis, the data will be treated as a set of *independent* measures[4].

Global discrimination results

The analysis of the post-shift recovery was made according to the structure displayed in Table 4. A weak tendency for differences across experimental conditions [$F(5,185)=1.890$, $p < 0.098$] was found, but there were no main age effects [$F(2,185)=0.133$, $p < 0.876$], nor any significant interaction between age and experimental condition [$F(10,185)$, $p < 0.286$]. However, a *post-hoc* comparison of each experimental condition with the control condition indicated significant differences for i/u [$F(1,185)=5.703$, $p < 0.018$] and for bA/dA [$F(1,185)=4.340$, $p < 0.039$]. None of the other comparisons with the control condition yielded significant differences (a/A, $F(1,185)=0.042$, $p < 0.837$; bA/ba, $F(1,185)=1.384$ $p < 0.241$; Ab/Ad, $F(1,185)=2.045$ $p < 0.154$). Contrasts of age subgroups within each condition relative to the control condition revealed a significant difference within the bA/dA group. Infants up to three months of age successfully discriminated bA from dA [$F(1,185)=8.675$, $p < 0.004$], but the older subjects did not [$F(1,185)=0.040$, $p < 0.843$].

4. DISCUSSION

Only two main aspects of the present results will be discussed here. One is the general difference observed between adult and infant results. The other is the indication of an age-related change in the infant's discrimination of these synthetic CV-syllables.

Adult subjects appear to have discriminated the stimuli on the basis of vowel differences. In contrast, they performed poorly when the acoustic difference was located at the point of maximum transition rate. The adult results may be accounted for by sensory smearing of the formant transitions (Lacerda, 1987a,b) and the ambiguity introduced by the static F3 and F4 formants. The discrimination pattern displayed by the infants is basically the opposite. Except for the large [i]/[u] contrast, which is in agreement with other infant studies (e.g. Kuhl, 1979; Trehub, 1973), the infants did not show evidence of vowel discrimination.

Interestingly, Jusczyk, Bertoncini, Bijeljac-Babic, Kennedy and Mehler's (1990) two-month-old and even newborn subjects could discriminate a [ba]/[b^] contrast in a modified HAS-paradigm. The acoustic difference in the contrast used by Jusczyk et al. was approximately equal to that of the present [ba]/[bA], when expressed in the tonotopical Bark scale. Otherwise, Jusczyk et al.'s stimuli provide a contrast along the high/low dimension instead of the current front/back. Thus, failure to discriminate along the front/back dimension should not, in principle, be attributed to lack of resolution in the infant's auditory system. Strictly, however, that cannot be taken for granted. Thus to address the issue directly, an additional experiment was set up in our laboratory in which a high-low contrast was created by applying to F_1 the same shift (in Bark) that had been used with F_2. The preliminary results seem to replicate Jusczyk et al.'s (1990) and support the notion of perceptual asymmetry between contrasts along the high/low and the front/back dimension (Lacerda, in preparation), at least when the present [A] vowel is used as a reference. If this asymmetry proves to be stable, it may be explained in acoustic terms by the fact that contrasts along the high/low dimension are emphasized by the larger concomitant changes in intensity, than those associated with corresponding front/back contrasts (Fant, 1960). Adult listeners compensate, however, for this variation and perceive vocal effort instead of physical vowel intensity (Ladefoged, 1967). Infants will have to learn to disregard intensity fluctuations as they acquire their ambient language. A serious problem with this explanation is to account for how the infant disregards intensity variation caused by non-phonetic variables like the speaker-to-listener distance. It is possible that one of the first equivalence problems faced by the young infant is just to learn how to disregard spurious intensity differences. Unfortunately, this avenue does not seem to have been pursued since intensity is traditionally one of the variables that is held constant as it is known to provide extra cues to the infants.

Regarding discrimination of the [bA]/[dA] contrast, the results indicated an advantage of the infants relative to the adults. In general, infant discrimination performance seems to improve with the dynamics in the stimuli but it only reached significance for the initial [b]/[d] contrast. It appears that fast formant transitions draw the infant's attention. It is not clear what causes the drop in the discrimination performance observed for the older infants (after three months of age). One possibility is that it is caused by an attentional shift, since by this age infants start displaying a qualitatively different pattern of interaction with their environment along with marked changes in their motor schemes (von Hofsten, 1986). Thus, at about this time the infant may start to process the [bA]/[dA] stimuli in a more adult-like fashion, i.e. lose its capacity to discriminate them on a more auditory basis and getting confounded by their ambiguous phonetic characteristics. The present decrement in the discrimination of the initial consonant contrast is similar to the picture provided by Jusczyk et al.'s (1989) and Eilers et al.'s (1981) results: while the younger infants tested by Jusczyk's team were able to perceive voicing contrasts signaled by single acoustic cues, Eiler's six-month-olds could not discriminate a voicing contrast cued by VOT differences only. However, while the discrepancy between Jusczyk's and Eiler's results might be attributed to procedural differences, the present drop in discrimination cannot. Yet, as pointed out by Jusczyk et al. (1989), "It is not obvious why infants should show decreased sensitivity to contrasts that *do* continue to appear in their native language environment" (p. 1748).

Clearly, additional research is needed in this area, but the present results seem to go against the simplistic notion that infants discriminate speech "even better" than adults. Infants and adults seem to attend to different aspects (maybe in different ways) of the speech signal. Presumably infants need more than single acoustic cues to perform discrimination of speech sounds, but their natural languages (and mothereses) surely provide enough redundancy to help them focus on the relevant differences.

Acknowledgments

The research upon which this paper was based was possible thanks to the cooperation of the parents, BVC personnel, and the support of The Bank of Sweden Tercentenary Foundation (Dnr 90-0150). The data collection would not have been possible without Ulla Sundberg's excellent collaboration.

Notes

1. Because these synthetic stimuli will be labeled by adult listeners, they are referred to by codes until the adult labels are known.

2. Pop music is in fact a more effective continuously masking music since it does not have so large and frequent intensity contrasts as classical music

3. A complete evaluation of the consequences of these different measures on the current results is being prepared for publication in the research reports from the Institute of Linguistics, University of Stockholm (PERILUS).

4. Treating the results as if they were independent measures has the advantage of making full use of all the collected data, which otherwise would be severely reduced by deleting the cases with missing cells in the results matrix. The failure to observe internal data structure when all the possible interactions between sessions were tested, legitimatizes the assumption of independence between the consecutive measurements.

References

Aslin, R., Pisoni, D., Hennessy, B., and Perey, A. (1981). Discrimination of voice onset time by human infants: New findings and implications for the effect of early experience, *Child Development*, 52, 1135-1145.

Bertoncini, J., Bijeljac-Babic, R., Blumstein, S., and Mehler, J. (1987). Discrimination in neonates of very short VCs, *JASA*, 82, 31-37.

Eilers, R., Gavin, W., and Wilson, W. (1979). Linguistic experience and phonemic perception in infancy: A cross-linguistic study, *Child Development*, 50, 14-18.

Eilers, R., Morse, P., Gavin, W., and Oller, D.K. (1981). Discrimination of voice onset time in infancy, *JASA*, 70, 955-965.

Eimas, P., Siqueland, E., Jusczyk, P., and Vigorito, J. (1971). Speech perception in infants, *Science*, 171, 303-306.

Fant, G. (1960). *Acoustic Theory of Speech Production*, Mouton, The Hague.

Fernald, A. and Kuhl, P. (1987). Acoustic determinants of infant preference for motherese speech, *Infant Behavior and Development*, 10, 279-293.

Hofsten, C. von (1986). The early development of the manual system, in Lindblom, B. and Zetterström, R. (Eds.), *Precursors of Early Speech*, Stockton, New York, 175-188.

Jusczyk, P. (1985a). On characterizing the development of speech perception, in: Mehler, J. and Fox, R. (Eds.), *Neonate Cognition: Beyond the Blooming Buzzing Confusion*, Erlbaum, New Jersey, 199-229.

Jusczyk, P. (1985b). The high-amplitude sucking technique as a methodological tool in speech perception research, in: Gottlieb, G. and Krasnegor, N. (Eds.), *Measurement of audition and vision in the first year of postnatal life: A methodological overview*, Albex, Norwood, N.J., 195-222.

Jusczyk, P., Pisoni, D., Walley, A., and Murray, J. (1980). Discrimination of relative onset time of two-component tones by infants, *JASA*, 67, 262-270.

Jusczyk, P., Rosner, B., Reed, M., and Kennedy, L. (1989). Could temporal order differences underlie 2-month-olds' discrimination of English voicing contrasts?, *JASA*, 85, 1741-1749.

Jusczyk, P., Bertoncini, J., Bijeljac-Babic, R., Kennedy, L., and Mehler, J. (1990). The role of attention in speech perception by young infants, *Cognitive Development*, 5, 265-286.

Jusczyk, P., Friederici, A., Wessels, J., and Svenkerud (1992). *Infants' recognition of foreign versus native language words*, in preparation, (personal communication).

Kelmer Nelson, D., Hirsh-Pasek, K, Jusczyk, P., and Wright Cassidy, K. (1989). How the prosodic cues in motherese might assist language learning, *Journal of Child Language*, 16, 53-68.

Kuhl, P. (1979). Speech perception in early infancy: Perceptual constancy for spectrally dissimilar vowel categories, *JASA*, 66, 1668-1679.

Kuhl, P., Williams, K., Lacerda, F., Stevens, K., and Lindblom, B. (1991). Linguistic experience alters phonetic perception in infants by 6 months age, *Science*, 255, 606-608.

Lacerda, F. (1987a). Effects of stimulus dynamics on frequency discrimination, in: Schouten, M.E.H. (Ed.), *The Psychophysics of Speech Perception*, Dordrecht, Martinus Nijhoff, 250-257.

Lacerda, F. (1987b). Effects of peripheral auditory adaptation on the discrimination of speech sounds, PERILUS VI, Stockholm University, Stockholm.

Ladefoged, P. (1967). *Three Areas of Experimental Phonetics*, Oxford University Press.

Siqueland, E. and DeLucia, C. (1969). Visual reinforcement of non-nutritive sucking in human infants, *Science*, 165, 1144-1146.

Studdert-Kennedy, M. (1986). Sources of variability in early speech development, in: Perkell, J. and Klatt, D. (Eds), *Invariance and Variability in Speech Processes*, Erlbaum, New Jersey, 58-84.

Trehub, S. (1973). Infant's sensitivity to vowel and tonal contrasts, *Developmental Psychology*, 9, 91-96.

Werker, J. and Tees, R. (1984). Cross-language speech perception: Evidence for perceptual reorganization during the first year of life, *Infant Behavior and Development*, 7, 49-63.

Auditory Analysis of Speech Gestures

Jean-Luc Schwartz,
Denis Beautemps,
Yonnel Arrouas,
Pierre Escudier
Institut de la Communication Parlée
U.R.A. CNRS n°368; INP-Université Stendhal
INPG, 46 Av. Félix-Viallet, 38031 Grenoble Cedex France

1. Towards an Articulatory Psychophysics: from Gibson to Repp... Passing by Marr and Poggio

In his contribution – and providing some kind of introduction – to our first meeting, Bruno Repp suggested that "the role of psychophysics in understanding speech perception" (Repp's contribution title) ought to be centered around

> an *articulatory psychophysics* based on the realization that speech is constituted of motor events (...). Its goal would be to describe the lawful relationships between a talker's articulations and a listener's perception or imitation of them. A first step in this enterprise would be to look at the speech signal not in terms of its acoustic properties, but in terms of the articulatory information that it conveys (Repp, 1987, p.19 - his underlining).

In an effort to support Repp's proposal, let us briefly examine how Gibson's heritage led to quite different histories in the fields of audition and vision. Gibson considered perception as recovery of the causes of the sensation, with a neural system able to "resonate" to the invariance imposed by the physical objects that produced the stimulus (Gibson, 1966). The first influence of this conception in audition is found in the Motor Theory of speech perception (Liberman and Mattingly, 1985). However, other considerations about the biological specificity of language and the fact that speech is both *perceived* and *produced* led Liberman to propose that *speech is special*, which made any work on auditory perception in general irrelevant for the understanding of speech perception. More recently, and in a more straightforward line from Gibson, Fowler defended a direct realist theory of event perception (Fowler, 1986). In her mind, the goal of auditory perception in general is supposed to be the recovery of the physical sources of the sound, speech perception being not specific in this respect (Fowler, 1990). However, not much is said by Fowler about *how* the recovery of causes could be realized by the auditory system. In the field of vision, Marr, in his famous book about vision (1982), acknowledged Gibson's view on human perception as quite deep and thoughtful. But he then insisted on the fact that recovery of physical sources from stimuli had to be considered as a true – and difficult – problem of *information processing*, needing all that is necessary in a computational framework, namely processing, representations, definition of a suitable architecture, etc. More recently, Poggio, a close colleague of Marr, proposed considering low-level perception in general as an *inversion* (from stimuli to objects, while physics deals with direct processes from objects to stimuli), and he noticed that inverse problems are generally "ill-posed" – which means that the solution of the inverse problem is not unique, and does not vary continuously with the input –, and hence that they must be *regularized* by adding *constraints* about the general properties of the objects to be recovered (Poggio, 1984).

Marr's processing and Poggio's constraints seem to us to provide the basic concepts for dealing with Repp's program, with an aim to understand both *biological principles of information processing* in the auditory system and *general properties of speech objects* coming from the fact that they are the product of a vocal tract and the consequences of articulatory gestures.

2. An Auditory Framework for Dealing with Speech Gestures

If a psychophysics of speech perception indeed exists, Ludmilla Chistovich is probably one of the pioneers and most influential researchers in this field. The series of works realized in the Pavlov Institute of Leningrad in the 70s led her to propose a basic architecture for auditory processing of speech sounds, with one system specialized in temporal processing and detection of acoustic events, and the other continuously delivering various analyses about the spectral content of the input (Chistovich et al., 1976; Chistovich, 1980). The system specialized in event detection could be based on so-called "phasic" units in the central nervous system, namely "on" and "off" units responding only to quick increases and decreases of the neural excitation in a given spectral region. The system specialized in spectral processing would need so-called "tonic" units responding continuously to a given stimulus, and then enabling precise statistics and computations about the variations of excitation depending on the characteristic frequency. This can be summarized in the schema of Fig. 1 – giving a very simplified idea of Chistovich's theory of speech perception – where the output of the phasic system would both provide the decoder with information about time ("when?", instants t_i) and control the flow of output of the tonic system so that spectra computed around the position of detected events would also feed the decoder ("what?", spectra S_i).

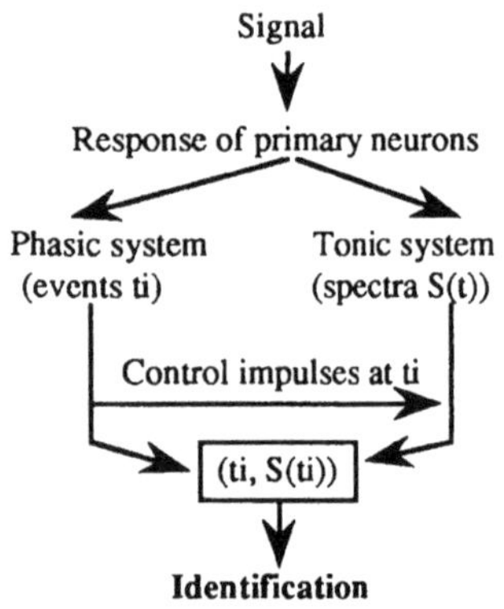

Fig. 1 Chistovich's basic architecture

This framework, though obviously simplified, can be defended on a double basis.

1. It receives physiological support with the differentiation between phasic and tonic cells in the cochlear nucleus, respectively with "on" cells on the one hand and "chopper" and "primary-like" cells on the other: see Young (1984), and Sachs et al. (this volume).
2. It is attractive from a functional point of view, considering the ability of human beings to be both good at time processing and spectral processing of sounds, in spite of the classical limitation provided by ($\Delta f.\Delta t$=constant). In fact, Fig. 1 provides a rather extreme and somewhat more sophisticated use of the classical double resolution in sonagram analysis with narrow or large bands.

However, our strategy – looking for auditory recovery of speech gestures – led us to slightly modify this architecture (Fig. 2). Indeed, we think that a key problem for future research about the auditory processing of speech concerns the *analysis of acoustic trajectories* (see Houtsma, this volume) considered as the surface (observable) consequences of articulatory gestures that obey general laws of human gestures, such as economy principles (leading to coarticulation; see Jordan, 1989; Bailly et al., 1991), control by dynamic systems (Kelso et al., 1986; Salzman and Munhall, 1989; Perrier et al., 1989), control of timing (Kelso et al., 1986; Abry et al., 1990). Such a system does not only need information about spectra, but also about dynamic parameters such as spectral variation with time, instantaneous and mean speeds, etc, in order to recover the attractors (the targets) of the gestures, be they reached, coarticulated, or not. It should be, as in the case of the tonic system in Fig. 1, under the control of the phasic system detecting articulatory events, since these events fix, in speech production, the sequence of attractors and gestures towards the attractors, and hence define in speech perception the time region in which a given gesture can be analyzed.

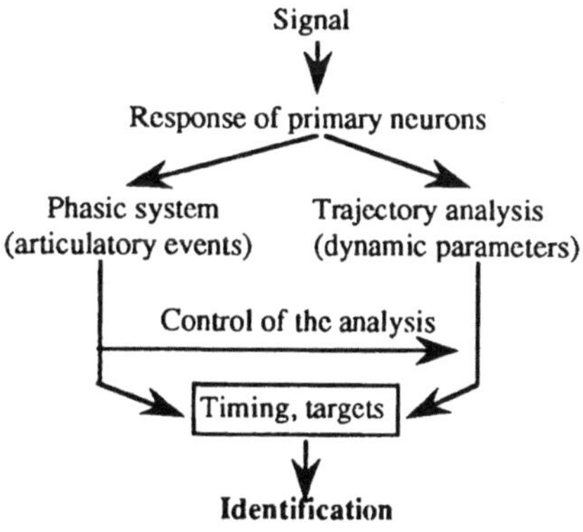

Fig. 2 A modified architecture

Finally, the architecture we propose in Fig. 2 mirrors in a nice way from the perceptual side a possible architecture for gesture control on the production side, with its two main components, namely *timing* and *targets*. Let us now enter each of the two sub-systems of this figure in some more detail.

3. Modelling the Phasic System: A Simulation and some Physiological, Psychological and Functional Support

3.1 A first modelling basis

Delgutte and Kiang (1984) presented very convincing data showing the role of neural adaptation in shaping the responses of primary auditory neurons to consonant-like speech stimuli. From these data, Delgutte (1986) adressed the problem of detecting Chistovich's "events" in a functional model of the auditory nerve with a neural adaptation component, and he obtained interesting results for the processing of French CVCV utterances, based on grouped responses in the low and high characteristic frequency regions (see also Chistovich et al., 1982).

We have been developing for four years a physiologically plausible module for detection of a set of articulatory-acoustic events defined in our laboratory by Abry et al. (1985) for the study of timing control in speech production. These events allow the labelling of every major discontinuity in the speech signal and provide a tool for the articulatory reading of a speech signal (Abry et al., 1990).

The first version of our model was realized by Wu (1990), and is based on a classical linear model of spectral analysis in the cochlea, a new model of neural adaptation in the auditory nerve (Wu, 1989), and a functional model of "on" cells in the ventral cochlear nucleus based on strongly reinforced neural adaptation. We (Wu et al., 1992) showed that this model was able to perform very well in the detection of "on" events (such as onset of voicing, onset of a vocalic state of the vocal tract or onset of burst friction) in CVCV French logatoms, with C a plosive and V a vowel within the set [a, i, u].

3.2 The role of inter-channel grouping mechanisms

A very important topic of modern psychophysics concerns grouping mechanisms and their possible auditory bases. However, Moore (this volume) notes that "the significance of these phenomena for speech perception remains unclear".

Within the series of data about inter-channel grouping and comparisons, our attention was specially raised by the experiment by Green and Forrest (1989), who showed that temporal gaps applied in a number of frequency components far apart from each other were easier to detect when they were applied *synchronously* to all frequency components. In our laboratory, Mizuno showed that the same kind of effect could be observed with short narrow-band pulses in noise: several pulses were easier to detect when they were synchronous (Mizuno et al., submitted). The reason could be, as Green and Forrest suggested for gaps, that individual pulses appear in their respective frequency channels as one more amplitude fluctuation superimposed on random noise fluctuations, which make them difficult to detect one by one, while synchronous pulses emerge as a coherent pattern superimposed on noise fluctuations not coherent from one channel to the other, so that their threshold is lower.

More generally, inter-correlation mechanisms between neighbouring channels in the cochlear nucleus (see Oertel's Type II units: Oertel, 1983; and noise-filtering models based

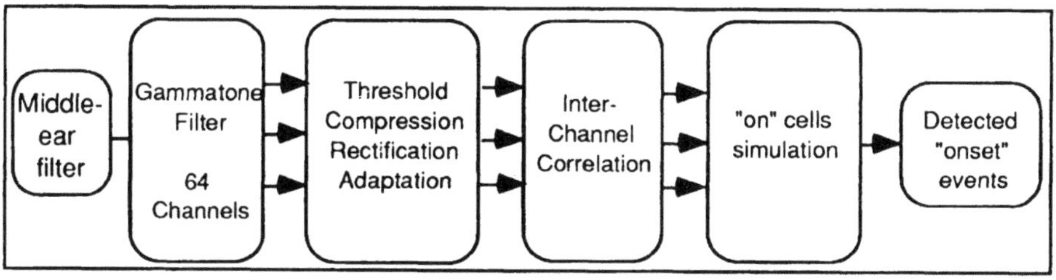

Fig. 3 A model schema for the detection of "onset" events

on inter-correlation, Berthommier, 1989, 1992) could provide an efficient mechanism for enhancing the representation of short wide-band pulses in noise, and thus make the phasic system more efficient. This led us to propose a new version of our model for the phasic system, with an inter-correlation stage at the output of the auditory nerve model (Fig. 3). The representation of such events as plosive bursts in noise is indeed rather robust (see Fig. 4): since the primary fibers have their "signal" response more correlated than their "noise" response, the friction bursts of the [k] (there are often two short close bursts in French for [k] because of its fricative character) appear clearly as vertical lines in Fig. 4d ("on" cells after inter-correlation pre-processing), which makes their detection easier. With the corpus used by Wu et al. (1992) for their study, we showed that the performance of our model of the phasic system was indeed consistently increased in the case of noisy signals thanks to this inter-channel grouping mechanism (Arrouas et al., 1991).

3.3 Phasic Units and Data Reduction

We have already presented the need for a phasic system, leading to what Terhardt (this volume) calls a "contourization" of the stimulus. But some more could be said in relation to one of the key difficulties in using auditory models as inputs to speech recognition systems, namely data reduction (Patterson et al., this volume). Indeed, a data reduction process operating linearly in time is certainly not optimal, considering that the amount of information conveyed by the signal varies with time. In our laboratory, Morris attempted to quantify these variations with classical tools of Information Theory.

He computed Mutual Information between the energy in a given frequency channel within a given time window and the underlying phonetic value of the signal. He was able to show that the amount of information about the place of articulation of an inter-vocalic voiced plosive in French was maximal precisely around two of the acoustic events defined by Abry et al. (1985), namely vocalic voicing offset – consonantal closure – and consonantal friction onset – burst – (Morris et al., 1991). This fact is easily understandable if one considers that closure and burst correspond to the portions of the signal where vocalic influence is smallest and the link between the signal and the articulatory consonantal gesture is strongest (see Stevens and Blumstein, 1978, vs Kewley-Port, 1986, for a strong discussion around auditory

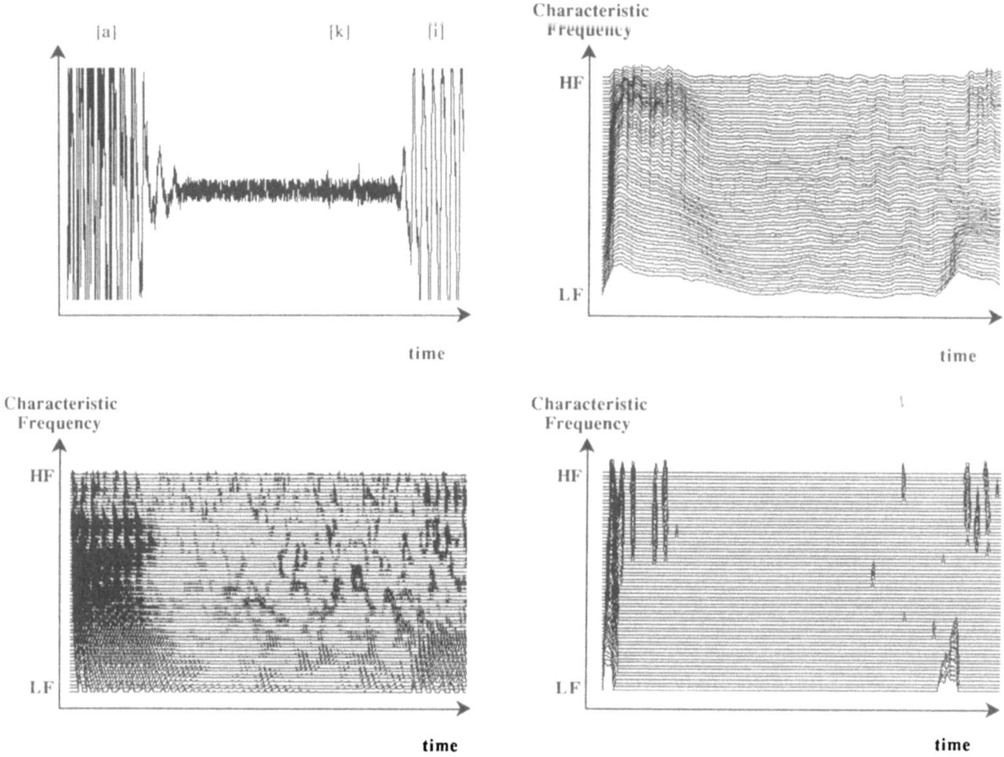

Fig. 4 Application of the model to a [baki] French logatom with noise
(a) a portion of the signal around the plosive [k] ; (b) output of the Gammatone filters
(c) output of the inter-channel correlation stage ; (d) output of the "on" cells stage

and acoustic data relevant to this problem). This seems to show that "on" and "off" units are able to detect "information bottlenecks" that could help to *focus the attention of higher decoding centres according to phonetic information density.*

3.4 Finally,...

In conclusion, our work converged towards a rather efficient model of detection of acoustic events, described in Fig. 3, compatible with well-known physiological mechanisms such as "on" units and intercorrelation mechanisms, supported by psychological data, and potentially important for efficient data reduction and organization of the processing at higher levels. This model has been integrated within the auditory software developed at MRC-APU Cambridge by Holdsworth (Patterson et al., this volume; Holdsworth et al., 1991).

4. Modelling the Trajectory Analysis System: a Case Study of Vowel Reduction

4.1 Vowel targets and vocalic gestures

In a controversial series of papers in the years 1976-1985, Strange, Verbrugge and colleagues at Haskins Laboratories tried to show that vowels uttered by an unknown speaker were easier to identify when inserted in a consonantal context than in isolation (Strange et al., 1976, 1983; Verbrugge et al., 1976). These data, though several times contested (Diehl et al., 1981; Macchi, 1980), seem to show that "dynamic acoustic information distributed over the temporal course of the syllable is utilized regularly by the listener to identify vowels" (Strange et al., 1976, p.213). Moreover, a lot of data about formant variability of vowels depending on context and speech conditions (rate, articulation,...) could not be understood without introducing the parameter *time* into the perceptual decoder.

Our present contribution to the problem of auditory analysis of acoustic trajectories is very preliminary. It consists of an acoustic analysis and search for discriminant parameters in a simple case of vowel reduction. This acoustic analysis should be accompanied in the future by both a psychophysical study (see Di Benedetto, 1989) and a biological simulation. Suffice it to say at present that all the variables considered in the following could be computed by the auditory system, either directly in the phasic-tonic structure of Fig. 1, or by more complex mechanisms of speed estimation, classical in several sensory systems (such as the somesthesic or vestibular systems, Buser and Imbert, 1982; the visual system, see the biological models proposed by Reichard, 1961; Barlow and Lewick, 1965) and very likely to exist also in the auditory system (see the data by Erulkar et al., 1968; Möller, 1974, which show cells presenting an optimal response for a given speed of frequency modulation in the cochlear nucleus or inferior colliculus).

4.2 A case study

The corpus considered in the present study consists of French vowels [a] vs [ɛ] in context [i=i] in the carrier sentences:

"Il y a immédiatement planté sa tente" ("He immediately put up his tent"),
beginning with the phonetic sequence [il**ia**ime], versus

"Il y est immédiatement retourné" ("He immediately came back"),

beginning with the phonetic sequence [il**iɛ**ime]. Two rate conditions (normal vs quick) and two stress conditions (normal vs focus on the studied vowel, e.g. "Il y **a** immédiatement..." or "il y **est** immédiatement...") were used, with three repetitions of each condition uttered by a single speaker, for a total number of 24 stimuli (8 conditions, namely 2 vowels x 2 rates x 2 stress conditions). The interest of this corpus is that it allowed us to consider articulatory gestures from the front unrounded high [i] to a front unrounded, either mid-low [ɛ] or low

[a], hence gestures more or less in the same direction, but with different intentional targets.

In Fig. 5 we have plotted, for each of the 24 logatoms, values of F1 and F2 at the maximally opened position in the trajectory from the first to the second [i], namely the position where F1 is maximal and F2 minimal. We can see in this figure that all acoustic trajectories reach positions that are more or less along the same line, typical of unrounded front vowels for this speaker. Moreover, we notice that, as expected, all three factors affect the reached position, which is pushed towards more open values (increasing F1, decreasing F2) for [a] vs [ɛ], normal vs quick rate and focus vs no focus. We interpret this by assuming that [a] and [ɛ] are respectively associated with more and less open *intentional targets*, while the quick-rate and no-focus conditions increase the trend to *miss the target* and thus to reach a less open position. The fact that some targets are not reached is obvious when one compares with isolated vowels uttered by the same speaker, with [a] from (F1 = 800 Hz, F2 = 1250 Hz) in isolation to (F1 = 400 Hz, F2 = 2250 Hz) in the quick-rate no-focus condition, and [ɛ] from (F1 = 650 Hz, F2 = 1800 Hz) in isolation to (F1 = 350 Hz, F2 = 2400 Hz) in the quick-rate no-focus condition (F3 values are not discriminant in the ambiguous cases). Notice, however, that in perceptual tests listeners could easily recognize [a] in all cases, though [ɛ] was more difficult to identify in the quick-rate conditions.

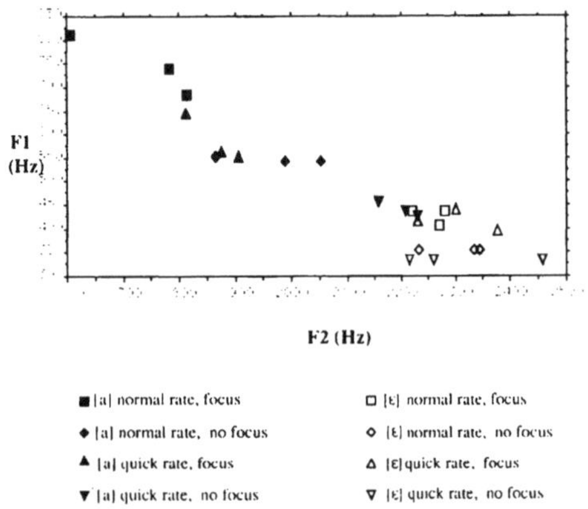

Fig. 5 [a] and [ɛ] reached positions in an (F1,F2) space for various conditions

These data show that the perceptual system uses *dynamic parameters* in order to disambiguate between [a] and [ɛ]. We shall now examine what these parameters could be. For all the logatoms of our corpus, we performed an automatic formant tracking (Feng, 1983) followed by a smoothing of F1, F2, and F3 by cubic spline functions (Marchouk, 1980). We shall only consider smoothed F1 trajectories on the rising portion between first and second [i], namely from initial [i] towards [a] or [ɛ], on which we computed various parameters such as speed, acceleration and plateau.

4.3 Local and mean speeds

The precise range of the transition from initial [i] towards [a] or [ɛ] was defined by applying a threshold criterion to local F1 speed (see Fig. 6). We then computed mean onglide speed during the transition, defined as $(F1_2 - F1_1) / (t_2 - t_1)$, according to the notation of Fig. 6, and maximal speed during the transition, defined as the maximum F1 speed value between t_1 and t_2. Data plotted in Fig. 7 show that (1) neither mean nor maximal speed increase significantly the [a] vs [ɛ] separation – the ambiguity between quick-rate no-focus [a] and focus [ɛ] remains – (2) the correlation between both variables is very high. Though the mathematical interpretation of point (2) is not at all trivial, this interesting fact shows that one or the other parameter could be used indifferently, at least in this case. Notice that the maximum local speed is better defined in the acoustic analysis, since it depends less on the spline smoothing, while the mean speed is likely to be easier to implement in auditory modelling.

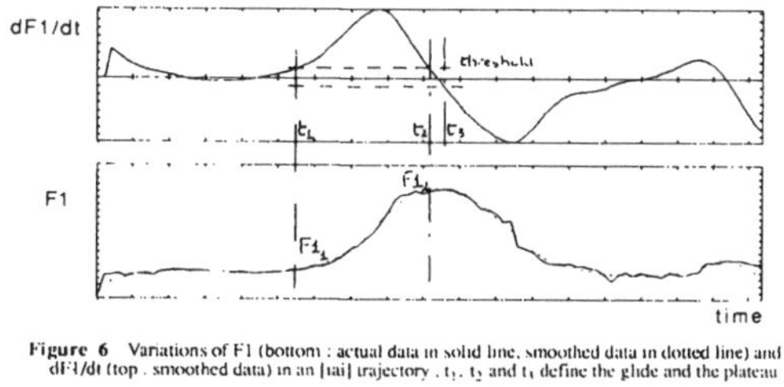

Fig. 6 Variations of F1 (bottom : actual data in solid line, smoothed data in dotted line) and dF1/dt (top : smoothed data) in an [iai] trajectory ; t_1, t_2 and t_3 define the glide and the plateau

4.4 Speed and plateau as two good candidates for dynamic parameters

Direct observation of the formant trajectories revealed that the occurrence of a plateau (flat region between the first transition from initial [i] and the second one towards final [i]) could be an interesting index of the departure between actually reached position and the intentional target: the target is more likely to have actually been reached with a long plateau than with a short one. This led us to think that the duration of the plateau relative to the first transition could be a good complementary parameter for disambiguation.

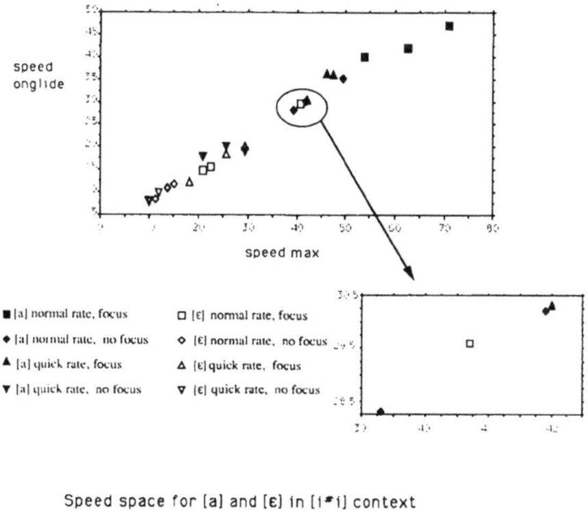

Fig. 7 Variations of max speed and mean speed onglide for [a] and [ε] in various conditions (same symbols as in Fig.5; speeds in Hz per temporal interwindow shift)

We defined the relative duration of the plateau in relation to the whole trajectory from the first [i] to the second vowel, by the formula: $(t_3 - t_2) / (t_3 - t_1)$ (see Fig. 6). As a matter of fact, we see in Fig. 8 that in a speed – plateau space, the separation between [a] and [ε] is much improved, in spite of one [ε] incorrectly classified as [a].

Therefore, we can assume that speed and plateau are two good candidates for the dynamic description of a vowel-to-vowel trajectory. In some sense, they signal the *range to be covered* between the initial position of the trajectory – here, the initial [i] – and the target to be reached: large speeds and small plateaus indicate in a rather complementary manner a distant target. Indeed, we verified that if we add as a third parameter the initial F1 value of the trajectory (around 250 Hz in our corpus), [a] and [ɛ] in context can be correctly grouped respectively with isolated [a] and [ɛ] for which the initial F1 value is equal to the final one (around 800 Hz for [a] and 650 Hz for [ɛ]); the speed is 0 and the pateau covers 100 % of the trajectory.

Such parameters as speeds and plateaus are likely to be good candidates for a general system of trajectory analysis, since they are the first kind of dynamic parameters that could be derived from a simple phasic / tonic architecture ("what?", "when?", "during how much time?",...).

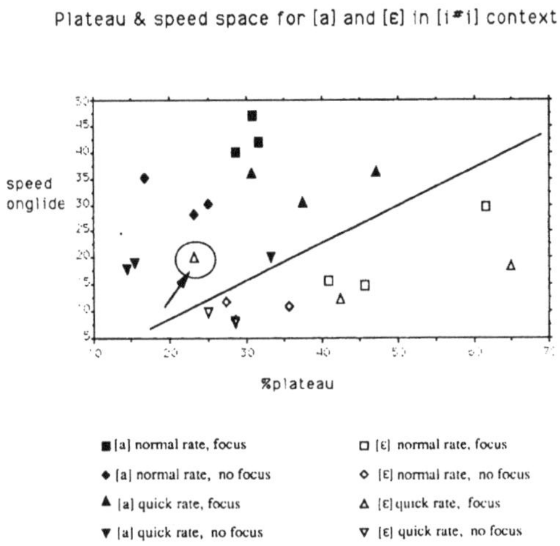

Fig. 8 Variations of plateau relative duration and mean speed onglide for [a] and [ɛ] in various conditions (same symbols as in Fig.5; speeds in Hz per temporal interwindow shift)

4.5 Towards a true inversion system

All present models of speech production introduce at some level the crucial concept of *dynamic systems driven towards an attractor* for the specification of the gesture from one target to the other. Thus, for example, the pilot work from Haskins Laboratories is based on second order dynamics in a target space, from which the articulator dynamics are "backwards" specified by classical principles of inverse dynamics (Saltzman and Munhall, 1989). The work in progress in our laboratory involves a low level of second-order articulatory gestures (mass-spring stiffness-driven model, Perrier et al., 1989) controlled at a higher level by complex optimization principles implemented by a non-linear dynamic system (Bailly et al., 1991). The important point here is that as soon as a gesture is defined as a dynamic system with the target as an attractor, the equation that specifies the dynamic system provides a constant link between cinematic articulatory variables (position x and speed dx/dt) and a limited set of control parameters with values fixed all along the gesture, which determine the gesture and hence the attractor (the "target", reached or not) (Schwartz and Escudier, 1991). Therefore, we feel that in order to take profit of the *lawful variability of speech* (Elman and McClelland, 1986), we perhaps need in the future a true system of trajectory analysis, performing all along the trajectory an estimation of its target from estimations of formant positions and speeds, and finally, after integration of these estimations for stabilization of the final result and noise filtering, making explicit what was the constant target "hidden" in this trajectory. This research program is ambitious, but a number of models and powerful tools now available (see Boë et al., 1992; Laboissière et al., 1991; Perrier et al., 1991) make it not completely unrealistic.

5. CONCLUSION

Curiously enough, the essential link between *human action and perception*, though acknowledged and very much taken into account in Cognitive Sciences in general, is not really considered in speech – obviously a part of Cognitive Sciences, however! In spite of its limitations, it was the interest of Gibson's thought to introduce a schema in which this link was installed in a central role. A few years later, Marr elaborated of a more complete framework in which the complexity of human perception was recognized, and the necessity of a link between the study of the physics of objects and the biology/psychology of human information processing was strongly recommended. This creates good conditions for a psychophysics of speech perception, which should aim in the future at providing a better insight into the *conditions of the negotiation between a listener and a speaker in Human Communication* (see Lindblom, 1990). Whatever its weaknesses and shortcomings, it is our hope that the present work may contribute to this exciting objective.

Acknowledgments

This work was supported by European Community contracts SC1.0044.c(H) and BRA ACTS 3207. Many thanks to G. Feng for his help in the signal processing of acoustic trajectories.

References

Abry, C., Benoît, C., Boë, L.J., & Sock, R. (1985). Un choix d'événements pour l'organisation temporelle du signal de parole. *14èmes Journées d'Etudes sur la Parole, Société Française d'Acoustique,* 133-137.

Abry, C., Orliaguet, J.P., & Sock, R. (1990). Patterns of speech phasing. Their robustness in the production of a timed linguistic task: single vs double (abutted) consonants in French. *European Bull. of Cogn. Psych.,* 10, 269-288.

Arrouas, Y., Escudier, P., Schwartz, J.L., & Wu, Z.L. (1991). Représentations auditives de signaux acoustiques - arguments physiologiques, algorithmiques et fonctionnels en faveur de l'existence d'un système phasique de détection d'événements, in: *Séminaire Traitements et représentations du signal de parole, Société Française d'Acoustique* 120-133. Le Mans.

Bailly, G., Laboissière, R., & Schwartz, J.L. (1991). Formant trajectories as audible gestures - An alternative for speech synthesis. *Journal of Phonetics,* 19, 9-23.

Barlow, H.B., & Levick, W.R. (1965). The mechanism of directionally selective units in rabbits retina. *J. Physiol.,* 178, 477-504.

Berthommier, F. (1989). Un modèle de la relation entre tonotopie et synchronisation du système auditif. *C.R.Acad.Sc.,* 309, 695-701.

Berthommier, F. (1992). Auditory processing based on temporal correlation between adjacent spikes trains. To appear in: B. Ainsworth (ed.) *Advances in Speech, Hearing and Language Processing (Vol. 3),* U.K.: JAI Press.

Boë, L.J., Perrier, P., & Bailly, G. (1992). What geometric variables of the vocal tract are controlled for vowel production? Some proposals for inversion. To appear in the *J. Phonetics*.

Buser, P., & Imbert, M. (1982). *Psychophysiologie sensorielle*. Paris: Hermann.

Chistovich, L.A. (1976). *Physiology of Speech: Human Speech Perception*. Leningrad: Nauka (in Rusian).

Chistovich, L.A. (1980). Auditory processing of speech. *Language and Speech*, 23, 67-72.

Chistovich, L.A., Lublinskaya, V.V., Malinnikova, T.G., Ogorodnikova, E.A., Stoljarova, E.I., & Zhukov, S.Ja. (1982). Temporal processing of peripheral auditory patterns of speech, in: R. Carlson & B. Granström (eds.) *The Representation of Speech in the Peripheral Auditory System* (165-180). Elsevier Biomedical.

Delgutte, B. (1986). Analysis of French stop consonants using a model of the peripheral auditory system, in: J.S. Perkell & D.H. Klatt (eds.) *Invariance and Variability in Speech Processes* (163-177). Hillsdale, N.J.: Erlbaum.

Delgutte, B., & Kiang, N.Y.S. (1984). Speech coding in the auditory nerve IV: sounds with consonant-like dynamic characteristics. *J. Acoust. Soc. Am.*, 75, 897-907.

Di Benedetto, M.G. (1989). Frequency and time variations of the first formant: properties relevant to the perception of vowel height. *J. Acoust. Soc. Am.*, 86, 67-77.

Diehl, R.L., Buchwald McCusker, S., & Chapman, L.S. (1981). Perceiving vowels in isolation and in consonantal context. *J. Acoust. Soc. Am*, 69, 239-248.

Elman, J.L., & Mc Clelland, J.L. (1986). Exploiting lawful variability in the speech wave, in: J.S. Perkell and D.H. Klatt (eds.) *Invariance and Variability in Speech Processes* (360-385). Hillsdale, N.J.: Erlbaum.

Erulkar, S.D., Butler, R.A., & Gernstein, G.L. (1968). Excitation and inhibition in the cochlear nucleus. II- Frequency modulated tones. *J. Neurophysiol.*, 31, 537-548.

Feng, G. (1983). Analyse cepstrale, visualisation sonographique et détection des formants. *Séminaire Traitement du Signal de Parole* (207-216). Groupement des Acousticiens de Langue Française.

Fowler, C. (1986). An event approach to the study of speech perception from a direct-realist perspective. *J. Phonetics*, 14, 3-28.

Fowler, C. (1990). Sound-producing sources as objects of perception: rate normalization and nonspeech perception. *J. Acoust. Soc. Am.*, 88, 1236-1249.

Gibson, J.J. (1966). *The senses considered as perceptual systems*. New-York, Boston: Houghton-Mifflin.

Green, D.M., & Forrest, T.G. (1989). Temporal gaps in noise and sinusoids. *J. Acoust. Soc. Am.*, 86, 961-970.

Holdsworth, J., Schwartz, J.L., Berthommier, F., & Patterson, R. (1991). A multi-representation model for auditory processing of sounds. *9th Int. Symposium on Hearing*. Carcans.

Jordan, M. (1989). Serial order: a parallel, distributed processing approach, in: J.L. Elman & D. E. Rumelhart (eds.) *Advances in connectionist theory: Speech*. Hillsdale, N.J.: Erlbaum.

Kelso, J.A.S., Saltzman, E.L., & Tuller, B. (1986). The dynamical perspective on speech production: data and theory. *J. Phonetics*, 14, 29-59.

Kewley-Port, D. (1986). Converging approaches towards establishing invariant acoustic correlates of stop consonants, in: J.S. Perkell & D. Klatt (eds.) *Invariance and Variability in Speech Processes* (193-197). New-York: Hillsdale, N.J.: Erlbaum.

Laboissière, R., Schwartz, J.L., & Bailly, G. (1991). Motor control for speech skills: a connectionist approach, in: D.Touretzky et al. (eds.) *Proceedings of the 1990 Connectionist Models Summer School*, 319-327. San Mateo, CA: Morgan Kaufmann.

Liberman, A.M., & Mattingly, I.G. (1985). The motor theory of speech perception revised. *Cognition,* 21, 1-36.

Lindblom, B. (1990). Explaining phonetic variation: a sketch of the H & H theory, in: W.J. Hardcastle & A. Marchal (eds.) *Speech Production and Speech Modelling.* Dordrecht: Kluwer Academic Publishers.

Macchi, M.J. (1980). Identification of vowels spoken in isolation versus vowels spoken in consonantal context. *J. Acoust. Soc. Am., 68,* 1636-1642.

Marchouk, G. (1980). *Méthodes de calcul numérique* (126-133). Moscou: Ed. Mir (French translation).

Marr, D. (1982). *Vision.* San Francisco, CA: Freeman & Company.

Mizuno, C., Schwartz, J.L., & Cazals, Y. (submitted). Detection of narrow-band pulses in low level noise: Some mixed effects of synchrony, occurrence-time uncertainty and overall duration.

Möller, A.R. (1974). Dynamic properties of the responses of single neurones in the cochlear nucleus of the rat. *J. Physiol.,* 259, 63-82.

Morris, A., Escudier, P., & Schwartz, J.L. (1991). On and off units detect information bottlenecks for speech recognition. Proc. of Eurospeech 91, 1441-1444.

Oertel, D. (1983). Synaptic responses and electrical properties of cells in brain slices of the mouse anteroventral cochlear nucleus. *J. Neurosc.,* 3, 2043-2053.

Perrier, P., Abry, C., & Keller, E. (1989). Vers une modélisation des mouvements du dos de la langue. *J. Acoust.,* 2, 69-77.

Perrier, P., Eck, L., & Laboissière, R. (1991). Modelling of speech motor control and articulatory trajectories. *Proc. of the XIIth ICPhS,* 2, 62-65.

Poggio, T. (1984). Low-level vision as inverse optics. *Symposium on Computational model of hearing and vision (Tallinn, USSR),* 123-127.

Reichardt, W. (1961). Autocorrelation, a principle for the evaluation of sensory information by the central nervous system, in: W. A. Rosenblith (ed.) *Sensory Communication.* New-York: John Wiley.

Repp, B.H. (1987). The role of psychophysics in understanding speech perception, in: M.E.H. Schouten (ed.) *The Psychophysics of Speech Perception* (3-27). NATO ASI Series, Dordrecht: Martinus Nijhoff Publishers.

Saltzman, E.L., & Munhall, K.G. (1989). A dynamical approach to gestural patterning in speech production. *Hask. Lab. SR,* 99/100, 38-68.

Schwartz, J.L., & Escudier, P. (1991). Integration for extraction: what speech perception researchers can learn from Gibson and Marr. *Proc. of the XIIth ICPhS,* 1, 68-72.

Stevens, K.N., & Blumstein, S.E. (1978). Invariant cues for place of articulation of stop consonants. *J. Acoust. Soc. Am.,* 64, 1358-1368.

Strange, W., Verbrugge, R.R., Shankweiler, D.P., & Edman, T.R. (1976). Consonant environment specifies vowel identity. *J. Acoust. Soc. Am.,* 60, 213-222.

Strange, W., Jenkins, J.J., & Johnson, T.L. (1983). Dynamic specification of coarticulated vowels. *J. Acoust. Soc. Am.,* 74, 695-705.

Verbrugge, R.R., Strange, W., Shankweiler, D.P., & Edman, T.R. (1976). What information enables a listener to map a talker's vowel space? *J. Acoust. Soc. Am.,* 60, 198-212.

Wu, Z.L. (1989). Simulating the adaptation phenomena in the response of auditory nerve fibers: a functional model, in: J.L. Lacoume, A. Chehikian, N. Martin & J. Malbos (Eds.) *Signal Processing IV: Theories and Applications* (1313-1316). Elsevier Science Publishers B.V. (North Holland).

Wu, Z.L. (1990). *Peut-on 'entendre' des événements articulatoires? Traitement temporel de la parole dans un modèle du système auditif.* PhD dissertation, INPG, Grenoble.

Wu, Z.L., Schwartz, J.L., Escudier, P. (1992). Physiologically-plausible modules and detection of articulatory-based acoustic events. To appear in B. Ainsworth (ed.) *Advances in Speech, Hearing and Language Processing (Vol. 3).* U.K.: JAI Press.

Young, E.D. (1984). Response characteristics of neurons of the cochlear nuclei, in: C.I. Berlin (ed.) *Hearing Science, Recent Advances* (423-460). San Diego: College Hill Press.

Perceiving Acoustic Components of Speech

Blas Espinoza-Varas
Department of Communication Disorders
Univ. Oklahoma Health Sciences Center
Oklahoma City, Oklahoma 73190
U.S.A.

1. Introduction

The general problem investigated in this paper is probably familiar to several participants of this workshop: namely, how performance in standard psychoacoustic tests relates to performance in speech identification tests (e.g., Festen and Plomp, 1983; Moore and Glasberg, 1987). In the past few years, a fairly large number of studies have addressed this question, but still there is debate about the relations between the two sets of performance measures. In previous work (e.g., Espinoza-Varas and Watson, 1988) we have investigated this question using a correlation approach that relies on inter-individual differences in test performance, similar to the approach of Festen and Plomp.

For example, performance on pure-tone intensity discrimination with a forced-choice procedure was correlated with performance in syllable identification. We studied a large number of correlations of this sort and practically all of them were negligible or insignificant. In the present work, we are investigating the above question with a different approach, which may help to identify factors that account for the low correlations obtained (Espinoza-Varas, 1987). The approach is illustrated in Table 1 for the case of level discrimination of noise bursts.

Table I

A:	Two-interval forced-choice level-discrimination of:
A.1:	random-noise bursts.
A.2:	stop-consonant bursts "in isolation."
A.3:	stop-consonant bursts "in context", with single word.
A.4:	stop-consonant bursts "in context", with set of words.
A.5:	Task A.4 preceded by word recognition.
B:	Syllable/word recognition, single-interval procedure.

Using a two-interval forced-choice procedure, we compare level discrimination for stimuli that range from non-speech bursts of random noise to stop-consonant noise bursts that occur naturally in spoken words. For example, Table I lists five level-discrimination tests with noise bursts (all of which employ a 2IFC procedure). Test A.1 uses bursts of random nonspeech noise (i.e., it is a standard psychoacoustic test of intensity discrimination). Test A.2 uses stop-consonant noise bursts presented "in isolation" (for example, the /t/ burst excerpted from the word "cat"). Test A.3 employs again stop-consonant noise bursts, but presented *in the context* of a *single* word such as the entire word "cat." Test A.4 uses stop-consonant noise bursts sampled from *a set of words* rather than from a *single word* (e.g., cat, pack, pat, etc.).

Test A.5 is the same as test A.4, but the listener must *identify or recognize* the word prior to making a discrimination of level. In brief, we are interested in finding out what happens to level discrimination for noise bursts as the stimulus and test procedure are made increasingly similar to the condition of identifying a spoken word. Note that the experimental tests (a 2IFC procedure) and the noise bursts are the same in task A.2 through A.5. We are especially interested in determining where in this progression the inter-test correlation falls apart. In this paper we will compare performance measured in tests A.1, A.2, and A.3 for level discrimination and for detection of temporal gaps.

2. Level Discrimination of Stop-Consonant Noise Bursts

2.1 Method

We shall begin with data on level discrimination of noise bursts (Espinoza-Varas, Jessee, and Cheung, 1990). The stimulus was a token of the word /kæt/ produced by a female talker. The utterance was digitized at 20 kHz and stored as a computer file. Three segments were defined in this utterance: a) the release-burst and aspiration noise of the initial stop consonant (75-ms duration); b) the vowel and silence preceding the final stop; and c) the release burst and aspiration noise of the final stop consonant (i.e., the 88-ms /t/ burst). All durations reported in this paper are nominal. The increments in the level of the bursts were specified according to Equation (1).

$$n(t) = n_o(t)\ (1+k) \tag{1}$$

Using a digital waveform editor, the RMS level of either the initial burst (including the aspiration noise) or of the final burst was increased by multiplication of the burst's sample points $n_o(t)$ by (1+k), where k ranges from 0.05 to 1.25 (the constant k has nothing to do with the /k/ burst). The resulting waveform n(t) had an increment in the burst RMS level ranging from 0.4 to 7.0 dB. The *difference* in RMS level, or "ΔL in dB," between the original and the amplified burst is equal to 20 log (1+k). This procedure has been described in detail by Forrest and Green (1987). In this manner, we obtained a series of tokens of the word /kæt/ that differed, *in one respect*, namely in terms of the RMS amplitude of the /t/ burst. The series ranges from the /kæt/ token in which the /t/ burst has the natural RMS amplitude, to a /kæt/ token in which the burst RMS level has an increment of 7.0 dB. Note that these stimuli are frozen noise bursts with fairly broad bandwidth (1.5-7.0 kHz). In addition, if one replaces the term (1+k) by (1-k) in the above equation, the result is an attenuation of the signal, and if k = 1 silence is obtained. That is, the same signal-processing procedure can be used to study discrimination of RMS-level increments and detection of temporal gaps. The tokens were output through a D/A converter and presented over earphones at an overall level of 82 dB SPL. The SPL of the bursts (without any RMS increment) was about 60 dB.

Fig. 1 shows the 2IFC test used in the experiments: one interval contains the /kæt/ token in which the /t/ burst has the "natural" RMS level, and the other interval contains the same /kæt/ token but with an increment in the RMS level of the /t/ (or the /k/) burst of variable magnitude. Subjects were asked to decide which interval contained the token with the louder burst. This we call the "speech condition," or the "in-context" condition.

Fig. 1.

Fig. 2.

In a second experimental condition, we used the waveform editor to excerpt one of the bursts from the syllable and only the burst was presented in each observation interval (Fig. 2 shows a trial with the /t/ burst). Again, the burst in the second interval has an increment in the RMS level. This we call the "isolation" or "nonspeech" condition. The waveforms and the level of the bursts were exactly identical in both conditions: either "in isolation" or "in context."

2.2 Results

Fig. 3 shows average psychometric functions (n=3) obtained with /t/ bursts presented "in context" and presented "in isolation." The bars show ±1.0 standard error of the mean. There is an orderly improvement in accuracy with the magnitude of the RMS-level increment. For /t/ "in isolation," increments ranging from 0.5-4.0 dB bracket the range from chance to perfect performance. For /t/ "in context" the range is 0.5-6.0 dB. There is more variability in the psychometric function for the /t/ burst *in syllable context*, and the slope is less steep than for the

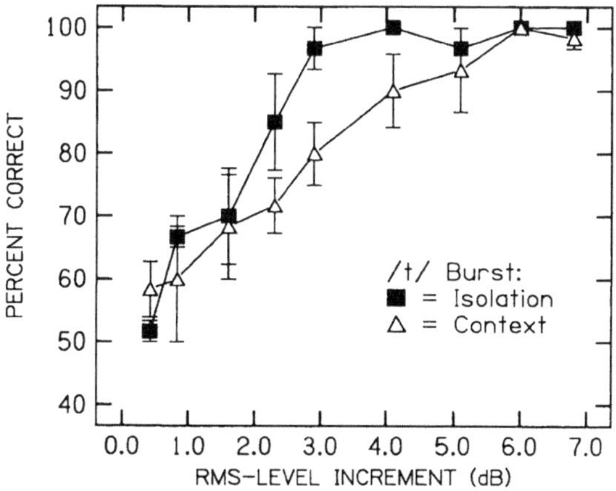

Fig. 3.

function "in isolation." Level discrimination is more difficult when the bursts are presented in context. Average thresholds estimated at the 75 percent correct level were 1.8 and 2.6 dB for the "isolation" and "context" conditions.

Fig. 4 shows average psychometric functions (n=3) obtained with the initial consonant burst /k/. Open triangles represent the "context" condition and solid squares the "isolation" condition. There is again a lower performance with the /k/ burst in context.

Fig. 5 compares the thresholds obtained in the present experiments to level discrimination thresholds for bursts of frozen noise reported by Raab and Goldberg (1975). The value of "ΔL in dB" is shown as a function of burst duration. Data with nonspeech bursts are shown by solid squares. Solid triangles show data for consonant bursts presented "in context" and open triangles are for consonant bursts presented "in isolation." In both conditions, the data points for initial and final burst (75 and 88 ms respectively) were arbitrarily connected. Florentine and Buus (1990) recently reported thresholds of 1.3 and 1.2 dB for conditions comparable to these. Thresholds for speech noise bursts are within 1.0 - 1.5 dB from those obtained with nonspeech bursts. Clearly, when the method described above is used, level discrimination performance for speech noise bursts looks quite similar to that observed for random noise bursts.

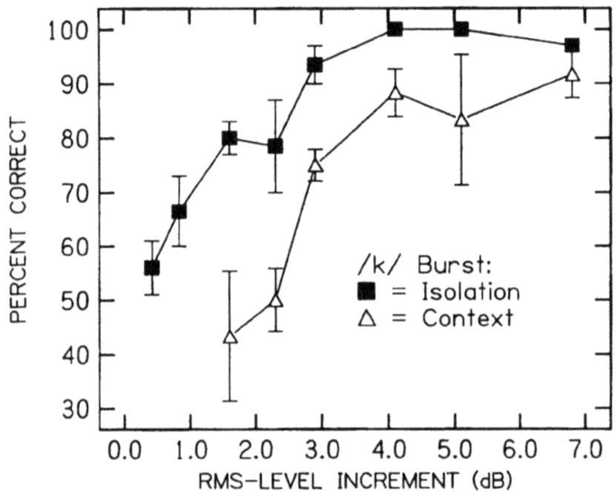

Fig. 4.

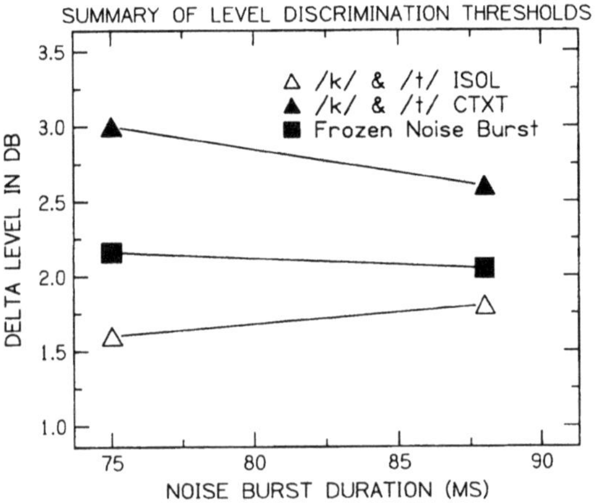

Fig. 5.

2.3 Summary of results

1. Level discrimination thresholds for stop-consonant noise bursts presented in isolation are 1.6-1.8 dB for the /k/ and the /t/ burst.
2. Level discrimination thresholds for stop-consonant bursts presented in syllable context are 2.6-3.0 dB. That is, discrimination in syllable context is less accurate than in isolation. These thresholds are obtained in listeners with moderate amounts of training.
3. Discrimination thresholds for speech noise bursts are within 1.0 -1.5 dB from those obtained for nonspeech noise bursts of comparable duration, level, and bandwidth.

3. Detection of Temporal Gaps in Frication Noise

3.1 Method

This section briefly describes data on detection of temporal gaps in the frication noise of the syllable /tʃa/ and of the word /watʃ/, produced by a female talker (Stein and Espinoza-Varas, 1990). To obtain temporal gaps, a 1-20 ms segment beginning at the temporal center of the frication noise was multiplied by either 0 or 0.2 (that is, k= -1.0 and -0.8 in Equation 1), for silent and partial gaps respectively. The stimuli were output through a D/A converter and presented monaurally to the right ear at 85 dB SPL. The overall level of the frication noise in the "isolation" condition was equal to the noise level in the "context" condition. Four listeners with normal hearing sensitivity, 29 to 42 years old, participated in the experiment.

3.2 Results

The results were summarized in terms of psychometric functions relating gap duration to percent correct. Gap-detection thresholds were interpolated from these psychometric functions at the 75% correct level using probit analysis. The thresholds are shown in Fig. 6 as a function of the value of k (i.e., the constant in Equation 1).

Open triangles and circles show the thresholds for frication noise in isolation for /tʃa/ and /watʃ/, respectively. Thresholds for frication noise in context are shown by solid circles and triangles (for /tʃa/ in context, we studied silent gaps only). Thresholds for silent gaps (k = 1.0) ranged from 3.1-3.6 ms, and for partial gaps (k = 0.8) the thresholds ranged from 3.3-4.6 ms. There were only small differences between "in context" and "in isolation" thresholds. For comparison, Fig. 5 (solid squares) shows gap-detection thresholds for broad-band noise reported by Green and Forrest (1989). Thresholds for frication noise, either in context or in isolation, are only 1-2 ms larger than for broad-band noise. Green and Forrest used highly trained listeners and defined the thresholds at the 71% correct level. In the present study, the listeners were not highly trained and the thresholds were defined at the 75% correct level. These procedure differences may account for the small differences in threshold between broad-band and frication noise.

3.3 Summary of results

1. Gap detection thresholds for frication noise are only 1-2 ms larger than thresholds for broad-band noise. 2. Thresholds for frication noise presented in isolation are virtually identical to thresholds for frication noise presented in context. This result was obtained with both partial and silent gaps. 3. The above results were obtained with the initial position affricate in the syllable /tʃa/, and also with the final position affricate of the word /watʃ/.

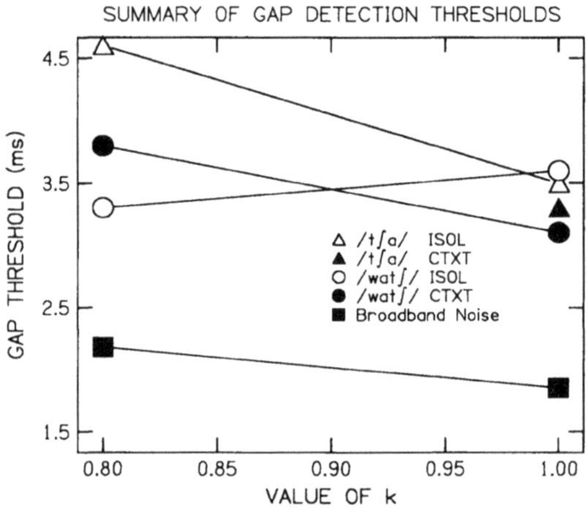

Fig. 6.

4. CONCLUSIONS

Considered together, the present results suggest that the ability to discriminate level increments and to detect temporal gaps in syllables or words is very similar to that observed with non-speech stimuli. In other words, psychoacoustic abilities involved in these tasks seem to be the same whether the sounds are speech or nonspeech. It is important to keep in mind the conditions in which this similarity is obtained: in the present study the utterances were presented in a 2IFC test format. The *same* syllable or word was presented throughout an experimental session, and an external reference was available to the subject to judge the stimuli. These conditions are very different from those existing in the identification of syllables or words. In the latter case, the subject must identify utterances sampled from a set of variable size, and no external reference is provided.

The low correlations observed between performance in psychoacoustic and speech-identification tests are probably caused by differences in the respective stimulus sets and/or task demands. Low correlations do not seem to result from fundamental differences in the psychoacoustic abilities involved in the processing of speech and nonspeech sounds. This conclusion is consistent with a hierarchical model of speech perception described at the 1986 workshop on the psychophysics of speech perception (Espinoza-Varas, 1987).

Acknowledgements

This work was supported by OCAST grant HSO-005 and the Presbyterian Health Foundation.

References

Espinoza-Varas, B. (1987). Levels of representation of phonemes and bandwidth of spectral and temporal integration, in: M.E.H. Schouten (ed.), *The Psychophysics of Speech Perception.* M. Nijhoff, The Netherlands, 80-90.

Espinoza-Varas, B. and Watson, C.S. (1988). Low communality between tests of auditory discrimination and speech perception, *J. Acoust. Soc. Am.* 84, S143.

Espinoza-Varas, B. Jessee, T. and Cheung Y.J. (1990). Hearing acoustic details of speech. I. Level discrimination of stop consonant noise bursts, *J. Acoust. Soc. Am.* 88, S170.

Festen, J.M. and Plomp, R. (1983). Relations between auditory functions impaired hearing, *J. Acoust. Soc. Am.* 73, 652-662.

Florentine, M. Buus, S. (1990). Level discrimination as a function of duration for normal and cochlearly impaired listeners, *J. Acoust. Soc. Am.* 88, S50.

Forrest, T.G. and Green, D.M. (1987). Detection of partially filled gaps in noise and the temporal modulation transfer function, *J. Acoust. Soc. Am.* 82, 1933-1943.

Green, D.M. and Forrest, T.G. (1989). Temporal gaps in noise and sinusoids, *J. Acoust. Soc. Am.* 86, 961-970

Moore, B.C.J. and Glasberg, B.R. (1987). Relationship between psychophysical abilities and speech perception for subjects with unilateral and bilateral cochlear hearing impairment, in: M.E.H. Schouten (ed.), *The Psychophysics of Speech Perception*, M. Nijhoff, The Netherlands, 449-460.

Raab, D.H. and Goldberg. I.A. (1975). Auditory intensity discrimination with bursts of reproducible noise, *J. Acoust. Soc. Am.* 57, 437-447.

Stein, R.L. and Espinoza-Varas, B. (1990). Hearing acoustic details of speech. II. Detection of temporal gaps in frication noise, *J. Acoust. Soc. Am.* 88, S171.

Chapter 4
Loss of Spectral and Temporal Resolution

Speech Recognition Using Only Temporal Cues

Robert V. Shannon,
Fan-Gang Zeng, and
John Wygonski
House Ear Institute
2100 W. Third St.
Los Angeles, CA 90057

1. Introduction

In the 1940s, J.C.R. Licklider and colleagues (e.g., Licklider and Pollack, 1948) presented a convincing demonstration that speech was highly intelligible when all amplitude information was removed by infinite clipping. Amplitudes in speech waveforms were converted to either plus or minus one, preserving zero-crossing information but removing all amplitude information. In spite of the spectral distortion caused by this manipulation, subjects were able to correctly recognize a high percentage of nonsense syllables. This remarkable observation convinced people that amplitude information in speech was unimportant and thus delayed research on the importance of amplitude information in speech for almost 25 years (Erber, 1972).

Only recently has research focussed on amplitude envelope cues in speech perception (van Tasell et al., 1987; Rosen, 1989), motivated primarily by cochlear implant research. In these studies, normal-hearing subjects were presented with a noise stimulus that was amplitude modulated by the overall speech envelope. Subjects achieved 30% to 40% correct in identification of consonants from a set of 12 to 19 alternatives, depending on the study. This level of performance was higher than most people expected, partly due to the implication of Licklider's experiment that amplitude information was not important.

Other recent research has studied the relative importance of amplitude and spectral cues in categorizing synthetic speech continua (Behrens and Blumstein, 1988; Diehl and Walsh, 1988; Nittrouer and Studdert-Kennedy, 1986). These studies found that formant frequency transitions are more important than envelope cues in signalling a /b/-/w/ or a /s,sh/-/f,th/ distinction. In general, amplitude cues are usually found to be less potent in altering speech classification boundaries than spectral cues.

However, this finding does not imply that amplitude cues do not contribute to speech discrimination. Although amplitude cues may be relatively less important than spectral cues for normal-hearing listeners, amplitude cues alone can convey a surprising amount of speech information for hearing-impaired listeners. In impaired ears which degrade spectral cues (Wightman et al., 1977; Turner and Nelson, 1982), amplitude cues can take on increased importance in providing perceptual information. In implant patients with no spectral resolution, temporal cues must carry all speech information. For effective transmission of speech information to these individuals, it becomes important to understand (1) if temporal resolution is also impaired with hearing impairment and (2) how much speech information can be conveyed by temporal cues alone.

2. Temporal Resolution and Hearing Impairment

Psychophysical research has addressed the question of whether temporal processing is impaired in hearing-impaired listeners. Gap detection and forward masking have been measured in normal and hearing-impaired listeners by several research groups.

One group (Nelson and Freyman, 1987; Henderson, et al., 1987) presented forward masking data in humans and animals that indicated that temporal processing was impaired with hearing loss. These researchers fitted a simple exponential decay function to their forward masking results and found that the time constants of recovery increased with increasing degree of hearing impairment. They concluded that hearing impairment reduced the effective level of the masker, and so the forward masking recovery time constant for a high-level masker was similar to the longer time constant typically found at a lower masker level.

Jesteadt et al. (1982) and Dubno et al. (1989) presented forward masking data from hearing-impaired listeners that showed normal threshold recovery following the masker. Jesteadt et al. (1982) found that the growth of masking function was abnormal, but the recovery functions following the masker were relatively normal when masker levels were equated in sensation level.

Florentine and Buus (1984) measured gap detection in hearing-impaired and normal listeners who were masked to simulate the hearing loss. These experiments demonstrated that masked normal listeners showed the same gap thresholds as hearing-impaired listeners, suggesting that the elevation in threshold in the hearing-impaired subjects explained the apparent differences in gap detection. No inherent damage to temporal resolution need be postulated to explain the differences between normal and hearing-impaired gap thresholds; differences in absolute threshold are adequate to account for the differences.

3. Temporal Resolution in Implanted Listeners

Recent psychophysical experiments in cochlear implant and auditory brainstem implant patients indicate that temporal resolution is normal, even in patients with no cochlea or VIII nerve (Shannon, 1983, 1986, 1989, 1991; Shannon and Otto, 1990; Moore and Glasberg, 1988). In these studies temporal resolution, as indicated by forward masking and gap detection results, was normal when plotted in physical units related to perceived loudness magnitude. Once acoustic and electrical amplitudes are normalized to a common perceptual scale, temporal resolution is comparable between electrical and acoustic stimulation.

This result suggests that the physiological mechanisms that determine temporal processing are located central to the cochlea and auditory nerve, and that these temporal mechanisms are unimpaired by damage to the cochlea and VIII nerve. We further suggest that if we preprocess the electrical signal so that the physiological response amplitude at the input to the central temporal mechanisms is equated with that of the normal auditory system, temporal processing of electrical stimulation would be indistinguishable from that of acoustic stimulation.

Patients with cochlear implants have no physiological mechanisms for spectral resolution. Their auditory nerves are directly stimulated electrically. Tonotopic information can be only crudely recreated in cochlear implant patients by multiple electrodes selectively stimulating different subpopulations of the nerve. On a single electrode, studies have shown that patients can detect frequency changes only up to about 300 Hz (Simmons, 1966; Eddington et al., 1979; Muller, 1983; Shannon, 1983; Tong et al., 1983; Hochmair-Desoyer et al., 1984), and that two frequency components cannot be separately resolved, even if they are several octaves apart (Shannon, 1983, 1991). Thus, only temporal information is available to provide speech information on a single electrode.

We suggest that there are two distinct classes of temporal information available to implant patients: (1) envelope information and (2) low-frequency rate pitch information. Envelope cues provide segmental information that aids in distinguishing consonants, as well as suprasegmental (prosodic) information that signals stress and rhythm. Low-frequency rate conveys voicing information and possibly some information about low-frequency first formants of vowels.

How does the ability to process these two types of temporal information compare between implanted and normal-hearing listeners? Psychophysical measures (Shannon, 1983, 1989, 1990, 1991; Moore and Glasberg, 1988; Dobie and Dillier, 1985) indicate that implant patients have normal ability to detect short gaps, normal recovery from adaptation, and normal ability to detect amplitude modulation. However, these temporal abilities are normal only if the reduced amplitude range of electrical stimulation is taken into account. Temporal rate discrimination in implanted patients is relatively normal for rates below 300 Hz (Simmons, 1966; Eddington et al., 1978; Muller, 1983; Tong et al., 1983), and modulation detection is relatively normal (Shannon, 1992).

4. A Model of Forward Masking

We propose the conceptual model in Fig. 1 to account for temporal processing differences between normal-hearing, hearing-impaired, and cochlear implant listeners. Forward masking is used as an example. The first stage of the model is a nonlinear amplitude mapping between physical amplitude (either acoustic or electrical) and the internal, perceived amplitude:

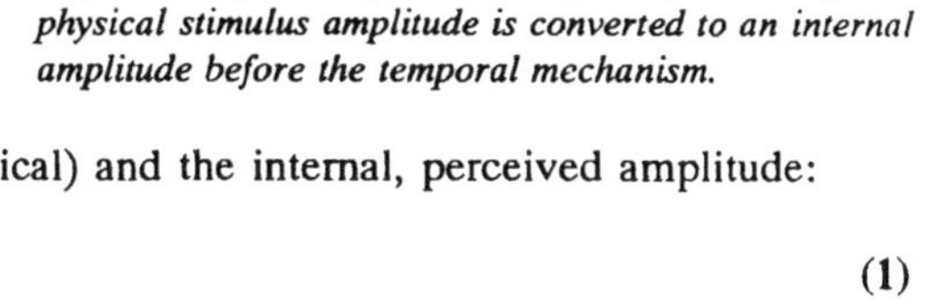

Fig. 1 Conceptual sequence of temporal processing. The physical stimulus amplitude is converted to an internal amplitude before the temporal mechanism.

$$\mathbf{Y = k * (X - T)^q} \quad (1)$$

where **X** is the physical stimulus amplitude, **Y** is the internal perceived amplitude, **T** is the absolute threshold in physical units, **k** is a scaling factor, and **q** is the exponent of the power-law relation. For example, the internal amplitude , $\mathbf{Y_0}$, produced by a masker of level $\mathbf{X_0}$ is

$$Y_0 = k * (X_0 - T)^q$$

The model then assumes that the internal amplitude decays exponentially with time constant a following stimulus offset. At time **t** following the offset of the masker, the internal excitation level decays to

$$Y = Y_0 * e^{-t/a} \quad (2)$$

If we combine Equations 1 and 2 for a particular masker level X_0 and solve for the input level, we obtain

$$X = T + (X_0 - T) * e^{-t/aq} \quad (3)$$

Fig. 2 plots the input level needed to achieve the same internal level as the decaying masker excitation at time **t** after the offset of a masker of input amplitude 100. A recovery time constant of 60 ms was used in all calculations. Recovery functions are plotted for several values of the intensity mapping exponent, **q**. As **q** increases, recovery apparently takes longer, even though the recovery time constant remains unchanged. Indeed, it is apparent from inspection of the exponent in Equation 3 that the recovery time constant and the intensity mapping exponent trade off with each other. If we double the time constant and halve the exponent, the recovery function would be unchanged because the exponential portion of Equation 3 would be unchanged. This is a simple demonstration of the inherent ambiguity between a change in time constant and a change in the intensity mapping. Penner (1978) demonstrated a similar uncertainty between intensity function changes and temporal processing changes in temporal integration.

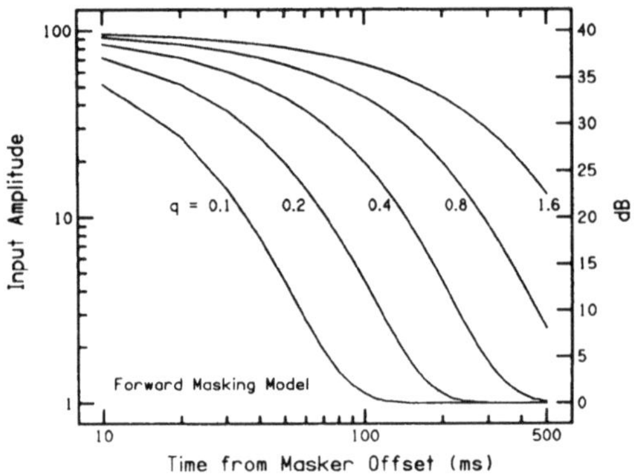

Fig. 2 Model predictions of forward masking as a function of signal delay following masker offset. Compressive exponent of the amplitude conversion is the parameter. All curves were calculated using the same temporal integration time constant.

We suggest that although a change in the amplitude function and a change in temporal processing are mathematically indistinguishable, the data from implanted listeners can be useful in resolving the ambiguity. The normal cochlea provides amplitude compression from acoustic power to neural spike transformation (e.g., Sachs and Abbas, 1974; Yates, 1990). Electrical stimulation bypasses this normal compression and stimulates the nerve directly. The dynamic range of loudness for electrical stimulation is only 10 to 20 dB compared to 100 to 120 dB for normal hearing. The loudness growth function is also steeper for electrical stimulation (Muller, 1983; Shannon, 1983; Tong et al., 1983). Fig. 2 demonstrates that one effect of this reduced dynamic range can be an apparent lengthening of the recovery time in forward masking. Forward masking functions from cochlear implant patients (Shannon, 1986) appear to have longer recovery times when plotted on the same axes as acoustic forward masking. Because a simple change in the amplitude function (which we know occurs) explains the apparent increase in recovery time, parsimony argues against the need to postulate damage to temporal mechanisms. Cochlear implants represent an extreme condition of reduced dynamic range (and thus steep loudness growth). The fact that their forward masking results can be understood simply by a change in the loudness function indicates that temporal mechanisms are relatively unaffected by cochlear damage and are thus located more centrally in the auditory system.

5. Single-Channel Speech Recognition by Implant Patients

Since implant patients have no spectral resolution and relatively normal temporal resolution, their performance on speech tasks can indicate how much speech recognition is possible with only temporal cues. Initial results with cochlear implant patients reported in the literature (Wilson et al., 1988, 1991) and recent results from our laboratory with brainstem implant patients indicate that relatively high levels of speech recognition are possible with temporal cues. Let us examine the speech recognition results from a patient with a single-channel brainstem implant. First, we will describe a speech processor designed to preserve temporal/envelope cues and then we will present results obtained using this processor.

Patients with auditory brainstem implants (ABI) have participated in speech recognition experiments in our laboratory. In these experiments patients are connected to a specially designed digital signal processing computer that can implement different speech processors in essentially real-time (Wygonski et al., 1989). Either microphone output (for live-voice testing) or the sound track from a laser video disk (for standardized test materials) is routed through this computer to the patient. The final output stage of the processor is an optically-isolated, constant-current source connected directly to the patient's percutaneous connector.

The processor design tested was developed by Wilson and colleagues (Wilson et al., 1988, 1991) and labeled the continuous interleaved sampler (CIS). (In the single-channel implementation of the processor, there is no need to interleave pulses on adjacent channels but we will use Wilson et al.'s terminology.) Fig. 3 presents a block diagram of the single-channel CIS processor. The analog acoustic signal is digitized and high-pass filtered (-6 dB/octave below 1200 Hz in the following data) to flatten the long-term spectral shape of the speech input. The resulting waveform is then half-wave rectified and low-pass filtered to obtain an envelope waveform. The low-pass filter cutoff frequency determines the temporal characteristics of the resulting envelope (-6 dB/octave above 800 Hz in the following data). The resulting waveform is then mapped from acoustic amplitude to electrical amplitude using the power function mapping

$$\mathbf{E - E_{th} = k * (A - A_{th})^p} \qquad (4)$$

The value of the constant $\mathbf{k}$ was chosen so that the output is $\mathbf{E_{max}}$ when the acoustic input level is $\mathbf{A_{max}}$. This mapping function is plotted for several values of $\mathbf{p}$ in Fig. 4. The mapped

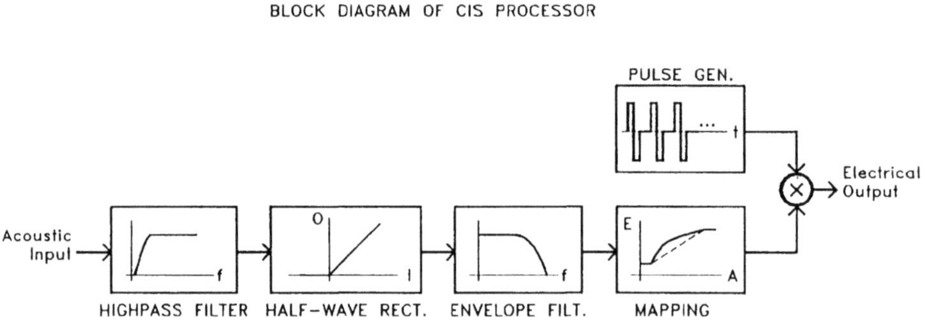

Fig. 3 Block diagram of the single-channel speech processor. The acoustic signal is high-pass filtered to equalize the energy between consonants and vowels. The signal is then half-wave rectified and low-pass filtered to produce an envelope waveform. The resulting acoustic envelope amplitude is mapped to electrical amplitude by the mapping function, and this transformed amplitude is used to modulate the amplitude of a continuous train of charge-balanced, biphasic pulses.

electrical waveform was then used to modulate the amplitude of a high-frequency train of biphasic pulses. For this ABI patient, a 100 μs/phase biphasic pulse was presented at a rate of 2000 Hz. The overall amplitude was then adjusted to a level that was comfortable for the patient.

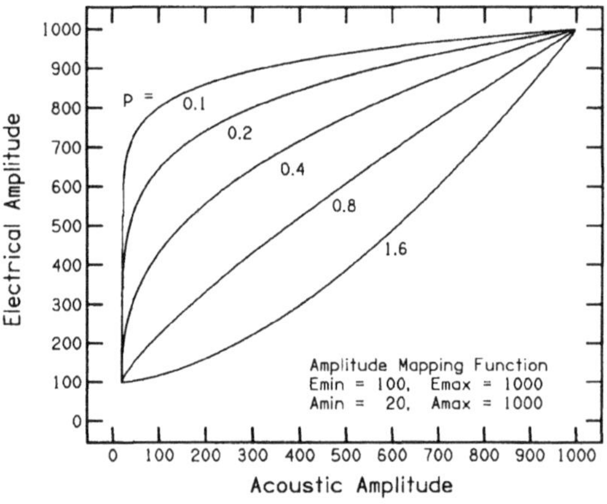

Fig. 4 Samples of the amplitude mapping function for different values of the exponent.

The patient was allowed to converse with the experimenter for several minutes to familiarize them with the specific processor and to ensure that the loudness adjustment was comfortable for a variety of sounds and voice levels. Then the sound track of the laser video disk was routed through the processor and the patient was presented with the test items several times for practice. The test was administered immediately thereafter, first with lip reading, then without lip reading.

In the Iowa Test of Medial Consonants (Tyler et al., 1983) used for this experiment, a male speaker produces consonants in the a/C/a format. The listener was presented with a list of alternatives from which to identify the item presented. The consonant stimulus set consisted of 16 items (m, n, f, v, s, z, sh, th, p, b, t, d, g, k, j, and l), each repeated 5 times in block-randomized order.

Fig. 5 presents the results for one ABI subject with the CIS processor. Filled bars represent performance with sound plus lip reading and open bars represent performance with sound only. Results for **p** = 0.1 are the average of four test runs of 80 trials each; all other results represent single 80-trial runs. Note that the performance of this subject was considerably better than that of normal-hearing listeners with modulated noise stimuli (Van Tasell et al., 1987; Rosen, 1989). Although the normal-hearing listeners were restricted to temporal cues by the use of noise-modulated stimuli, their performance was not as good as that of this ABI patient. This difference suggests that there are more temporal cues available in speech signals than are used by normal-hearing listeners with a modulated noise stimulus.

The ABI patient using sound alone correctly identified 62% of the items in the 16 consonant set. Of this total, 97% correct was obtained on voicing distinctions, 89% correct on manner distinctions, and 68% correct on place distinctions.

Fig. 6 presents the percentage of correct consonants as a function of the value of the exponent, **p**, of the amplitude mapping function. As the exponent approached 1.0 (which would be linear compression from acoustic to electrical amplitudes), performance deteriorated. Best performance was achieved with the most compressive exponents, **p** = 0.1 and 0.2.

This patient's speech perception was also measured using open-set materials in the sound-only condition. He was able to recognize 12% correct monosyllabic words from the NU-6 word list and 25% correct words in sentences on CID sentence material. Thus, some open-set speech recognition is possible using only temporal cues on a single-channel implant.

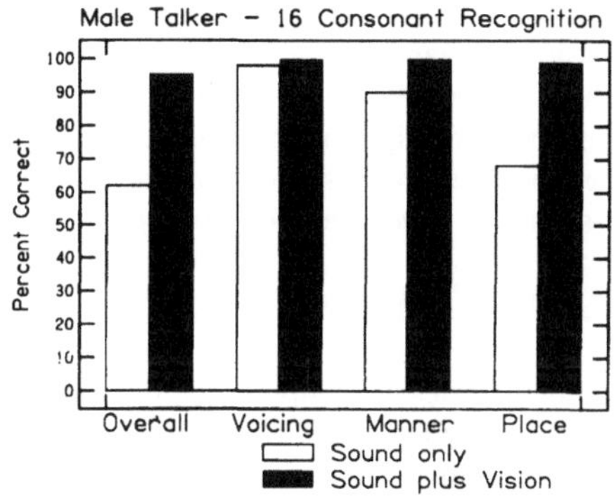

Fig. 5 Percent correct recognition of 16 consonants from a male speaker, presented either in sound only or sound-plus-vision conditions.

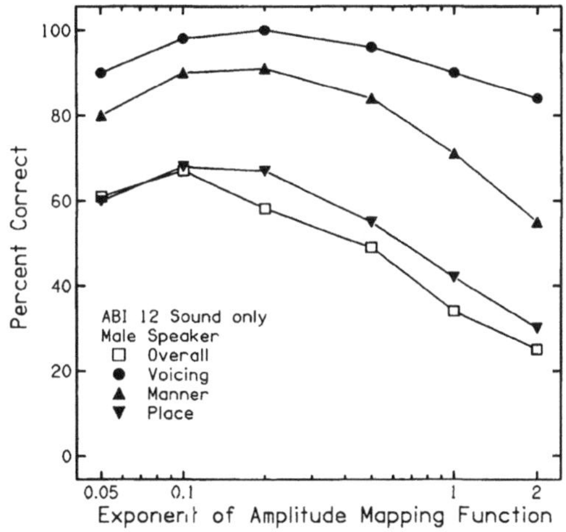

Fig. 6 Percent correct recognition of 16 consonants in the sound-only condition as a function of the exponent of the amplitude mapping function.

6. Comparison with Cochlear Implant Listeners

The overall recognition performance of this ABI patient both in sound-only and sound-plus-vision conditions is comparable to that of patients with multi-electrode cochlear implants (Dorman et al., 1990). There is also a similarity between the ABI and multi-electrode CI performance in that electrical stimulation provides mostly voicing and manner information, whereas the high-frequency place information is only partially conveyed. Nevertheless, compared to listeners wearing 3M/House single-channel implants (Rosen et al., 1989), the transmission of place information is greatly increased. We attribute this to differences in the processing strategy. Traditional 3M/House strategy processes speech waveforms in a manner that conveys primarily fundamental frequency information. The current CIS strategy preserves both the envelope profiles and low-frequency periodicity information to allow discrimination of fine-structure envelope cues in speech waveforms.

7. Loudness Mapping

Fig. 6 demonstrates the importance of correct loudness mapping for speech recognition by implant listeners. The more linear the loudness mapping (**p** = 1), the poorer the recognition performance. Why does a compressive mapping function preserve the fine-structure envelope cues in speech waveforms? This seems counterintuitive in that more compression leads to less envelope fluctuation in speech waveforms. We address this question in the following two ways. First, one function of a normal cochlea is to perform a nonlinear compression so that the wide psychophysical range is reduced to the narrow dynamic range of nerve fibers. Such a compression function no longer exists in either CI or ABI patients. Therefore, an external intensity transformation, simulating the normal compressive cochlear function, is needed to compensate for the narrow dynamic range using direct electrical stimulation. Second, it is known from implant psychophysical studies that the near-miss to Weber's law in intensity discrimination also applies to implant ears (Shannon, 1983; Pfingst, 1984). Intensity discrimination studies in implanted ears indicate that a 3 to 4 dB difference in the lower portion of the loudness range is just noticeable, whereas only 0.3 to 0.4 dB difference is needed in the upper range. Therefore, a large intensity difference in the stimulus domain may be unnoticeable in the response (loudness) domain if it is mapped to the lower portion of the loudness range. A nonlinear compression function will amplify low-amplitude speech sounds (i.e., consonants) far more than high-amplitude sounds, so that the soft consonants are boosted to the upper loudness range, where the intensity DL is much smaller. In other words, implant patients can use the fine-structured envelope cues more efficiently.

We hypothesize that amplitude compression differentially affects the envelope cues and the low-frequency rate cues. Voicing can be signalled effectively by presence or absence of a periodic waveform. This information may be relatively unaffected by strong compression. The segmental cues conveyed by the amplitude envelope, however, may depend more critically on the relative levels of the phonetic components and thus on the shape of the amplitude compression function. For this information to be effectively received, the amplitude compression function must convert the relative envelope information into a perceptual region in which intensity discrimination is best, but too much compression would eliminate the salient envelope differences.

8. Addition of Spectral Cues

Some cochlear implant patients achieve much higher levels of performance than those reported in Fig. 6. In general, multi-channel implants provide some spectral information by multiple bandpass filters applied to the speech signal. The output of each filter is presented to a different electrode, presumably stimulating distinct neural populations related to tonotopic location. Performance in multi-channel cochlear implant patients has been documented as high as 80% correct on recognition of monosyllabic words in isolation (NU-6). Perfect performance using sound only has been measured in the consonant recognition task for some subjects (Wilson et al., 1991).

We have demonstrated that high levels of speech recognition are possible using only temporal cues when stimuli are delivered to a single electrode in the cochlea or cochlear nucleus. When crude spectral information is added to this temporal information, dramatically high levels of speech recognition are possible (Wilson et al., 1988). Both of these results suggest that many of the detailed response properties of the cochlea and auditory nerve are not essential for speech recognition. Even crude representations of temporal and spectral information are sufficient for surprisingly good speech recognition. To optimize reception of temporal cues by implanted patients, we need to understand in more detail the acoustic factors that contribute to the important temporal distinctions in speech. The CIS processor may be only a step in the right direction in this regard; better performance with only temporal cues might be possible with a better processor design.

Another observation that lies outside the scope of the present discussion is the tremendous variability in performance across implanted patients. Some patients perform as well as the ABI patient in Fig. 6, while others benefit mainly from lipreading enhancement and receive relatively little information without lipreading (Rosen et al., 1989). If the temporal information is present to allow the brainstem implant patient in Fig. 6 to correctly identify consonants, why do other patients using the same processor perform at a significantly lower level? Interestingly, Van Tasell et al. (1987) also observed large variability in the performance of normal-hearing listeners with modulated noise stimuli. There may be some individual factor that causes such a wide variation in performance using only temporal cues that is not apparent when redundant and dominant spectral information is present.

We present the data from the ABI patient as a demonstration that high levels of performance are possible with a single electrode, even when stimulating the cochlear nucleus. The results from this patient are not intended to represent all ABI patients; his performance is clearly among the best. But the results from this patient demonstrate that significant speech recognition is possible using only temporal cues. The exact nature of the temporal acoustic cues and temporal patterns that contribute to this level of performance remains to be understood.

Acknowledgements

We appreciate Dewey Lawson for providing software to administer the LVD test materials and perform some of the data analysis. Albert Maltan and Phil Mobley helped in the design and construction of the real-time speech processing system. Blake Wilson provided many helpful discussions in the implementation of the CIS processor. We are indebted to John Petito for his invaluable contributions to this research.

References

Behrens, S. and Blumstein, S.E. (1988). On the role of the amplitude of fricative noise in the perception of place of articulation in voiceless fricative consonants, *J. Acoust. Soc. Am.*, 84, 861-867.

Diehl, R.L. and Walsh, M.A. (1989). An auditory basis for the stimulus-length effect in the perception of stops and glides, *J. Acoust. Soc. Am.*, 85, 2154-2164.

Divenyi, P.L and Shannon, R.V. (1983) Auditory time constants unified, *J. Acoust. Soc. Am.*, 74, S10.

Dobie, R.A. and Dillier, N. (1985) Some aspects of temporal coding for single-channel electrical stimulation of the cochlea, *Hearing Research*, 18, 41-55.

Dorman, M.F., Soli, S. Dankowski, K., Smith, L.M., McCandless, G., and Parkin, J. (1990). Acoustic cues for consonant identification by patients who use the Ineraid cochlear implant, *J. Acoust. Soc. Am.*, 88, 2074-2079.

Dubno, J.R. and Dirks, D.D. (1989). Associations among frequency and temporal resolution and consonant recognition for hearing-impaired listeners, in: *Hearing Impairment and Signal-Processing Hearing Aids, Acta Oto-Laryngologica*, Supplement 469, 23-29.

Eddington, D.K., Dobelle, W.H., Brachman, D.E., Mladevosky, M.G., and Parkin, J.L. (1978) Auditory prosthesis research with multiple channel intracochlear stimulation in man, *Ann. Otol. Rhinol. Laryngol.*, 87, Suppl. 53, 1-39.

Erber, N. (1972). Speech envelope cues as an acoustic aid to lipreading for profoundly deaf children, *J. Acoust. Soc. Am.*, 51, 1224-1227.

Florentine, M. and Buus, S. (1984). Temporal gap detection in sensorineural and simulated hearing impairment, *J. Speech Hear. Res.*, 27, 449-455.

Fourcin, A.J., Rosen, S.M., Moore, B.C.J., Doueck, E.E., Clarke, G.P., Dodson, H., and Bannister, L.H. (1979). External electrical stimulation of the cochlea: Clinical, psychophysical, speech-perceptual, and histological findings, *Br. J. Audiol.*, 13, 85-107.

Henderson, D., Arehole, S., and Salvi, R.J. (1987). The relation between hearing level, frequency selectivity, and forward masking, *Abstr. ARO Midwinter Mtg.*, D. Lim (ed.), 38.

Hochmair-Desoyer, I.J., Hochmair, E.S., and Stiglbrunner, H.K. (1984) Psychoacoustic, temporal processing, and speech understanding in cochlear implant patients, in: R.A. Schindler and M.M. Merzenich (eds.), *Cochlear Implants: Current Status and Future*, Raven Press, New York.

Jesteadt, W. (1980). Effects of masker level and signal delay on forward masking in normal and impaired listeners, *J. Acoust. Soc. Am.*, 68, Suppl. 1, S28.

Jesteadt, W., Bacon, S.P., and Lehman, J.R. (1982). Forward masking as a function of frequency, masker level, and signal delay, *J. Acoust. Soc. Am.*, 71, 950-962.

Licklider, J.C.R. and Pollack, I. (1948). Effects of differentiation, integration, and infinite peak clipping on the intelligibility of speech, *J. Acoust. Soc. Am.*, 20, 42-51.

Moore, B.C.J. and Glasberg, B.R. (1988). Gap detection with sinusoids and noise in normal, impaired, and electrically stimulated ears, *J. Acoust. Soc. Am.*, 83, 1093-1101.

Muller, C.G. (1983) Comparison of percepts found with cochlear implant devices, in: C.W. Parkins and S.W. Anderson (eds) *Cochlear Prostheses: An International Symposium, Annals of the N.Y. Academy of Sciences*, 405, 412-420.

Nelson, D.A. and Freyman, R.L. (1987). Temporal resolution in sensorineural hearing-impaired listeners, *J. Acoust. Soc. Am.*, 81, 709-720.

Nittrour, S. and Studdert-Kennedy, M. (1986). The stop-glide distinction: Acoustic analysis and perceptual effect of variation in syllable amplitude envelope for initial /b/ and /w/, *J. Acoust. Soc. Am.*, 80, 1026-1029.

Penner, M.J. (1978). A power law transformation resulting in a class of short-term integrators that produce time-intensity trades for noise bursts, *J. Acoust. Soc. Am.*, 63, 195-201.

Pfingst, B.E. (1984). Operating ranges and intensity psychophysics for cochlear implants. Implications for speech processing strategies, *Arch. Otolaryngol.*, 110, 140-144.

Rosen, S., Walliker, J., Brimacombe, J.A., and Edgerton, B.J. (1989). Prosodic and segmental asppects of speech perception with the House/3M single channel implant, *J. Speech Hear. Res.*, 32, 93-111.

Rosen, S. (1989). Temporal information in speech and its relevance for cochlear implants, in: B. Fraysse and N. Cochard (eds.), *Cochlear Implant: Acquisitions and Controversies*, Toulouse Implant Conference Procedings, Toulouse, 3-26.

Sachs, M.B. and Abbas, P.J. (1974). Rate versus level functions for auditory-nerve fibers in cats: Tone-burst stimuli, *J. Acoust. Soc. Am.*, 56, 1835-1847.

Salvi, R.J., Giraudi, D.M., Henderson, D., and Hammernik, R.P. (1982) Detection of sinusoidally amplitude modulated noise by the chinchilla, *J. Acoust. Soc. Am.*, 71, 424-429.

Shannon, R.V. (1983) Multichannel electrical stimulation of the auditory nerve in man: I. Basic psychophysics, *Hearing Research*, 11, 157-189.

Shannon, R.V. (1986). Temporal processing in cochlear implants, in: M.J. Collins, T.J. Glattke, and L.A. Harker (eds.), *Sensorineural Hearing Loss: Mechanisms, Diagnosis, and Treatment*, Univ. of Iowa Press, 349-368.

Shannon, R.V. (1989) Detection of gaps in sinusoids and biphasic pulse trains by patients with cochlear implants, *J. Acoust. Soc. Am.*, 85, 2587-2592.

Shannon, R.V. (1992). Temporal modulation transfer functions in patients with cochlear implants, *J. Acoust. Soc. Am.*, (in press).

Simmons, F.B. (1966) Electrical stimulation of the auditory nerve in man, *Arch. Otolaryngol.*, 84, 2-54.

Tong, Y.C., Blamey, P.J., Dowell, R.C., and Clark, G.M. (1983). Psychophysical studies evaluating the feasibility of a speech processing strategy for a multiple-channel cochlear implant, *J. Acoust. Soc. Am.*, 74, 73-80.

Turner, C.W. and Nelson, D.A. (1982). Frequency discrimination in regions of normal and impaired sensitivity, *J. Speech Hear. Res.*, 25, 34-61.

Tyler, R.S., Preece, J.P., and Lowder, M.W. (1983). The Iowa cochlear implant test battery, Laboratory Report, Department of Otolaryngology, University of Iowa, Iowa City.

van Tasell, D.J., Soli, S.D., Kirby, V.M., and Widin, G.P. (1987) Speech waveform envelope cues for consonant recognition, *J. Acoust. Soc. Am.*, 82, 1152-1161.

Wightman, F., McGee, T., and Kramer, M. (1977). Factors influencing frequency selectivity in normal and hearing-impaired listeners, in: E. Evans and J. Wilson (eds.), *Psychophysics and Physiology of Hearing*, Academic Press, New York.

Wilson. B.S., Finley, C.C, Lawson, D.T., Wolford, R.D. (1988). Speech processors for cochlear prostheses, *Proc. I.E.E.E.*, 76, 1143-1154.

Wilson. B.S., Finley, C.C, Lawson, D.T., Wolford, R.D., Eddington, D.K., and Rabinowitz, W.M. (1991). Better speech recognition with cochlear implants, *Nature*, 352, 236-238.

Wygonski, J., Maltan, A., and Mobley, J.P. (1989). A DSP-based system for electrical stimulation, *Proc. IEEE Eng. in Med. and Biol. Soc., 11th Annual International Conference*, 1067-1068.

Yates, G.K. (1990). Basilar membrane nonlinearity and its influence on auditory nerve rate-intensity functions, *Hearing Res.*, 50, 145-162.

Auditory Pattern Perception in the Profoundly Hearing Impaired

Nic van Son
Arjan Bosman
Pieter J.J. Lamoré and
Guido F. Smoorenburg
Laboratory for Experimental Audiology
Department of Otorhinolaryngology
University Hospital Utrecht
The Netherlands

1. Introduction

In designing signal-processing schemes for the profoundly hearing-impaired we may, in principle, propose the presentation of sounds that are gross transformations of the incoming acoustic speech signals. There is some freedom to relate any physical aspect of sound to any perceptual sensation in the listener, creating new optimal relations between physical and perceptual dimensions in profoundly impaired hearing (Smoorenburg, 1990). It is at least required that the coded information should match the limited auditory capacities. It is of crucial interest, therefore, to obtain insight into what acoustic (speech) information the residual hearing can deal with. In general, profoundly hearing-impaired listeners are able to process only temporal and low-frequency information in speech (Erber, 1972; Boothroyd, 1984; Shannon, Zeng and Wygonski, this volume), which cues may be used in perceiving suprasegmental speech structures, and certain aspects of consonants, such as voicing and manner of articulation. Detailed spectral information is often reported to be hardly transmitted, though, implying that the perception of vowels and consonant place of information is severely hampered.

It is often argued that spectral information can hardly be processed by the profoundly hearing-impaired and deaf, but that they mainly rely on temporal cues. In recent years, good results have been reported on the use of only voicing and envelope cues with cochlear implants and signal-processing hearing aids (Walliker, Rosen, Douek, Fourcin and Moore, 1983; Boothroyd, 1988; Boothroyd, Hnath-Chisolm, Hanin and Kishon-Rabin, 1988; Faulkner, Fourcin and Moore, 1990), leaving consonant place information to the visual sense, as used in lipreading. However, it has also been shown that presentation of crude spectral information may be used successfully in order to reach above-chance levels of overall consonant and vowel recognition (Dowell, Martin, Tong, Clark, Seligman and Patrick, 1982; Tyler, Tye-Murray, Moore and McCabe, 1989; Shannon et al., this volume), even without lipreading.

In our approach to signal-processing schemes we intend to incorporate both temporal and spectral information. In investigating the information-processing capacities of the profoundly hearing-impaired, with reference to speech perception, we will therefore study the relative contributions of both temporal and spectral aspects of sounds. At this moment, however, we are mainly concerned with spectral information contained in static harmonic sound patterns. Dynamic patterns will be studied in future stages of the research.

In this paper we report on the results from a pilot study in which various auditory patterns were presented to a group of profoundly hearing-impaired listeners. We were not interested in studying systematic variations among patterns using only one physical parameter, but rather in a more general approach. We used a few different physical parameters, and studied the global relations that exist between these parameters and the perceptual cues that our subjects use in processing the patterns. A more detailed and systematic study will be based on the results of this general approach.

In this pilot phase the following questions were posed:

(1) To what extent are profoundly hearing-impaired listeners able to indicate (dis)similarities among eight different static harmonic patterns ?

(2) Which perceptual dimensions underlie their judgments of (dis)similarity ?

The physical differences among the patterns were mainly of a spectral kind, although the inherently different amplitude waveforms may be used as cues in perceiving differences. The crucial point in this study is the interpretation of the relations between physical cues and perceptual dimensions in the profoundly hearing-impaired.

2. Auditory Pattern Perception

2.1 Stimulus Material: Complex Harmonic Patterns

In Fig. 1 schematic spectra of the auditory patterns used in this study are given. Pattern 1 is a summation of 12 sine waves with components at multiples of the fundamental frequency of 125 Hz. All sine waves are in phase. The other signals were derived by removing certain components from this pattern. All signals were designed to elicit a pitch sensation equal to that of a 125 Hz sine wave.

The patterns were constructed applying three criteria:

(1) *Number of sine wave components*, ranging from 2 to 12.

(2) *Spectral distribution*. Components were spread regularly over the spectrum (signals 1 and 2), or in a grouped fashion, either using two 'peaks' (signals 3, 4, 5, and 6) or only one (signals 7 and 8).

(3) *Presence of adjacent harmonics*. Spectral 'peaks' may be represented by adjacent harmonics (signals 3, 5, 7 and 8) or by single harmonics (4 and 6).

All spectra were shaped to each individual's dynamic range (see next section), in such a way that all signal components fell within the subject's dynamic range while at the same time the overall sensation level was acceptable. The steady state part of each stimulus was 300 msec, with a 100 msec cosine-shaped onset and offset.

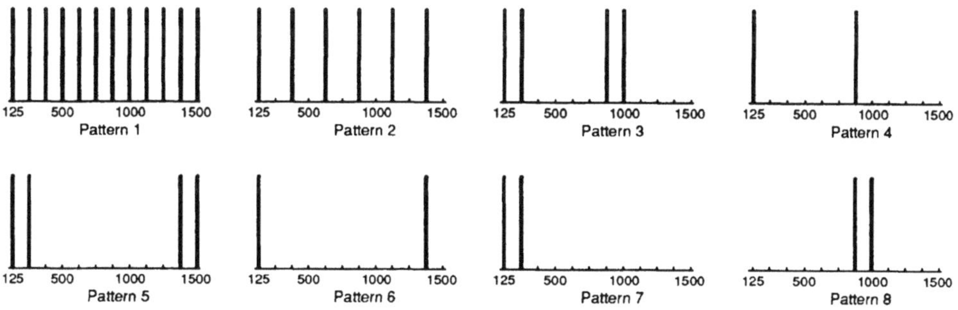

Fig. 1 Schematic spectra of 8 complex harmonic signal patterns

2.2 Subjects

11 postlingually sensorineurally hearing-impaired subjects participated in the experiment. Ages ranged from 19 to 68 years. Subjects were paid for their co-operation. For all subjects thresholds and loudness discomfort levels were measured for pure tones between 125 and 1500 Hz, at multiples of 125 Hz. The threshold was measured by means of a simple up-down procedure using the Von Békésy paradigm (Levitt, 1971). Loudness discomfort was measured by presenting a series of tones, with increasing intensity, using 1 dB steps. Increasing the level was ended when the subject indicated that loudness became uncomfortable. That point was taken as the estimate of the loudness discomfort level (LDL). In most cases LDL could not be established as the headphone (TDH 39P) output was the restrictive factor (maximum level about 140 dB SPL). In Fig. 2 the distribution of thresholds is expressed in 10, 25, 50, 75 and 90% percentiles.

2.3 Design and Procedure

Two experimental sessions were held, with a two-month interval, the second being a repeated measurement in order to check consistency of responses. Subjects had to give assessments of similarity/dissimilarity among the complex harmonic signals. These ratings were acquired by means of triadic comparisons (Levelt, van de Geer, and Plomp, 1966). In each of 56 triads the subject had to indicate, in this order, which were the two *most similar* and which were the two *least similar* signals of the three. The ratings of each subject were gathered in a dissimilarity matrix. For each session separately, the matrices of all subjects were analysed together using an INDSCAL technique after Carroll and Chang (1970).

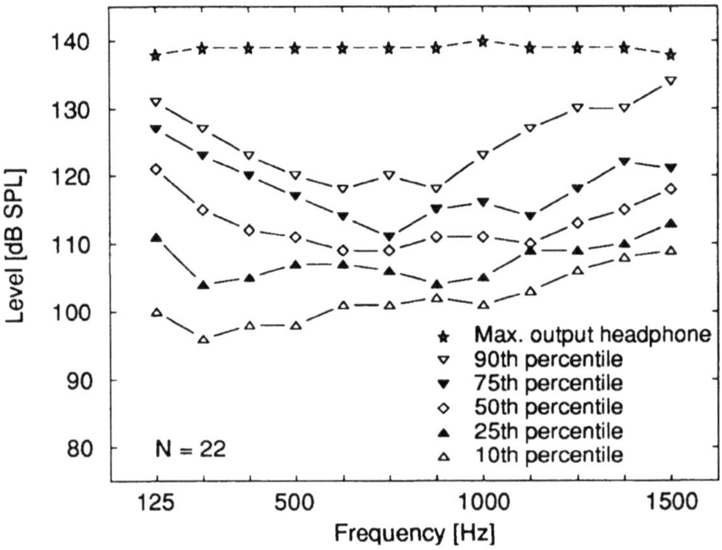

Fig. 2 Threshold distribution expressed in 10, 25, 50, 75 and 90% percentiles.

We expected subjects to base their assessments solely on perceived timbre differences. However, one perceptual cue possibly confounding the results was the perceived loudness of the stimuli, although the signals were meant to be equally loud. In preparing the stimuli, the following procedure was adopted. First, the intensity contour, as described by the levels of the individual components, was set halfway the dynamic range. If the loudness of a signal was uncomfortable for the subject, the contour was situated at a lower level, reducing each component proportionately to the dynamic range at that frequency, until the loudness was acceptable. Finally, the subject had to indicate whether all signals were about equally loud. If possible, an outlying signal was computed anew by determining a new contour.

During *session I* it appeared that the subjects were not always able to indicate reliably whether stimuli were equally loud. Therefore, in *session II* we asked them to rate the loudness of the signals on a 10-point scale. In interpreting the results, these loudness rankings provided some insight into the importance each subject attached to this percept.

One of the subjects experienced loudness discomfort with signal 1 (all components present) even when the contour was at a level just above threshold. As a consequence, he did not take part in the triadic comparisons. The results discussed below apply to 10 subjects only.

3. Results and Conclusions

In Fig. 3 the INDSCAL plots of the *session I* data are given. The left panel shows the two-dimensional stimulus space of the eight patterns, while the right panel displays the subject space, showing the relative weights that individual subjects attach to the two dimensions. Fig. 4 shows similar INDSCAL plots for the *session II* data. The two-dimensional INDSCAL configurations accounted for 63% (*session I*) and 70% (*session II*) of the variance in the data. Three-dimensional solutions raised the portion of explained variance by about 10%, but the third dimension could hardly be interpreted in terms of perceptual or physical cues.

There are differences between the two solutions. Some signals hold the same positions relative to each other, but in general signals tend to shift somewhat along one or both dimensions. In order to give a global quantitative measure for the equality of both solutions, we adopted the following procedure. We compared, for each dimension independently, the positions of signals in the solutions of both sessions, computing correlation coefficients. For dimension I the correlation proved highly significant (Pearson's $r = .89$, $p < .01$), for dimension II the correlation just failed the .05 level of significance (Pearson's $r = .54$). These results indicate that the subjects rated pattern similarity quite reliably, making use of the perceptual cue(s) represented by dimension I. Dimension II, however, appears to represent one or more cues which cannot be used very reliably by the subjects.

Dimension I cannot be interpreted unambiguously. First of all, rank order correlations between loudness ratings and pattern order along this dimension suggested that four of the subjects (1, 2, 6 and 10) chiefly used loudness cues in their discrimination of the patterns. Removing their data from the INDSCAL analyses of both sessions did not yield very different solutions, though, suggesting that a second cue was used. The solutions hint at the importance of adjacent frequency components in the higher frequency region as a cue for auditory discrimination between patterns 1, 2, 3, 5 and 8 on the one hand, and patterns 4, 6 and 7 on the other hand. The information provided by these adjacent components may involve temporal cues (*beats*) rather than spectral cues, as we suppose that a profoundly impaired ear cannot resolve high-frequency components lying only 125 Hz apart. So, the presence of *beats*, resulting from two adjacent frequency components in the (high-frequency region of the) spectrum, seems an important cue in auditory discrimination by the profoundly hearing impaired, although there is some confounding influence from loudness perception.

Dimension II is more difficult to interpret, especially so considering the substantial differences in the stimulus spaces between *session I* and *session II*. If we only consider the peaked spectra, leaving patterns 1 and 2 aside, we come to the following interpretation. To one side of the plot we find patterns 5 and 6, having high-frequency peaks that are separated substantially from the low-frequency components, and pattern 8, which has no low-frequency components at all. To the other side of the plot patterns 3 and 7 are situated. Pattern 7 only contains low-frequency components, whereas pattern 3 also contains a peak in the mid-frequency region. Apparently, this mid-frequency information cannot be separated perceptually from low-frequency information. Pattern 4 is not very stable along this dimension. It seems that the presence of a high-frequency peak may be used as a cue for distinguishing patterns 5, 6 and 8 (and possibly 4) from patterns 3 and 7. Note that in both INDSCAL solutions, pattern 7 (only low-frequency components) and pattern 8 (only high-frequency components) are as far apart from each other as possible.

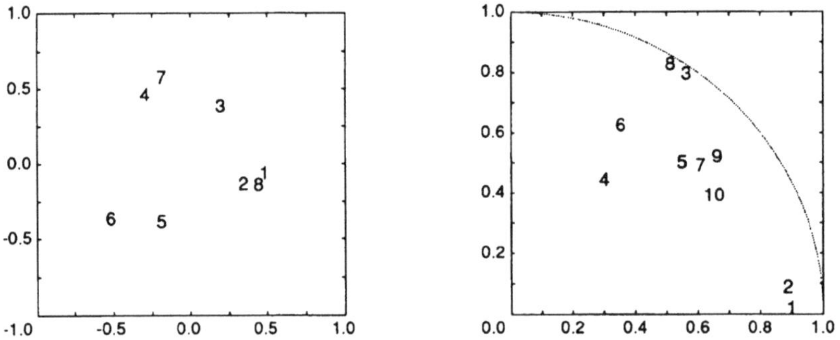

Fig. 3 INDSCAL solution from session I. Left panel: stimulus space. Right panel: subject space. Explained variance: 37.0% (dimension I) and 26.5% (dimension II).

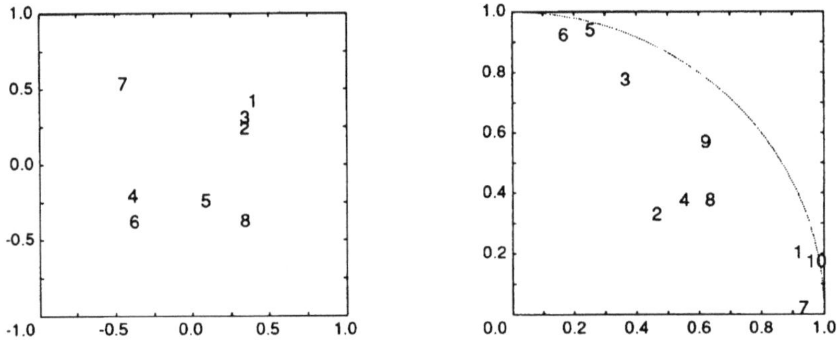

Fig. 4 INDSCAL solution from session II. Left panel: stimulus space. Right panel: subject space. Explained variance: 40.2% (dimension I) and 29.4% (dimension II).

4. Discussion

It is obvious that the profoundly hearing-impaired in our study are able to perceive differences among spectrally different patterns. This ability may be mainly based on spectral cues, but we cannot exclude the importance of other physical cues such as the time-intensity envelope. The results strongly suggest that the profoundly hearing-impaired base their distinctions on different information in low-frequency and high-frequency components. Our global results suggest that the cross-over area between low and high frequencies is somewhere between 800 and 1000 Hz.

The first perceptual dimension was shown to be related (at least partly) to the presence of adjacent harmonics in the high-frequency region. This evoked a percept that we interpreted as 'beats', audible amplitude fluctuations (even the non-adjacent high-frequency components of pattern 2 may be close enough to evoke 'beats'). Contrastively, adjacent harmonics in the low-frequency region, as in pattern 7, do not seem to evoke this percept: pattern 7 is grouped together with patterns 4 and 6 along this dimension.

In the second perceptual dimension this high-low difference also plays a role. Patterns with high-frequency components are clearly distinguished from patterns with low-frequency components, as long as there is a substantial separation between the two regions. In our study this separation implies a 'spectral gap' of 5 to 6 harmonics. The fact that the high-frequency component of pattern 4 lies within the cross-over area may explain why it holds such different positions in the INDSCAL plots from two sessions. Also, the spectral gap of pattern 3 may be too small to make the pattern sound differently from the dense spectra of patterns 1 and 2.

All in all, there are two important cues that profoundly hearing-impaired listeners use in processing complex harmonic signals:

(1) Primarily, the presence of adjacent harmonics in the high-frequency region of the spectrum, possibly leading to audible *beats*. This is a *temporal cue*; however, loudness seems to be a confounding percept.

(2) Secondarily, the presence of *high-frequency peaks*, provided the separation from low-frequency components is substantial (5 to 6 missing harmonics). This is clearly a *spectral cue*.

Having some idea about these perceptual cues, we now need to study them more systematically and in more detail. In our next experiments, our major concern will be the question as to how loudness cues can be controlled, in order to rule out loudness differences among the patterns. A loudness matching paradigm, in order to equalize all patterns, will be considered. However, the fact that not all subjects were able to give reliable indications for loudness causes some doubts as to how well loudness cues can be kept under control.

The main question in future is how perceptual cues can be used in making certain speech features discriminable from each other when applying signal-processing schemes. In proposing such schemes for presentation of certain speech elements, spectral cues, e.g. in the form of vowel formants, may be considered together with temporal cues, in the form of gross amplitude envelope variations. Appreciating the fact that substantial separation between high-frequency and low-frequency information is required, simultaneous presentation of two formants may not be profitable. Integration of auditory and visual cues (lipreading) may be deemed necessary in order to reach good vowel perception. How the 'beat' cue, if indeed it is strong when not confounded with loudness cues, can be used is not clear so far. Informal observation by the authors (normal-hearing !) suggests that the two-component representation of peaks leads to a more speech-like quality of sounds. This cue may then be used for sound quality reasons rather than for establishing speech pattern contrasts. This observation needs substantiating in further research with hearing-impaired listeners.

References

Boothroyd, A. (1984). Auditory perception of speech contrasts by subjects with sensori-neural hearing loss, *Journal of Speech and Hearing Research*, 27, 134-144.

Boothroyd, A. (1988). Perception of speech pattern contrasts from auditory presentation of voice fundamental frequency, *Ear and Hearing*, 9, 313-321.

Boothroyd, A., Hnath-Chisolm, T., Hanin, L., and Kishon-Rabin, L. (1988). Voice fundamental frequency as an auditory supplement to the speechreading of sentences, *Ear and Hearing*, 9, 306-312.

Carroll, J.D. and Chang, J.-J. (1970). Analysis of individual differences in multidimensional scaling via an n-way generalization of "Eckart-Young" decomposition, *Psychometrika*, 35, 283-319.

Dowell, R.C., Martin, L.F.A., Tong, Y.C., Clark, G.M., Seligman, P.M., and Patrick, J.F. (1982). A 12-consonant confusion study on a multiple-channel cochlear implant patient, *Journal of Speech and Hearing Research*, 25, 509-516.

Erber, N.P. (1972). Speech-envelope cues as an acoustic aid to lipreading for profoundly deaf children, *Journal of the Acoustical Society of America*, 51, 1224-1227.

Faulkner, A., Fourcin, A.J., and Moore, B.C.J. (1990). Psychoacoustic aspects of speech pattern coding for the deaf, *Acta Oto-Laryngologica*, Suppl.469, 172-180.

Levelt, W.J.M., Geer, J.P. van de, and Plomp, R. (1966). Triadic comparisons of musical intervals, *British Journal of Mathematical and Statistical Psychology*, 19, 163-179.

Levitt, H. (1971). Transformed up-down methods in psychoacoustics, *Journal of the Acoustical Society of America*, 49, 467-477.

Smoorenburg, G.F. (1990). Physical versus perceptual dimensions in cochlear implants, in: J.M. Miller and F.A. Spelman (eds.), *Cochlear implants: models of the electrically stimulated ear*, New York: Springer-Verlag, Inc.

Tyler, R.S., Tye-Murray, N., Moore, B.C.J., and McCabe, B.F. (1989). Synthetic two-formant vowel perception by some of the beter cochlear implant users, *Audiology*, 28, 301-315.

Walliker, J.R., Rosen, S.M., Douek, E.E., Fourcin, A.J., and Moore, B.C.J. (1983). Speech signal presentation to the totally deaf, *Journal of Biomedical Engineering*, 5, 316-320.

Effect of Spectral Envelope Smearing on Phoneme Identification

Mariken ter Keurs,
Joost M. Festen, and
Reinier Plomp
Dept. of Otolaryngology
Free University Hospital
P.O. Box 7057
1007 MB Amsterdam
The Netherlands

1. Introduction

In recent studies ter Keurs et al. (1991a,b) measured the extent to which the intelligibility of speech in noise depends on the ear's (limited) resolution of spectral contrast. Loss of frequency resolution of the auditory system was simulated by smearing the short-term spectral envelope of the speech signal with a Gaussian-shaped filter, while preserving the signal's phase and harmonic structure. The results suggest that the ear's high selectivity in frequency is of particular importance to understanding speech in the presence of interfering sounds; the masked speech-reception threshold for sentences increases markedly as spectral energy is smeared over bandwidths exceeding the ear's critical bandwidth. In the present paper data are presented on how vowel and consonant identification suffers from spectral envelope smearing.

2. Signal Processing

The signal processing is based on an analysis-resynthesis scheme which permits modification of the short-term spectrum in either its phase or amplitude content without introducing undesired distortion in the resynthesized signal (Allen and Rabiner, 1977). It consists of short-time fast Fourier transforms and overlapping additions to reconstruct a continuous signal. Spectral contrasts are reduced by convolving the short-term spectral envelope on a log-frequency scale with a Gaussian-shaped filter of fixed relative bandwidth. The degree to which the envelope is smeared is given by the equivalent rectangular bandwidth of the filter. In this way spectral energy is smeared - that is spectral contrast is reduced - but the signal's phase and harmonic structure are preserved. As far as speech intelligibility is concerned, this smearing process is assumed to be a reasonable simulation of the ear's limited resolution of frequency. Fig. 1 gives an example of the effect of spectral envelope smearing on an arbitrary speech segment in 3 conditions. From top to bottom the figure shows the original log-power spectrum and the log-power spectrum of the same segment smeared over 1/8, 1/2, and 2 octaves, respectively.

3. Listening Experiment: Phoneme Identification

3.1 Stimuli

All stimuli were pronounced by a female speaker. The vowel stimuli consisted of 8 utterances of 11 different Dutch monophthongs: /a, ɑ, e, ɛ, i, I, o, ɔ, u, y, œ/. The vowels were equalized in SPL and duration. Total duration of the stimuli was 115 ms, including 12.5-ms rise and fall times.

The consonant stimuli consisted of 16 lists of 12 meaningless Dutch syllables of the consonant-vowel-consonant type as designed by Bosman (1989). In order to avoid a bias towards sense responses, subjects were asked to identify only the initial or the final consonant of the syllables. The set of initial consonants consisted of: /t, k, b, d, X, v, z, n, l, j, w, h/, the set of vowels of: /a, ɑ, e, ɛ, i, I, o, ɔ, ɸ, u, au, ɛi/, and the set of final consonants of: /p, t, k, f, s, X, m, n, n, l, j, w/. The syllables were normalized for RMS level.

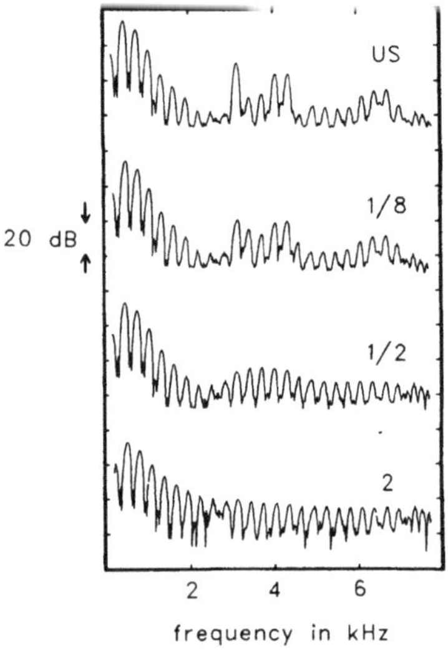

Fig. 1 Log-power spectra of an arbitrary speech segment as a function of spectral envelope smearing. From top to bottom : the original log spectrum and the log spectra after smearing over 1/8, 1/2, and 2 octaves, respectively.

3.2 Test procedure

For both vowel and consonant identification, unsmeared stimuli and stimuli smeared over 1/8, 1/2, and 2 octaves were presented in quiet and in noise to 16 normal-hearing subjects in balanced order. All stimuli were presented diotically through headphones at a level of 65 dBA. In the masked conditions noise was used with the long-term average spectrum of sentences as pronounced by the same speaker. The level of the noise was fixed at 60 dBA. In each condition both the stimuli and the noise were subjected separately to the same degree of spectral smearing. Prior to both the vowel and consonant identification tests, subjects were familiarized with the experimental task by means of two test lists. Subjects wrote down their responses. A closed-response set was used in the vowel identification task and an open one in the consonant identification task.

In this way 128 identifications (16 subjects x 8 utterances) were obtained for each vowel in eight conditions (4 smearing bandwidths both in quiet and in noise). For each initial and final consonant 64 identifications (16 subjects x 4 repetitions of the syllables) were obtained in each condition.

3.3 Results

Vowel identification

Fig. 2 gives the overall vowel-identification scores in quiet and in noise for original vowels, and vowels smeared over 1/8, 1/2, and 2 octaves, respectively. Identification scores for the long vowels /e/ and /o/ are not included as these vowels were systematically confused with their short counterparts /I/ and /ɛ/. Overall identification for unsmeared vowels and for vowels smeared over 1/8 and 1/2 octave is 97%. Identification drops to 32% in the 2-octaves condition. Unfortunately, the ceiling effect in the first three conditions makes it impossible to estimate the bandwidth at which spectral envelope smearing starts affecting vowel identification.

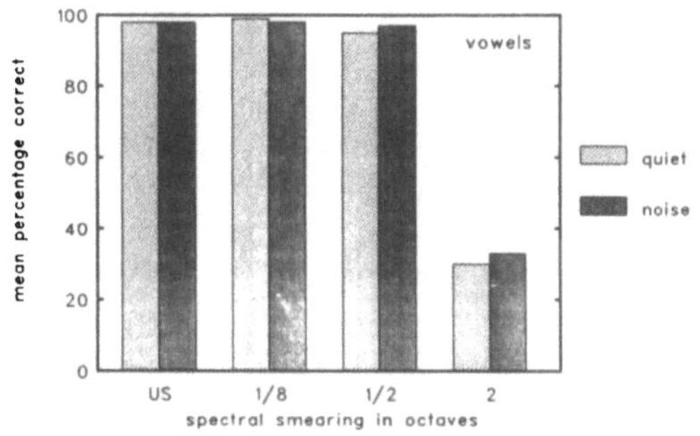

Fig. 2. Overall vowel-identification score in quiet and in noise for unsmeared vowels and vowels spectrally smeared over 1/8, 1/2, and 2 octaves, respectively.

The pattern of confusions for vowels smeared over 2 octaves is very similar in quiet and in noise. Therefore, in the analysis these two conditions have been combined. Table I gives the resulting confusion matrix in percentages. In this smearing condition a predominant proportion of vowels is identified as the back vowels /ɔ/ and /u/. Generally, the responses correspond to vowels with low first and second formants (F1 and F2), and within this subset, vowels are chosen whose F1 is closest in frequency to the F1 of the target vowel [formant frequencies of Dutch vowels (female) as given by van Nierop et al., 1973] (cf. for similar results with two-formant vowels Delattre et al., 1952, and Dubno and Dorman, 1987). In the 2-octave condition F2 and higher formants have generally been smoothed out, leaving primarily a broadened F1 to determine identification. Stated in terms of deteriorated auditory analysis, limited frequency resolution will lead to fewer vowel formants being resolved individually. The resolution of higher formants is first to suffer. The results suggest that at least F1 and F2 of a vowel should be resolvable to warrent correct identification.

Consonant identification

Fig. 3 gives the overall identification score for the original initial and final consonants in quiet and in noise, and for consonants smeared over 1/8, 1/2, and 2 octaves. Identification of initial consonants in quiet shows a ceiling effect for the original, 1/8 and 1/2 octave condition. Scores for the other three consonants conditions - final consonants in quiet, masked initial and final consonants - drop as the smearing bandwidth is increased from 1/8 to 1/2 octave. This bandwidth, for which scores start to drop, agrees rather well with the inflection bandwidth found for the speech-reception threshold for sentences in noise, which is between 1/3 and 1/2 octave (ter Keurs et al., 1991a,b). In the 2-octave condition the average identification score for consonants in quiet drops to 69% and for masked consonants to 52%. This is nearly twice the average vowel identification score (32%) in the same condition. Apparently, consonant identification is much less susceptible to reduced spectral contrast than vowel identification. This confirms the relative importance of other than spectral cues in consonant identification, such as temporal and voicing cues (harmonic structure).

The pattern of confusions is very similar for initial and final consonants in quiet and in noise. Therefore, only the confusion matrices for initial and final consonants in quiet are given in Table II. Spectral envelope smearing of the consonants consistently results in place-of-articulation errors. Thus, plosives, fricatives, nasals, and semi-vowels are predominantly confused with consonants within their respective categories (cf. Miller and Nicely, 1954). The degree to which each individual consonant suffers from spectral smearing depends on how its energy is distributed over the spectrum. For example, consonants characterized by energy at higher frequencies, such as /d/, suffer more than consonants characterized by energy at lower frequencies, such as /b/.

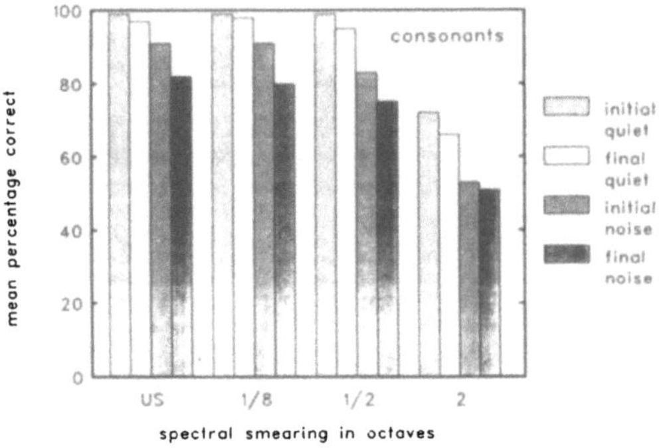

Fig. 3. Overall identification score for initial and final consonants in quiet and in noise for unsmeared consonants and consonants spectrally smeared over 1/8, 1/2, and 2 octaves, respectively.

Table I. Confusion matrix in percentages for vowels smeared over 2 octaves.

	responses							VOWELS			
stimuli	a	ɑ	e	ɛ	i	I	o	ɔ	u	y	œ
a	24	28	.	4	.	2	5	32	3	.	2
ɑ	6	32	.	1	.	.	4	48	7	1	1
e	1	1	1	5	.	7	9	62	10	2	2
ɛ	5	22	.	7	.	2	3	56	4	.	1
i	.	.	.	.	14	3	2	9	67	4	1
I	.	1	.	3	2	11	5	51	20	4	3
o	.	2	.	.	.	.	16	61	18	1	2
ɔ	.	1	.	.	.	.	6	73	18	2	.
u	.	.	.	.	.	.	1	2	97	.	.
y	.	.	.	.	7	1	1	6	68	15	2
œ	.	.	.	1	1	3	9	45	23	9	9

4. CONCLUSION

In the present paper we investigated the extent to which phoneme identification depends on limited resolution of spectral contrast. The results suggest that a reduction in spectral contrast affects vowel identification more than consonant identification. Vowels were primarily confused with the back vowels /ɔ,u/, and consonants were confused where place of articulation is concerned.

Table II.

TABLE II Confusion matrices in percentages for initial and final consonants smeared over 2 oct.

	responses																
												INITIAL CONSONANTS IN QUIET					
stimuli	t	k	p	b	d	v	f	z	s	X	n	m	l	w	j	h	r
t	94		6	.	.	.	.	.		.	.	.	.	.	.	.	.
k	13	42	44	.	.	.		.	.	.	.	.	.	.	1	.	.
b			.	99	1	.	.	.	.	.	.	.	.	.	.	.	.
d			.	44	56			.	.	.	.	.	.	.	.	.	.
v	.		.	.	.	88	3	.	.	.	.	.	.	9	.	.	.
z			.	.	.	39	3	50	3	.	.	.	.	5	.	.	.
X				.	.	14	22	.	.	64	.	.	.	.	.	.	.
n			.	.	.	.	.	.	.	.	97	1	1	1	.	.	.
l	.		.	.	.	.	.	.	.	.	10	.	85	3	.	1	1
w			.	.	.	1	.	.	.	.	.	.	.	98	.	.	1
j	.	.	.	.	.	1	.	.	.	.	.	.	.	46	51	1	1
h		.	.	.	.	56	.	.	.	.	.	.	.	5	.	39	.

	responses													
										FINAL CONSONANTS IN QUIET				
stimuli	t	k	p	b	d	f	s	X	n	n	m	l	j	w
t	78	1	21	.	.	.	.	.	.	.	.	.	.	.
k	1	27	71	1	.	.	.	.	.	.	.	.	.	.
p	.	.	97	3	.	.	.	.	.	.		.	.	.
f	.	.	.	.	.	99	.	.	.		.	.	.	1
s	.	.	.	.	.	45	54	.	.	.	.	.	.	1
X	.	.	.	.	1	50	.	49	.	.	.	.	.	.
n	1	.	.	.	1	.	.	.	89	3	1	5	.	.
n	.	.	.	.	.	1	.	.	19	64	9	6	.	1
m	.	.	.	.	.	.	.	.	13	44	34	9	.	.
l	.	.	.	.	.	.	.	.	3	3	.	78	5	11
j	.	.	.		.	1	.	.	5	.	.	6	85	3
w	.	.		.	.	.	.	.	.	.	.	59	.	41

References

Allen, J.B. and Rabiner, L.R. (1977). A unified approach to short-time Fourier analysis and synthesis. *IEEE* 65 (11), 1558-1564.

Bosman, A.J. (1989). *Speech Perception by the Hearing Impaired*, doctoral thesis, Utrecht, The Netherlands.

Delattre, P., Liberman, A.M., Cooper, F.S., and Gerstman, L.J. (1952). An experimental study on the acoustic determinants of vowel color; Observations on one- and two-formant vowels synthesized from spectrographic patterns, *WORD*, 8 (3), 195-210.

Dubno, J.R. and Dorman, M.F. (1987). Effects of spectral flattening on vowel identification, *J. Acoust. Soc. Am.*, 82 (5), 1503-1511.

Miller, G.A. and Nicely, P.E. (1954). An analysis of perceptual confusions among some English consonants, *J. Acoust. Soc. Am.*, 27 (2), 338-352.

Nierop van, D.J.P.J., Pols, L.C.W., and Plomp, R. (1973). Frequency analysis of Dutch vowels from 25 female speakers, *Acoustica*, 29, 110-118.

Ter Keurs M., Festen, J.M, and Plomp, R. (1991a). Effect of spectral envelope smearing on speech reception in noise and in competing speech, *J. Acoust. Soc. Am.*, 89 (4).

Ter Keurs M., Festen, J.M, and Plomp, R. (1991b). Effect of spectral envelope smearing on speech reception. I. *J. Acoust. Soc. Am.* (in press).

Chapter 5
Phoneme Perception

Effects of Token Variability on Vowel Identification

Rosalie M. Uchanski,
Kathleen M. Millier,
Charlotte M. Reed, and
Louis D. Braida

Research Laboratory of Electronics
Massachusetts Institute of Technology
Cambridge, MA 02139
U.S.A.

1. INTRODUCTION

Our ability to identify speech segments is determined by the physical properties of the segments, by limitations on auditory resolution for salient differences between segments, and by limitations on the processes required to remember the segments. The goal of this research is to understand the limitations associated with natural variations in the utterances of the same speech sound produced by a given speaker. Although the difficulties posed by such variation for automatic speech recognition systems are increasingly appreciated (Perkell and Klatt, 1986; Pisoni, 1990), their effects on human speech reception have not been studied systematically. While we are seldom aware of these effects in everyday communication situations, they may be particularly severe when speech reception is restricted by noise or hearing loss. Under such conditions, the variations in the utterances may consume a proportionally larger fraction of the available perceptual space.

An important motivation for our research on token variability arises from practical concerns in conducting research on speech intelligibility. While various investigators have employed widely different type-token ratios in their experiments, there has been very little study of the effect of this variable on experimental results. For example, in the case of studies of the reception of lowpass-filtered speech, Miller and Nicely (1955) employed a fresh utterance of each stimulus on each experimental trial, while Wang *et al.* (1978) used three pre-recorded utterances of each phoneme throughout their experiment. Most recorded materials used in clinical audiometry include only a single utterance for each speech item. In order to make comparisons across studies employing different numbers of tokens, the dependence of intelligibility on the number of tokens must be established. Furthermore, such research is necessary to determine the levels of token variability that must be employed in order to ensure that listeners focus on general, rather than artifactual, characteristics of recorded speech materials. Specification of necessary levels of token variability is particularly important to the development of speech training procedures (Logan, Lively and Pisoni, 1991).

Ultimately this research will consist of three components: 1) measuring the perceptual effects of token variability on intelligibility in normal and hearing-impaired listeners, 2) characterizing the variability in the acoustic properties of the speech sounds, and 3) developing a model that relates perceptual effects to acoustical properties. In this paper we present data that address the perceptual consequences of token variability for vowel identification for listeners with normal hearing. Identification performance is examined for conditions both with and without feedback.

2. Stimuli and Methods

The speech corpus consists of vowels produced in CVC context by one female talker. This corpus includes 16 repetitions of 10 American English monophthongs in 6 consonant contexts, for a total of 960 utterances. The CVC's consist of all possible combinations of initial consonant {b, p, h}, vowel {ae, ah, aw, ee, eh, er, ih, oo, uu, uh}, and final consonant {t, d}. Table I provides the phonetic equivalents for these orthographic symbols. For each vowel and context the utterances are arbitrarily labelled #1 through #16. The entire set of syllables was spoken in random order in citation style and recorded over a two-day period. The experiments reported in this paper focus on the /h/-V-/d/ context. For this context, the average vowel duration was 264 ms and the average fundamental frequency was 214 Hz. Preliminary analysis indicates that the coefficient of variation for these parameters is roughly 9% (Maney, 1989). In quiet these vowels can be identified with better than 99% accuracy by listeners with normal hearing.

Orthographic	Phonetic	Example
ae	æ	had
ah	ɑ	father
aw	ɔ	bought
ee	i	heed
eh	ɛ	head
er	ɝ	herd
ih	ɪ	hid
oo	u	hoot
uu	ʊ	hood
uh	ʌ	bud

Table I Phonetic equivalents of orthographic symbols.

To make the vowel identification task non-trivial, each utterance was distorted by a process described by Schroeder (1968). Unlike simple additive noise, which provides different amounts of masking for each utterance, this distortion is self-adjusting relative to the level of each utterance. In the Schroeder distortion each sample of the resultant, distorted speech signal, r(t), is related to the corresponding sample of the original, undistorted speech signal, s(t), by the scaled addition of a signal-dependent noise, n(t). That is,

$$r(t) = \frac{s(t) + \alpha n(t)}{\sqrt{1 + \alpha^2}} \tag{1}$$

where

$$n(t) = \varepsilon(t)s(t) \tag{2}$$

and $\varepsilon(t)$ is a random pulse train with values 1 or -1 occurring with equal probability. The parameter α specifies an equivalent instantaneous signal-to-noise ratio (SNR)

$$SNR = 10 \log \frac{S}{N} - 20 \log \frac{1}{\alpha} . \tag{3}$$

Each utterance was distorted once. All the distorted signals were then normalized to the same overall RMS level. The stimuli were presented monaurally over TDH-39 headphones at a level of 74 dB SPL to listeners seated in a sound-treated room. In pilot experiments a SNR of -12 dB ($\alpha \approx 4.0$) was found to yield a useful range of identification scores for the 10 vowels tested. For this distortion, the primary cues for distinguishing between the vowels in the set appear to be fundamental frequency, first formant frequency, and duration.

Our identification tests used a single-interval paradigm. In each interval, one of the 10 vowels was presented. In each condition, the number of utterances used to represent each vowel was varied.

3. Vowel Identification with Feedback

Although speech identification experiments are often conducted with relatively little training and without providing feedback to subjects, it is important to know how performance improves when extensive training and trial-by-trial correct response feedback are provided. For experiments with only a single-token of each speech sound, it might be possible for a listener to focus on and learn characteristics of little phonetic value rather than general speech characteristics.

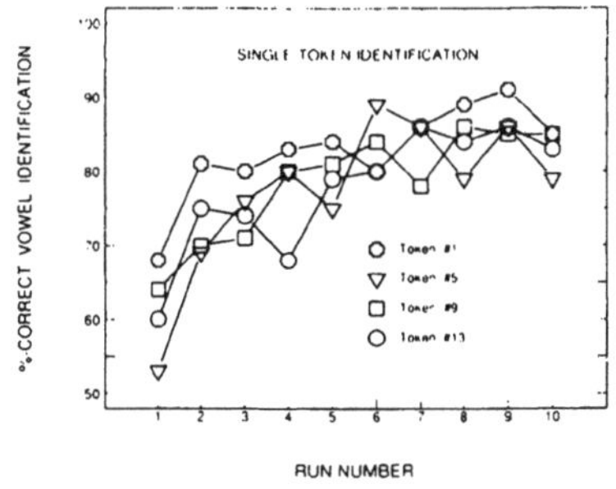

Fig. 1 Learning curves for the identification of 10 vowels in /h/-V-/d/ syllables for four different single-token sets. Performance on the first run for each set was obtained without the use of feedback; all subsequent runs employed trial-by-trial correct-answer feedback. There were 80 trials per run.

In these experiments feedback was given and percent correct performance was measured until an asymptote was reached. The first run for each set did not employ feedback; subsequent runs employed trial-by-trial correct-answer feedback. Data were collected from a single listener. The task was identification for 10 vowels in the /h/-V-/d/ context. Data were obtained for four different single-token sets (tokens #1, #5, #9, and #13), two different four-token sets ({#1, #5, #9, and #13} and {#2, #6, #10, #14}), and the complete sixteen-token set.

Experimental results from the four single-token sets are shown in Fig. 1. Initial performance (run #1, without feedback) varies over a 15 percentage point range; from 53 to 68% correct. By contrast, asymptotic performance (an average of runs 7 through 10) only varies over a 5 percentage point range; from 83 to 88% correct. For these single-token sets, it appears that 1) there is a substantial effect of training on performance and 2) asymptotic identification performance is roughly independent of the particular single-token set.

Experimental results from sets with different numbers of tokens are shown in Fig. 2. Learning curves are presented for an average of four single-token sets, one four-token set, and the sixteen-token set. Asymptotic performance on the single-token set (roughly 84-86% correct) was higher than asymptotic performance on the four-token and sixteen-token sets (roughly 72-75% correct in both cases). Unlike the substantial improvement in performance with training for single-token sets, little consistent change was observed in scores for the four-token and sixteen-token sets. In the single-token conditions, confusion between specific pairs of vowels was reduced, presumably due to the learning of cues associated with the specific utterances in a given set. For example, with single-token set #13, initially /ae/ and /ah/ were confused with each other (and not with any other vowels) such that each was identified correctly approximately 70% of the time. At asymptotic performance, /ae/ and /ah/ were identified correctly about 91% of the time. By contrast, for the four-token set, /ae/ and /ah/ were confused with each other 62% of the time, initially, and 65% of the time after 2000 trials. Even when training is provided, the memory requirements for a strategy based on learning specific cues are evidently too great for it to be effective with the multiple-token sets. Similar improvements have been reported for training on consonant identification (Reed *et al.*, 1991). Listeners can learn to identify a set of 24 consonants lowpass filtered to 500 Hz with an accuracy of roughly 78% when only one utterance of each syllable is used and extensive training is provided. Accuracy drops to 64 and 58% when three- and nine-token sets are used.

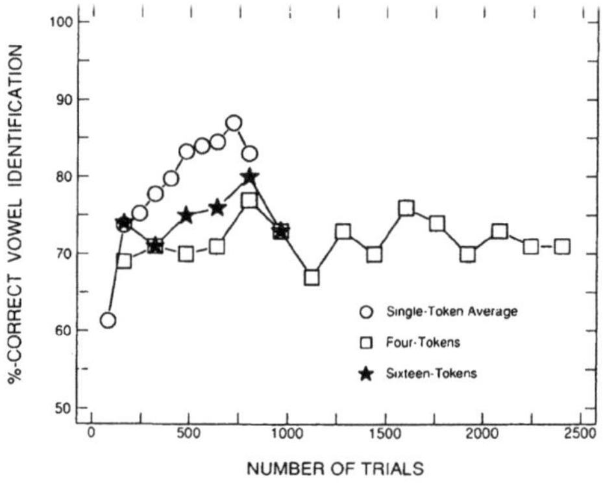

Fig. 2 Learning curves for the identification of 10 vowels in /h/-V-/d/ syllables for three different sets of tokens: single-token, a four-token set, and a sixteen-token set. The single-token curve is the average of 4 separate single-token training tests using tokens #1, #5, #9, and #13 individually. The four-token set consisted of tokens #1, #5, #9, and #13 together. Training results from the other four-token set (tokens #2, #6, #10, and #14 together) are very similar. For clarity data from only one four-token set are shown here. Performance on the first run for each set was obtained without the use of feedback; all subsequent runs employed trial-by-trial correct-answer feedback. The number of trials per run was 80 for the single-token tests and 160 for the four- and sixteen-token sets.

4. Vowel Identification without Feedback

Three normal-hearing listeners, none of whom participated in the previous experiment, identified vowels drawn at random from the set of 10 vowels in /h/-V-/d/ context. Although some initial training was given to familiarize the listeners with the procedure, trial-by-trial feedback was not provided. Vowel responses were collected in 80-trial runs. In separate experiments the number of tokens used to represent each of the vowels was one (tokens #1,

Token(s)	Raw Scores KM	MA	ML	listener ave.	Modified Scores KM	MA	ML	listener ave.
#1	82	59	65	69	77	61	78	72
#5	80	59	48	62	81	60	59	67
#9	66	32	58	52	66	66	77	70
#13	66	63	67	65	77	69	70	72
single-token ave.	74	53	60	65	75	64	71	70
four-tokens	74	50	52	60	74	54	57	62
sixteen-tokens	68	51	54	58	68	54	56	59

Table II Percent correct vowel identification scores for each token condition for each of three listeners. The four-token set consists of tokens #2, #6, #10, and #14. The relation between raw and modified scores is described in Section 4.

#5, #9, and #13 tested separately), four (tokens #2, #6, #10, and #14 tested together), or sixteen. To minimize the effect of token variability, all single-token tests were completed before the four-token experiment was begun, and these were completed before the sixteen-token experiment was begun. In all cases, each vowel *type* was presented 48 times to each listener. This is equivalent to 48, 12, and 3 presentations of each vowel *token* to each listener for the single-, four-, and sixteen-token conditions respectively.

Vowel identification scores for each condition and each listener are summarized in the left-hand columns of Table II (raw scores). These scores are not necessarily good indications of the listeners' abilities to distinguish between vowels, particularly in the single-token experiments. In several cases subjects consistently misidentified pairs of vowels. For example, MA and ML identified token #1 of /ah/ as /aw/ and vice versa more than 90% of the time, and KM identified token #13 of /ae/ as /ah/ (and vice versa) roughly 70% of the time. It seems likely that if feedback were provided such "reversals" would not occur. To estimate scores more representative of the subjects' abilities to assign labels consistently we permuted the responses assigned by each listener in each experiment so as to maximize the percentage of correct responses, assuming that the *a priori* probabilities of stimulus presentations are equal. The permuted response is the identity of the stimulus for which the conditional probability of the observed response is greatest (*e.g.*, Braida, 1991). The percentages of correct responses corresponding to these permutations are shown in the right-hand columns of Table 2 (modified scores). Subsequent discussion concerns these modified scores.

Averaged across listeners, there is little difference between scores for the four single-token experiments. Across conditions, on average there are performance decreases of 8 and 11 percentage points for the four- and sixteen-token conditions relative to the single-token condition. However, individually the performance changes are not the same as number of tokens increases. Listener KM's scores dropped very little as the number of tokens increased from one to four, but the scores on the sixteen-token set were further reduced. Listeners MA and ML achieved scores on the single-token sets that were consistently higher than on the multiple-token sets, but there was little difference between scores on the four- and sixteen-token sets for these listeners. The three listeners also differ in overall level of performance. Subject KM has the highest overall scores followed by listeners ML and MA, in that order.

In summary, the decrease in scores from the single-token conditions to the sixteen-token condition is 7, 10, and 15 percentage points for listeners KM, MA, and ML, respectively. These differences are roughly comparable to those found for the vowel identification with feedback experiment where 10 percentage points separated asymptotic performance in the single-token conditions from that in the sixteen-token condition. Finally, for these identification experiments, it is essential to look beyond the percent correct scores to determine how the number of tokens interacts with vowel confusions.

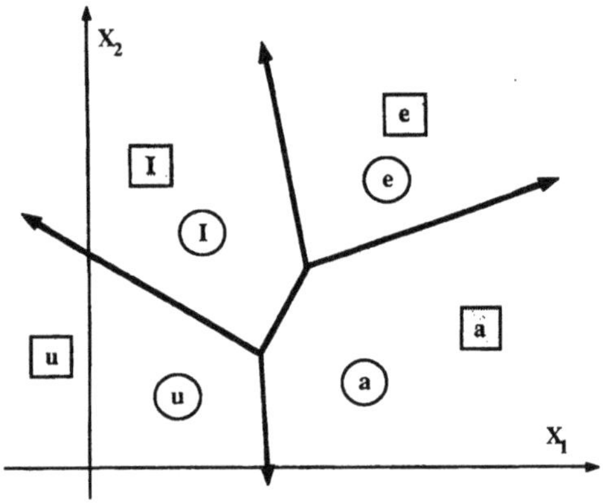

Fig. 3 Two-Dimensional (X_1,X_2) cue space for a hypothetical identification experiment with the four vowels /a, e, I, and u/. Location of the stimulus centers (circles) relative to response prototypes (squares) is arbitrary in this figure. Response regions are bounded by line segments (extended bold lines), each of which coincides with a segment of the perpendicular bisector of a line connecting two response prototypes. The region corresponding to the response "e" is shaded. All the points in a given response region are closer to the prototype in that region than to any other prototype. In general $P(R_j|V_i)$ is computed by integrating the multidimensional Gaussian density with mean V_i over the response region that contains R_j.

4.1 Analysis of Identification Experiments

In vowel identification experiments perceptual confusions cannot generally be attributed to the use of a single cue that can be characterized by a scalar decision variable. In order to analyze performance in such experiments we use a generalization of the scalar model (Braida, 1988; Braida, 1991) that is a multidimensional extension of the theory of signal detection. Each presentation of one of the N possible stimuli (vowels) V_i is assumed to generate a D-dimensional vector of cues $X=[x_1,x_2,...,x_D]$ described by the conditional probability density

$$p(X|V_i) = \prod_{k=1}^{D} p(x_k|V_i) = \prod_{k=1}^{D} \frac{1}{\sqrt{2\pi}} \exp\left(\frac{-(x_k-v_{ik})^2}{2} \right) . \quad (4)$$

Alternately, the cue vector **X** may be thought of as displaced from the stimulus center $V_i=[v_{i1},v_{i2},...,v_{iD}]$ by an additive noise vector whose components are independent Gaussian random variables with zero means and common unit variance.

Corresponding to each response there is a *prototype* $\mathbf{R}_i=[r_{i1},r_{i2},...,r_{iD}]$. (We do *not* assume that $\mathbf{R}_i=\mathbf{V}_i$.) The listener responds R_k if and only if the distance from the vector of cues **X** to $\mathbf{R}_k$ is smaller than the distance to any other prototype, *i.e.*, $\|\mathbf{X}-\mathbf{R}_k\| < \|\mathbf{X}-\mathbf{R}_j\|$ for all $j \neq k$. This rule has the effect of partitioning the *D*-dimensional space of cue vectors into *N* compact "response regions" that are bounded by hyperplanes (see Fig. 3). All the points in each region are closer to the prototype in that region than to any other prototype. The probability that R_j is the response when the stimulus is V_i is the probability that the vector of cues $\mathbf{X}$ is closer to $\mathbf{R}_j$ than to any other prototype when V_i is presented. Since the density $p(\mathbf{X}|V_i)$ weights the relative likelihood of occurrence of cue vectors in these conditions, $P(R_j|V_i)$ is determined by integrating the density with mean $\mathbf{V}_i$ over the response region containing $\mathbf{R}_j$.

The decision process in an identification experiment is thus assumed to reflect the listener's comparison of cue vectors with prototypes. Errors result from the assumed noisiness of the cue vector and the distribution of error responses reflects the relative locations of stimulus centers and prototypes. The boundaries of the response regions are analogous to the scalar decision criteria of signal detection theory. The locations of the prototypes, which determine these boundaries, are assumed to be at least partially under the control of the listener reflecting the effects of instructions and payoffs. A listener's sensitivity $d'(i,j)$ in distinguishing stimulus V_i from stimulus V_j, is given in the multidimensional case by

$$d'(i,j) = \|V_i - V_j\| = \sqrt{\sum_{k=1}^{D} (v_{ik} - v_{jk})^2} \ . \tag{5}$$

Given a set of $\mathbf{V}_i$ and a set of $\mathbf{R}_j$, a confusion matrix can be predicted by numerical integration. The inverse problem of estimating the set of $\mathbf{V}_i$ and $\mathbf{R}_j$ that are most consistent with a given confusion matrix has not yet been solved completely. Braida (1988) described a procedure for estimating values of these parameters (*i.e.*, the coordinates of the set of $\mathbf{V}_i$ and $\mathbf{R}_j$) corresponding to a given confusion matrix for a specified value of *D*. In this method, initial estimates of the stimulus centers are obtained by nonmetric multidimensional scaling (Kruskal and Wish, 1978) and the response centers are initially aligned with the stimulus centers. Subsequent estimates of both sets of centers are obtained iteratively by attempting to improve the match (as specified by a χ^2-like measure) between the predicted matrix and the observed matrix.

4.2 Sensitivity in Vowel Identification Experiments

The vowel responses were collected into confusion matrices and analyzed with the model described in Section 4.1 to obtain estimates of $d'(i,j)$ (with $D=2$ or $D=3$ chosen to achieve the best fit to each confusion matrix) for each pair of vowels in the experiment. These values of d' were then averaged across subjects for each condition.

To evaluate the quality of the parameters derived from estimated configurations, model parameters derived from the empirical confusion matrices were used to create new confusion matrices using Monte Carlo simulation techniques consistent with the assumptions of the decision model. Each stimulus was presented 48 times in a given simulation, and each condition was simulated 16 times. For each simulation, new model parameters were estimated and used to compute values of d' for the simulation. The bias (less than 10% on average) and

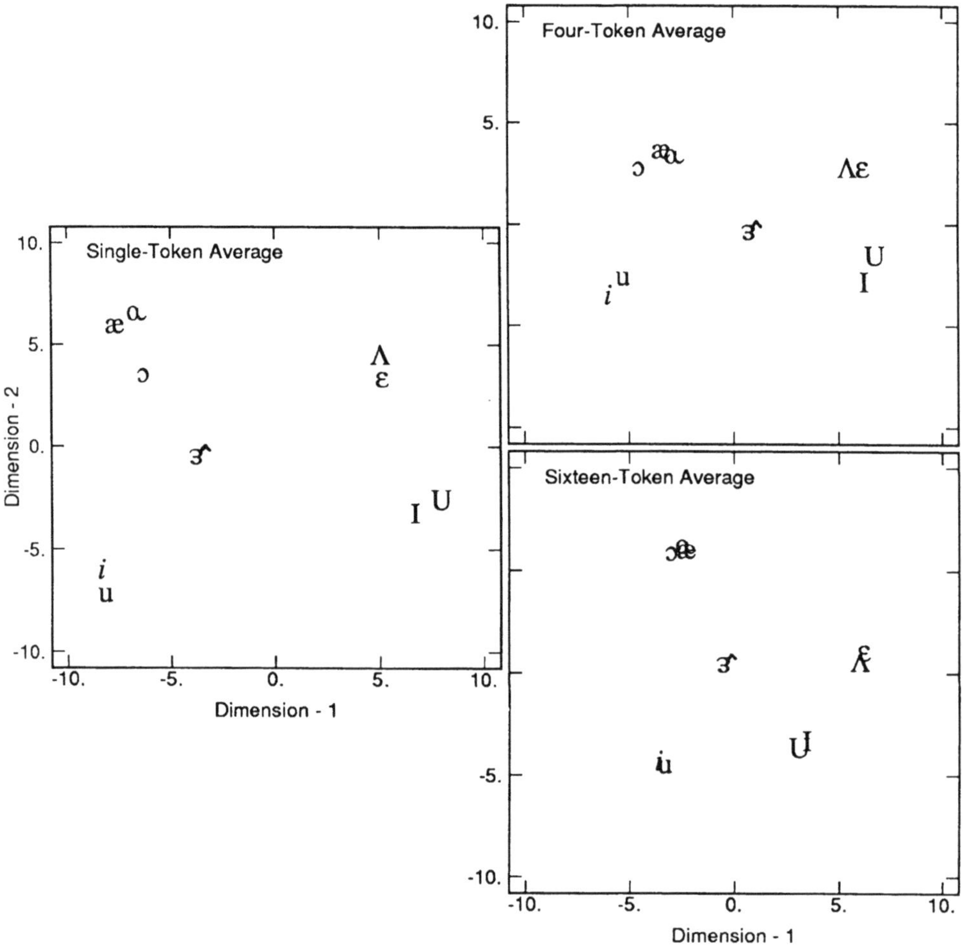

Fig. 4 Configuration of stimulus points for single-, four-, and sixteen-token experiments. The leftmost configuration was derived by fitting the model of Section 4.1 to each confusion matrix obtained in a single-token experiment from each subject, estimating distances between stimulus points, averaging these distances across tokens and subjects, and constructing a new configuration of stimulus points corresponding to the resulting distances. Similar configurations, derived from the four-token and sixteen-token results, are shown on the right-top and right-bottom, respectively.

variability of these estimates (including the effects of both the Monte Carlo simulation and the estimation procedure) were used to evaluate the robustness of changes in sensitivity across conditions.

To provide a visual display of the cue space, conventional multidimensional scaling was applied to the average values of *d'* (averaged across tokens in the case of the 1-token data) and two-dimensional configurations were derived. The scale of these configurations was adjusted so that distances in these spaces correspond to the estimated values of *d'*. The resulting configurations are shown in Fig. 4. Note that the scale unit in each of the panels of this figure corresponds roughly to one standard deviation of the Gaussian cue density. Generally, stimuli whose points are separated by four standard deviations or more are well distinguished, while those separated by two standard deviations or less are confused.

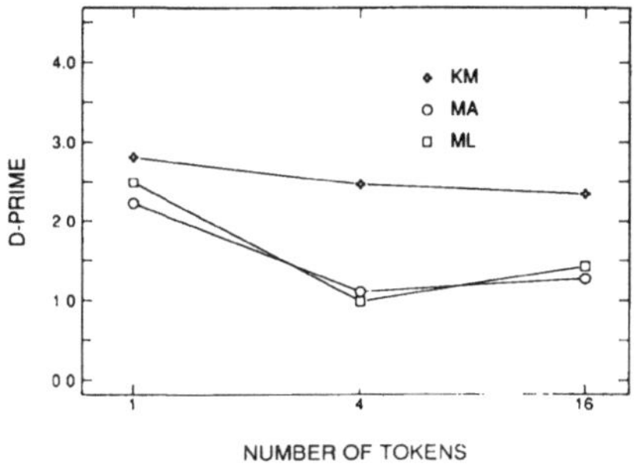

Fig. 5 Vowel identification d' as a function of number of tokens for the three subjects KM, MA, and ML. Estimates of sensitivity were averaged across data obtained from the six vowel-pairs {ee,oo}, {ae,ah}, {uh,eh}, {ih,uu}, {ae,aw}, and {ah,aw}.

The configuration of points is very similar in all three panels. Confusions are largely confined to subsets of the vowels with relatively few confusions occurring across subsets. For example, in this 2-dimensional space the vowels /uh/ and /eh/ are close to each other and thus easily confused, but are far away from, and not confused with, any other vowel cluster or singlet. Although the structure of the cue space is relatively invariant to the number of tokens that represent the vowel, there is a general tendency for the span of the points to shrink as the number of tokens increases.

To a first approximation, we can treat the distances between the points representing the vowels in the different cue spaces as differing by a single scale factor for each space. The reduction in separation between vowels as the number of tokens increases presumably reflects the effect of increasing variability in the representation of each vowel. Six vowel pairs ({ee,oo}, {ae,ah}, {uh,eh}, {ih,uu}, {ae,aw}, and {ah,aw}), with estimated values of *d'* less than 5.0 for all three conditions, are examined. Fig. 5 is a plot of vowel identification *d'*, averaged over these six pairs, as a function of number of tokens. The data for each of the three listeners are shown separately. Our methods are only sensitive enough to have confidence that subjects MA and ML exhibited less sensitivity in the four- and sixteen-token experiments than in the single-token experiment, and do not detect any difference between sensitivity in the four- and sixteen-token experiments for any subject.

Average (over listener) *d'*s for the same six vowel pairs are presented in Fig. 6 for the pairs of conditions {single-token, four-token} and {single-token, sixteen-token}. On average, sensitivity in the four- and sixteen-token experiments is roughly 27% and 35% less, respectively, than that in the single-token experiment, although not all subjects experienced

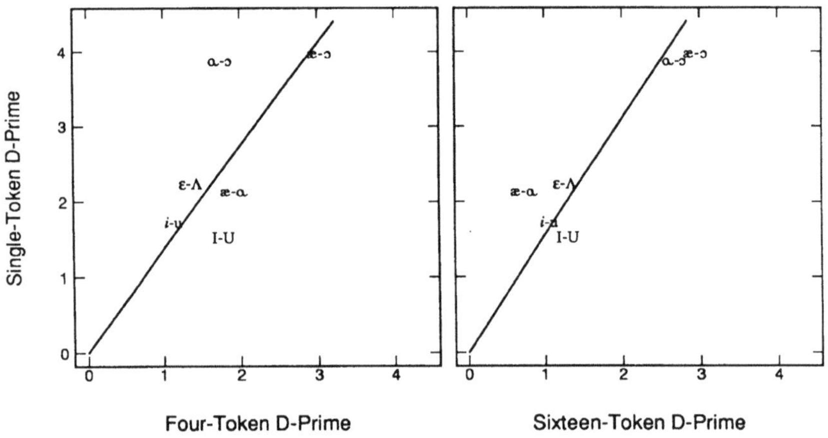

Fig. 6 Vowel identification d's for the six vowel pairs {ee,oo}, {ae,ah}, {uh,eh}, {ih,uu}, {ae,aw}, and {ah,aw}. The values of single-token sensitivity are averages of estimates of sensitivity over the four single-token experiments. All estimates of sensitivity were derived using the model discussed in Section 4.1.

the same degree of reduction (as seen in Fig. 5). The reduction in sensitivity is fairly uniform across vowel pairs, although our estimation methods are not sensitive enough to detect changes in *d'* for the pairs {ae,aw} and {ah,aw}.

5. DISCUSSION

For a given vowel, the utterance-to-utterance variability studied in these experiments is only one component of the variation that occurs in natural speech. The physical characteristics of a given vowel are known to vary substantially across speakers (*e.g.*, Peterson and Barney, 1952) and consonant contexts (*e.g.*, House and Fairbanks, 1953; Klatt, 1976), as well as lexical stress and speaking style (*e.g.*, Picheny *et al.*, 1986; Huang, 1991). However, even this restricted utterance-to-utterance variability can have substantial perceptual effects. In an experiment with feedback, asymptotic identification performance is roughly 10 percentage points greater for single- than for sixteen-token vowel sets. In experiments without feedback we found comparable changes in the modified percent correct scores (11 percentage points) although changes in raw scores were smaller. We also found significant changes in *d'*, for two of our three listeners, as token variability increased (see Fig. 5). For identification of 24 consonants with feedback, an even larger effect of token variability has been reported. Reed *et al.* (1991) report a decrease in identification score from 78% to 58% as the number of tokens increased from one to nine. Others have examined the effects of less restricted utterance variability, such as inter-talker variability, on speech perception. For example, van Velden and Smoorenburg (1991) measured the speech reception threshold (SRT, *i.e.*, the 50%-correct-level) for identification of 15 Dutch vowels in a /t/-V-/t/ context, by normal listeners in different level noise backgrounds. They recorded utterances from 15 speakers; 5 adult male,

5 adult female, and 5 children. In a pilot experiment they found ranges of more than 9 dB in SRT across the vowels for one speaker and more than 12 dB across speakers for one vowel. A much smaller range of SRT's was found across different talker groups: on average, the SRT was 2 dB lower for the intra-group vowel sets than for the inter-group vowel set. For an open-set word identification task, Mullennix, *et al.* (1989) obtained scores of 33.9% and 40.6% in single- and mixed-talker conditions. Although these studies differ in many details from this one, it appears that for humans the perceptual effect of utterance-to-utterance variation is comparable to that of talker-to-talker variation, at least for degraded speech signals. This result contrasts with the performance of automatic speech recognition systems on undegraded speech, for which utterance-to-utterance variation has a much smaller effect than talker-to-talker variation.

The variability of our stimuli includes both the utterance-to-utterance variation in the production of the speech sounds and the waveform-dependent variability of the distortion applied to each utterance (*e.g.*, Equation 1). The experiments reported in this paper do not permit us to separate the effects of these two types of variability. This separation is essential to our goal of relating perceptual measures of variability to variations in the physical characteristics of the utterances of vowels. To this end we plan to measure resolution under conditions that include controlled variation in the distortion as well as across tokens.

Our results shed some light on the question of how many tokens of speech stimuli must be used to obtain representative results. In the case of identification, four tokens appear to provide a reasonable sample of variability and reasonable protection from reliance on specific characteristics, at least when the stimulus set consists of ten distinct speech items.

In these identification experiments, most confusions between vowels occurred within clusters of two or three elements. This suggests that future studies may be more efficient if discrimination rather than identification tasks are employed. In general, discrimination tasks are simpler to describe to listeners and impose smaller memory loads, so that effects of token variability on performance are expected to be more pronounced. Moreover, the cues that permit discrimination between small groups of tokens may be substantially different from those that must be monitored to identify vowels from a large set. Thus, although we expect discrimination studies to yield large token-variability effects, it may be difficult to relate these effects to those seen in identification experiments.

Acknowledgement

This work was supported by the N. I. H. (Grants DC00010 and DC00117). We are grateful to J. Besing for help preparing the speech corpus. We also appreciate thoughtful discussions with J. Besing, S. Dubois, C. B. Huang, J. W. Maney, Jr., D. B. Pisoni, M. H. Power, and W. M. Rabinowitz.

References

Braida, L.D. (1988). Development of a model for multidimensional identification experiments, *J. Acoust. Soc. Am.*, 84, S142.

Braida, L.D. (1991). Crossmodal integration in the identification of consonant segments, *Q. J. Expt. Psych.*, 43 A(3), 647-677.

House, A.S. and Fairbanks, G. (1953). The influence of consonant environment upon the secondary acoustical characteristics of vowels, *J. Acoust. Soc. Am.*, 25(1), 105-113.

Huang, C.B. (1991). *An Acoustic and Perceptual Study of Vowel Formant Trajectories in American English*, PhD thesis, Massachusetts Institute of Technology.

Klatt, D.H. (1976). Linguistic uses of segmental duration in English: Acoustic and perceptual evidence, *J. Acoust. Soc. Am.*, 59, 1208-1221.

Kruskal, J.B. and Wish, M. (1978). *Multidimensional Scaling, Quantitative Applications in the Social Sciences*, Sage Publications, Inc., 07-011.

Logan, J.S., Lively, S.E., and Pisoni, D.B. (1991). Training Japanese listeners to identify English /r/ and /l/: A first report, *J. Acoust. Soc. Am.*, 89(2), 874-886.

Maney, J.W., Jr. (1989). *Token variability of intra-speaker speech.* S.B. Thesis, Massachusetts Institute of Technology.

Miller, G.A. and Nicely, P.E. (1955). An analysis of perceptual confusions among some English consonants, *J. Acoust. Soc. Am.*, 27(2), 338-352.

Millier, K.M. (1990). *Intelligibility of vowels represented by multiple intra-speaker tokens.* S.B. Thesis, Massachusetts Institute of Technology.

Mullennix, J.W., Pisoni, D.B., and Martin, C.S. (1989). Some effects of talker variability on spoken word recognition, *J. Acoust. Soc. Am.*, 85(1), 365-378.

Perkell, J.S. and Klatt, D.H., editors, (1986). *Invariance and variability in speech processes*, Lawrence Erlbaum Associates, Hillsdale, NJ.

Peterson, G.E. and Barney, H.L. (1952). Control methods used in a study of the vowels, *J. Acoust. Soc. Am.*, 24(2), 175-184.

Picheny, M.A., Durlach, N.I., and Braida, L.D. (1986). Speaking clearly for the hard of hearing II: Acoustic characteristics of clear and conversational speech, *Journal of Speech and Hearing Research*, 29(4), 434-446.

Pisoni, D.B. (1990). Effects of talker variability on speech perception: Implications for current research and theory, in Fujisaki, H., editor, *Proceedings of the 1990 International Conference on Spoken Language Processing*, Kobe, Japan.

Reed, C.M., Power, M.H., Durlach, N.I., Braida, L.D., Foss, K.K., Reid, J.A., and Dubois, S.R. (1991). Development and testing of artificial low-frequency speech codes, *J. Rehabilitation Research and Development*, 28(3), 67-82.

Schroeder, M.R. (1968). Reference signal for signal quality studies, *J. Acoust. Soc. Am.*, 44(6), 1735-1736.

van Velden, J.G. and Smoorenburg, G.F. (1991). Vowel recognition in noise for male, female and child voices, in *Proceedings of the IEEE International Conference on Acoustics, Speech and Signal Processing*, Toronto, Canada.

Wang, M., Reed, C., and Bilger, R. (1978). A comparison of the effects of filtering and sensorineural hearing loss on patterns of consonant confusions, *Journal of Speech and Hearing Research*, 21, 5-36.

Evaluation of Prototypes and Exemplars in Perceptual Space for Place Contrast

Xiaofeng Li,
Richard E. Pastore
Center for Cognitive and Psycholinguistic Sciences
State University of New York at Binghamton
Binghamton, New York 13902-6000 USA

For several decades one of the recurrent themes in the speech perception literature has been that phonetic categories are perceived on the basis of category prototypes. With the exception of several studies involving selective adaptation (Miller, Connine, Schermer and Kluender, 1983; Samuel, 1982) and dichotic listening (Repp, 1976), very little research has attempted to evaluate the notion of prototypes and the related notion of the nature of the perceptual structure of phonetic categories (e.g., Kuhl, 1991). The goal in the current research is to provide such an evaluation in a matrix of stop consonants varying in categories of place of articulation.

Much modern research on perception of phoneme categories has used labeling techniques which are used to define category boundaries. From the perspective of psychophysics, such labeling research is providing little more than a possibly biased estimate of perceptual thresholds. The research described here is based upon three different experiments, two of which borrow techniques developed and validated in the cognitive literature.

The first experiment uses a typical labeling technique to map out the general boundaries of perceptual space for a matrix of stimuli varying factorially in F2- and F3-onset frequency. This first study represents a partial replication and expansion of the work by Harris, Hoffman, Liberman, Delattre and Cooper (1958; also, Harris and Hoffman, 1958). The remaining two experiments use measures of classification, reaction time and stimulus similarity to evaluate the perceptual space of subjects and then to evaluate two models of categorization based respectively upon prototypes and exemplars. Reaction time measures have been used to study phonetic categories (e.g., Pisoni and Tash, 1974; Summerfield and Haggard, 1975). Also, multidimensional scaling (MDS) has been used to investigate phoneme (usually vowel) perception based upon confusion matrices (e.g. Krull, 1990; van der Kamp and Pols, 1971; Sidwell and Summerfield, 1986), although some studies have used similarity ratings (e.g., Bladon and Lindblom, 1981). The models for MDS-based prototypes and exemplars are derived from the extensive cognitive literature investigating categorization (Nosofsky, 1991). Our research brings together these strategies and techniques to investigate the perceptual phoneme space and the notion of categorization by prototypes and exemplars for a place contrast in a specific vowel context /a/. The results therefore should be interpreted in terms of this specific vowel context.

1. Current Investigation

All of our subjects were students in our introductory psychology course, with 14 to 18 different subjects participating in each experiment. All were native speakers of American English and reported normal hearing.

We began with a 56 synthetic stimulus matrix factorially crossing seven values of F2-onset frequency with eight values of F3-onset frequency. The onset frequencies for stimuli can be found as the axis coordinates in the figures summarizing results. In the first experiment subjects labeled the 56 stimuli in terms of the categories "B," "D," "G," and "other." Since "other" was almost never used, the results are discussed only in terms of three phonetic categories. Fig. 1 provides the summary of the stimuli and the most frequent category response for each stimulus. The "B" category is defined by a low F2-onset frequency and is independent of F3-onset frequency. This finding is generally consistent with the early research by Harris and Hoffman (cited above). When F2-onset frequency is high, the perceptual category can be described as "not B," with the actual phonetic category ("D" or "G") determined by an interaction of F2- and F3-onset frequency. An unexpected result is the existence of two regions for the category "G."

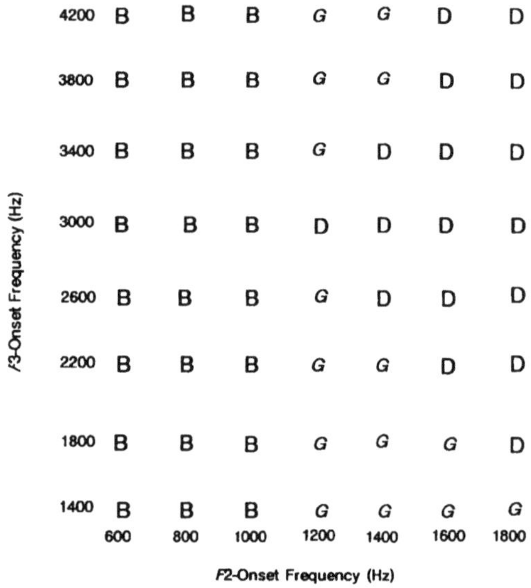

Fig. 1 The matrix (7x8) of stimuli used in Experiment 1 varying 7 levels of F2-onset frequency and 8 levels of F3-onset frequency. The letters (B, D, and G) designate the most frequent categories to which subjects classified each stimulus (the lattice in the matrix).

The remaining two experiments focus solely on stimuli within and across the "B" and "D" categories. The stimuli for each experiment were sampled from the initial set of the 56 stimuli, with additional stimuli inserted between the original stimuli to provide a better mapping of the narrower stimulus space, especially focusing on the prototypes and the ambiguous stimulus region between the categories.

Experiment 2 was a speeded classification task where response category and response time (RT) were measured for each of the 38 stimuli. After practice, each subject classified each stimulus twenty times. Fig. 2 summarizes the most frequent category response (Fig. 2a) and the mean RT (Fig. 2b). The stimuli also used in Experiment 3 are underscored and designated by a digit or letter. In general, the stimulus with the fastest RT for each category is located near the center of the given category. These stimuli (3 and e) will be used as an approximation of the category prototypes.

In Experiment 3 subjects used a 5-point scale to rate the similarity between each of the 169 pairs of stimuli (each stimulus paired with every stimulus including itself). The similarity ratings for stimulus pairs were treated as distances and a multidimensional space was

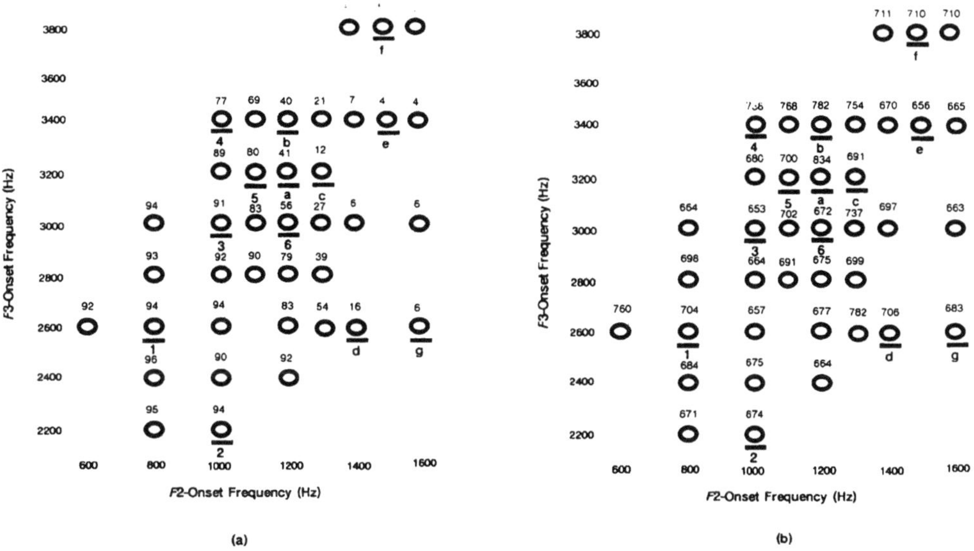

Fig. 2 The circles in the matrix are the stimuli used in Experiment 2. Unfilled circles are categorized as "B", while filled circles are categorized as "D". In panel a, the numbers indicate the percentages of responses to category "B". In panel b, the three-digit numbers are the response times. The underscored stimuli are those also used in Experiment 3. The single digit ("B") or letter "D" is used to draw the parallel between this figure and Fig. 3.

computed. Fig. 3 is the two-dimensional configuration with a stress value of 0.092 and accounts for 96% of the variance. Note that all of the "B" stimuli are located in the left half of the Fig. and all of the "D" stimuli are located in the right half of the figure, indicating that the horizontal dimension represents a decision axis between "B" and "D."

The two prototype stimuli (3 and e) with the fastest RTs from Experiment 2 are located near the ends of this dimension. The ambiguous stimuli tend to be located in the middle of the Fig. and are distributed along the vertical dimension. RT in Experiment 2 seems to be a function of horizontal distance from the prototype and also vertical distance from the centered horizontal axis. Therefore, it appears that the horizontal dimension defines category membership and the vertical dimension defines category goodness for each degree of category membership. This observation is supported by a canonical correlation analysis. The canonical correlation analysis between the F2- and F3-onset frequencies and the coordinates from the multidimensional scaling solution indicated a high loading between F2-onset frequency and the horizontal dimension, and also between F3-onset frequency and the vertical dimension.

Finally, a MDS version of a prototype-based model was used to evaluate the classification of the phonemes for place of articulation (Nosofsky, 1991). We computed the predicted percentages of classification for categories "B" and "D" in the 13 stimuli in Experiment 3. Table 1 shows the comparison between the observed (second column) and predicted (third column) percentages for each stimulus. The correlation between the observed and predicted results is 0.97, indicating that the prototype model seems to provide an excellent representation of the perception of these stimuli by the subjects.

Despite the excellent predictions of the MDS based prototype model, we also computed the predictions based upon a MDS-based exemplar model, which states that category membership is determined by computing the similarity of the test stimulus with all members in a particular category. The predictions from the exemplar model are reported in the fourth column of Table 1. The correlation of 0.97 between the predictions of the exemplar model and the observed data indicates that the exemplar model is equally qualified to predict the classification for place contrast. The exemplar model better predicts classification of ambiguous stimuli, whereas the prototype model better predicts classification of stimuli within each category.

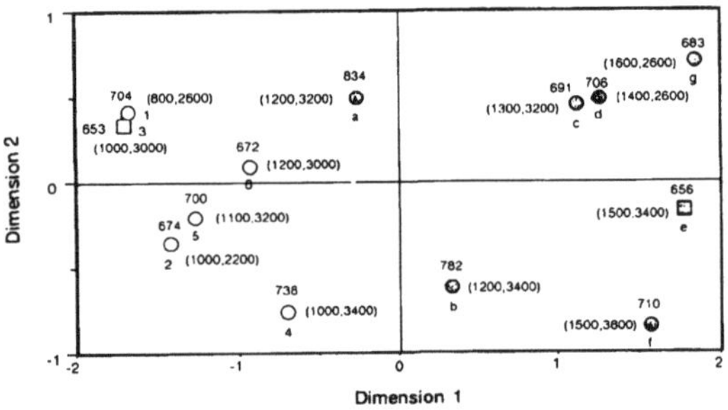

Fig. 3 The two-dimensional perceptual configuration is derived from a MDS of similarity ratings. Category "B", represented by filled symbols, is located on the right. The response time for categorization is shown above each stimulus. The two squares are the category prototypes defined according to the fastest response times. The numbers and letters under each stimulus correspond to the stimulus designation in Fig. 2. The actual onset frquencies are indicated in parentheses.

2. General Discussion

These different techniques investigating the perceptual space of subjects have provided (1) an indication of the possible role played by the different physical dimensions, (2) the organization of the various stimuli in terms of perceptual dimensions, and (3) the role played by those perceptual dimensions for the subjects. The results in Figs. 2 and 3 also provide an important insight into a problem with phonetic trading relations which typically use only standard labeling procedures (e.g., Best, Morongiello and Robson, 1981; Repp, 1982). Begin with stimuli 4 and b in Fig. 2a; by increasing F2-onset frequency, perception of the stimulus changes from the "B" to a marginal member of the "D" category without improving categorical goodness (see Fig. 3). Now consider stimuli b and 6; decreasing F3-onset frequency causes a major perceptual change in categorical goodness, which also restores the stimulus to the "B" category (see Fig. 3). Looking only at category membership, these results would be claimed to be a phonetic trading relation between the F2- and F3-onset frequency cues. However, we already have seen that the two cues play very different roles for the "B" category, with the change in the F3-onset frequency cue being primarily a shift in perceived goodness. It is not obvious that there is any advantage to claim that these two cues have a trading relation for the "B" category, or for the "B/D" contrast, with each cue playing an equivalent role. In fact, this conclusion would seem to be incorrect.

Table I The Observed and Predicted Percentages of Classification to Category /b/ On the Basis of Prototype and Exemplar Models

Stimulus Code	Observed	Prototype	Exemplar
1	.94	.96	.87
2	.94	.92	.85
3	.91	.96	.87
4	.77	.77	.72
5	.80	.90	.83
6	.56	.85	.75
a	.41	.64	.46
b	.40	.37	.33
c	.12	.14	.13
d	.16	.12	.11
e	.04	.04	.09
f	.05	.07	.11
g	.06	.06	.08

Note. Stimulus codes correspond to those in Figs. 2 and 3 with the numbers representing category "B" and letters representing category "D".

3. Conclusions

We have found new evidence supporting conclusions about F2-and F3-onset frequency drawn in some of the early research in place categories. We also have found evidence which is consistent with the use of prototypes in the judgement of speech categories, although the distinction from other models of categorization, especially exemplar models, needs to be further evaluated. Finally, the continuing use of alternative measures to investigate the perception of phonemes may provide different or alternative insights into the nature of perceptual relationships among stimuli and dimensions.

Acknowledgements

This research was supported in part by the National Science Foundation under Grant BNS8911456 to the second author. Any opinions, findings and conclusions expressed in this paper are those of the authors and do not necessarily reflect the views of the National Science Foundation.

References

Best, C.T., Morrongiello, B., and Robson, R. (1981). Perceptual equivalence of acoustic cues in speech and nonspeech perception, *Perception and Psychophysics*, 29, 191-211.

Bladon, R.A. and Lindblom, B. (1981). Modeling the judgement of vowel quality differences, *J. Acoust. Soc. Am.*, 69, 1414-1422.

Delattre, P.C., Liberman, A.M., and Cooper, F.S. (1955). Acoustic loci and transitional cues for consonants, *J. Acoust. Soc. Am.*, 27, 769-773.

Harris, K.S., Hoffman, H.S., Liberman, A.M., Delattre, P.C., and Cooper, F.S. (1958). Effect of third-formant transitions on the perception of the voiced stop consonants, *J. Acoust. Soc. Am.*, 30, 122-126.

Hoffman, H.S. (1958). Study of some cues in the perception of the voiced stop consonants, *J. Acoust. Soc. Am.*, 30, 1035-1041.

Kamp, van der L.J. Th. and Pols, L. C. W. (1971). Perceptual analysis from confusions between vowels, *Acta Psychologica*, 35, 64-77.

Krull, D. (1990). Relating acoustic properties to perceptual responses: A study of Swedish voiced stops, *J. Acoust. Soc. Am.*, 88, 2557-2570.

Kuhl, P.K. (1991). Human adults and human infants show a "perceptual magnet effect" for the prototypes of speech categories, monkeys do not, *Perception and Psychophysics*, 50, 93-107.

Miller, J.L., Connine, C.M., Schermer, T.M., and Kluender, K.R. (1983). A possible auditory basis for internal structure of phonetic categories, *J. Acoust. Soc. Am.*, 73, 2124-2133.

Nosofsky, R.M. (1991). Tests of an exemplar model for relating perceptual classification and recognition memory, *Journal of Experimental Psychology: Human Perception and Performance*, 17, 3-27.

Pisoni, D.B. and Tash, J. (1974). Reaction times to comparisons within and across phonetic categories, *Perception and Psychophysics*, 15, 285-290.

Repp, B. (1976). Identification of dichotic fusions, *J. Acoust. Soc. Am.*, 60, 456-469.

Repp, B. (1982). Phonetic trading relations and context effects: New evidence for a phonetic mode of perception, *Psychological Bulletin*, 92, 81-110.

Samuel, A.G. (1982). Phonetic prototypes, *Perception and Psychophysics*, 31, 307-314.

Sidwell, A. and Summerfield, A.Q. (1986). The auditory representation of symmetrical CVC syllables, *Speech Communication*, 5, 283-297.

Summerfield, A.Q. and Haggard, M.P. (1975). Vocal tract normalization as demonstrated by reaction times, in G. Fant and M.A.A. Tatham (Eds.), *Auditory Analysis and Perception of Speech*. NY: Academic.

Different Discrimination Strategies for Vowels and Consonants

Bert Schouten
Arjan van Hessen
Research Institute for Language and Speech
University of Utrecht
Trans 10
3512 JK Utrecht
The Netherlands

Fig. 1 contains plots of two-step categorization (called "identification" here) and discrimination functions for a consonant continuum /p-t-k/ (top) and a vowel continuum /i-e-a/ (bottom). The 15 stimuli in each continuum were obtained by spectral interpolation between the words *pak, tak, kak* and between *pit, pet, pat,* as pronounced by a male native speaker of Dutch; this interpolation process, which is described in detail by Van Hessen (1988), resulted in stimuli that were completely natural. We did not have the tight parametric control over our stimuli that is usual in speech perception experiments: the differences between our stimuli were multi-dimensional. However, the advantage was that subjects had to judge the complete percept, since it did not pay to concentrate on one or two parameters. We hoped that the use of natural-sounding, multidimensional stimuli would bring us closer to normal speech perception: apart from being encouraged to listen to overall timbre, subjects would also be able to refer each stimulus to their own internal phoneme representations, rather than to the continuum endpoints.

There were 14 subjects. They had to perform four tasks:

- Identification of each stimulus as one one of the three relevant phoneme categories. The identification scores are shown in Fig. 1 as d' values for the "predicted discrimination" of stimuli that are two steps apart; for example, at stimulus pair 7 in the top panel, p(H) was the proportion of /t/-responses to stimulus 6 and p(FA) was the proportion of /t/-responses to stimulus 8. The "prediction" here is that stimuli can only be discriminated to the extent that they are labelled differently; this prediction is known as the categorical perception hypothesis (see Macmillan, Kaplan, and Creelman, 1977). If the results from the real discrimination tasks differ significantly from this prediction, perception is not fully categorical.
- AX same-different. Subjects had to indicate whether the two stimuli in a trial were identical or different. The two stimuli were always two continuum steps apart, and presentation was fixed, i.e. in blocks of the same pairs.
- Two-interval, two-alternative forced choice (2IFC), fixed. Subjects had to indicate in which of two possible orders (AB or BA) the two stimuli in a trial had been presented. The distance between them was again two stimulus steps. Presentation was fixed, i.e. in separate blocks for each pair of stimuli.
- Two-interval, two-alternative forced choice (2IFC), roving. This was the same as 2IFC

fixed, but without the blocked presentation: stimulus pai's were chosen randomly from the whole continuum.

In the discrimination tasks, correct-response feedback was given after each trial, and subjects were punished or rewarded financially for each incorrect or correct response. The d' values in Fig. 1 were, for the three discrimination tasks, calculated in accordance with the standard assumptions about optimum decision strategies (Macmillan et al., 1977). As can be seen in the bottom panel, discrimination of the vowel stimuli was reasonably, but certainly not fully, categorical: the identification and discrimination functions have the same shape and they are rather close together. The order of the functions is the usual one: identification yields the lowest d'-values, 2IFC roving is higher, and fixed discrimination is best of all (where the two fixed-discrimination functions do not coincide, 2IFC is always higher than AX same-different).

The top panel is more surprising. Identification and forced-choice discrimination of stop

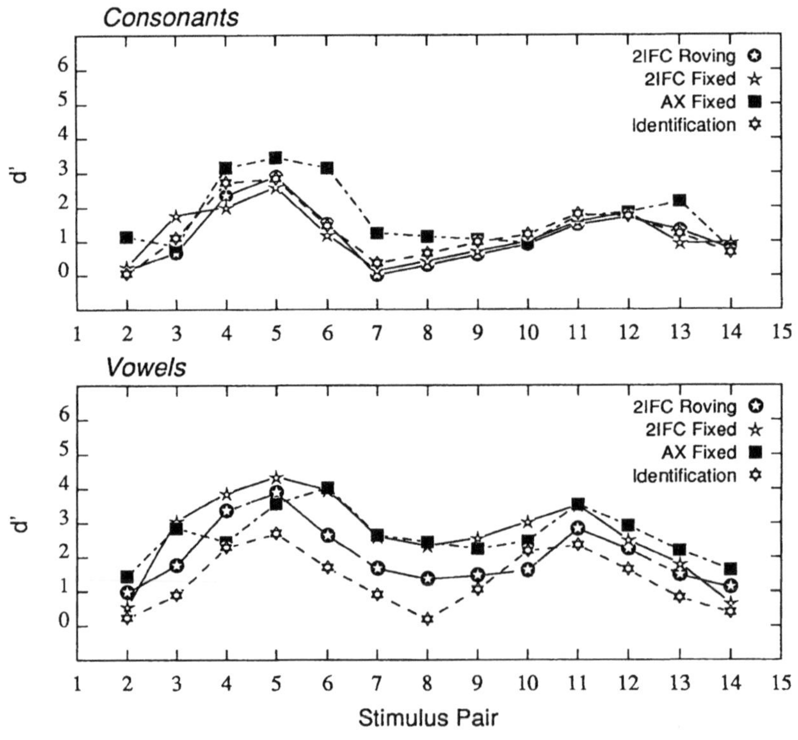

Fig. 1 2IFC discrimination calculated according to standard assumptions

consonants coincide completely, which means that perception was fully categorical, but the AX discrimination function is considerably higher. This is an anomalous result, since it implies that subjects can use only category label information in 2IFC, but that other information is available to them in AX. We therefore have to reconsider our assumptions about subjects' decision strategies, at least in the case of stop consonants.

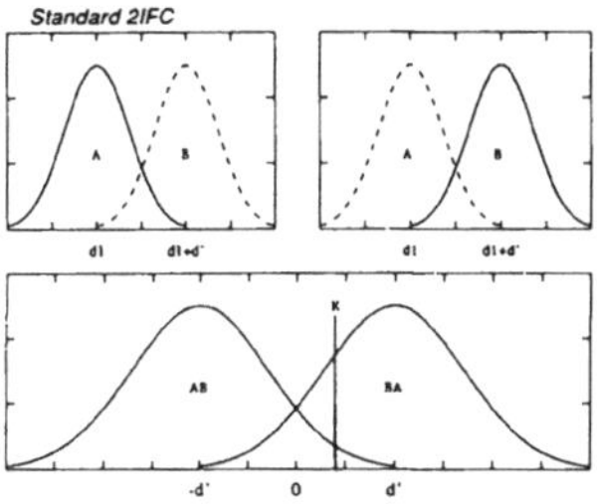

Fig. 2 Standard 2IFC decision model.

$$H_{AB} = \Phi[\frac{(k+d')}{\sigma}] \qquad (1)$$

$$FA_{AB} = \Phi[\frac{(k-d')}{\sigma}] \qquad (2)$$

$$d_{2IFC} = \frac{(k+d')-(k-d')}{\sqrt{2}} = \sqrt{2}d' \qquad (3)$$

$$d' = \frac{d'_{2IFC}}{\sqrt{2}} = 0.5\sqrt{2} * \{z(H_{AB})-z(FA_{AB})\} \qquad (4)$$

The standard assumptions about 2IFC are shown graphically in Fig. 2. The top two panels show the two possible orders in which stimuli A and B can be presented, with the dashed curve representing the second interval in a trial. Stimulus A is assumed to be at position d1 along the sensation axis (called "stimulus axis" here), and stimulus B at position (d1+d'). The distributions of the sensations caused by A and B are assumed to be normal and to have an equal variance of 1. The subject subtracts the sensation caused by the stimulus in the second interval from that in the first interval; this results in the two difference distributions shown in the bottom panel. The one on the left is caused by presentation AB; its mean is d1-(d1+d')=-d', and its variance is 2. The one on the right is caused by presentation BA; its mean is (d1+d')-d1=d', and its variance also equals 2. If the difference between the two sensations exceeds criterion k, the subject responds "BA"; if it does not, he responds "AB". Since his decision involves two difference distributions which are 2d' apart and each of which has a variance of 2, subtraction of z(H) and z(FA) leads to an overestimation of "true" d' by a factor of √2, so the resulting d' values must be divided by √2 in order to establish the resolution of the original stimuli.

These assumptions about the optimum decision strategy do not cause any clear anomalies in vowel discrimination; the conclusion seems to be that subjects base their vowel discrimination judgments on the differences between the two intervals, and that vowel discrimination therefore does not differ greatly from e.g. intensity resolution. It remains surprising and even paradoxical, however, that vowel discrimination should be based on phoneme label differences to such a great extent.

For stop-consonant discrimination, we propose a different decision strategy, based on what subjects told us and on our own experience when trying to perform the 2IFC task. The important question is: what does a subject do when he hears two /p/-like or /t/-like or /k/-like stimuli and has to decide whether they were presented in the order /p-k/ or the order /k-p/?

Our answer is that, as soon as the first stimulus in a trial has been presented, the subject attempts to calculate its distance to one or more of the phoneme prototypes; he codes this distance in such terms as "reasonably good /p/" or "poor /t/". The same happens to the second stimulus, after which the subject subtracts the two distances in order to reach a decision.

Fig. 3 is a graphical representation of this process. The top left panel shows the distribution of sensations caused by stimulus A, which is positioned at a distance of d1 from the mean of a category (phoneme) prototype; the variance of the category is unknown. The top right panel shows the same for stimulus B, which is positioned at (d1+d') from the prototype mean. Subtraction of the prototype from each of the two stimuli results in two difference distributions, which are shown in the middle panel of Fig. 3. These distributions are at a distance of (d1+d')-d1=d' from each other, and have a variance which is the sum of stimulus variance σ_s^2 and category variance σ_p^2. The next step is to subtract the recoded stimuli from each other; this is shown in the bottom panel, where each stimulus presentation order has its own distribution with a variance of $2(\sigma_s^2 + \sigma_p^2)$.

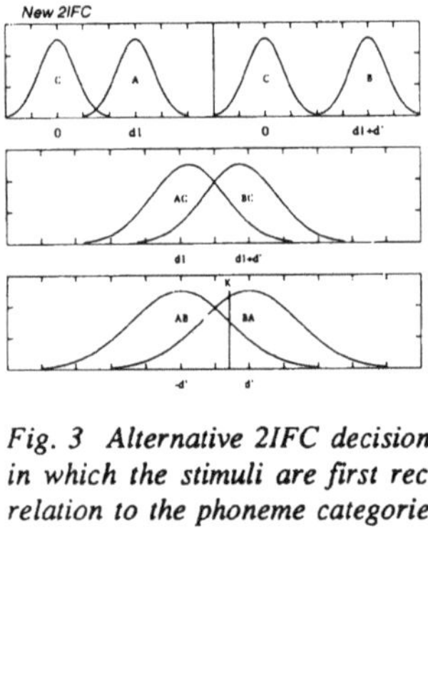

Fig. 3 Alternative 2IFC decision model, in which the stimuli are first recoded in relation to the phoneme categories

$$H_{AB} = \Phi\left[\frac{(k+d')}{\sqrt{(2(\sigma_p^2+\sigma_s^2))}}\right] \quad (5)$$

$$FA_{AB} = \Phi\left[\frac{(k-d')}{\sqrt{(2(\sigma_p^2+\sigma_s^2))}}\right] \quad (6)$$

$$d'_{2IFC} = \frac{2d'}{\sqrt{2(\sigma_p^2+\sigma_s^2)}} = \sqrt{\frac{2}{(\sigma_p^2+\sigma_s^2)}} * d' \quad (7)$$

$$d' = \{z(H_{AB})-z(FA_{AB})\} * 0.5\sqrt{2(\sigma_p^2+\sigma_s^2)} \quad (8)$$

$$if\ \sigma_p^2 = 0,\quad d'_{2IFC} = z(H)-z(FA) = \sqrt{2}\, d' \quad (9)$$

$$if\ \sigma_p^2 = 1,\quad d'_{2IFC} = z(H)-z(FA) = d' \quad (10)$$

The two distributions are 2d' apart. The net result of substituting the new assumptions for the old ones, and of assuming that category variance is the same as stimulus variance (formula (10)), is that d' becomes √2 times as high as in Fig. 1: z(H)-z(FA) now yields straight d'-values. This is shown in Fig. 4, where these assumptions have been incorporated in both the consonant and the vowel data. The anomaly has been removed from the stop-consonant discrimination data, but perception remains highly categorical. It is less clear what can be said about the vowels: it remains paradoxical that vowel perception is fairly categorical if we follow standard psychophysical assumptions (Fig. 1), but is much less categorical as soon as phoneme categories are included in the assumptions, as is the case in the bottom panel of Fig. 4. Category variance is the unknown factor here: if it were zero (formula (9)), we would be back at Fig. 1 and the standard assumptions. We think it lies between zero and unity, probably closer to unity.

Finally, our assumptions predict that subjects should benefit from increased inter-stimulus time in 2IFC discrimination, since an operation has to be performed on the first stimulus before the second stimulus is presented. Other data (Van Hessen and Schouten, forthcoming) show that this is indeed the case: up to a particular optimum ISI, performance improves with time.

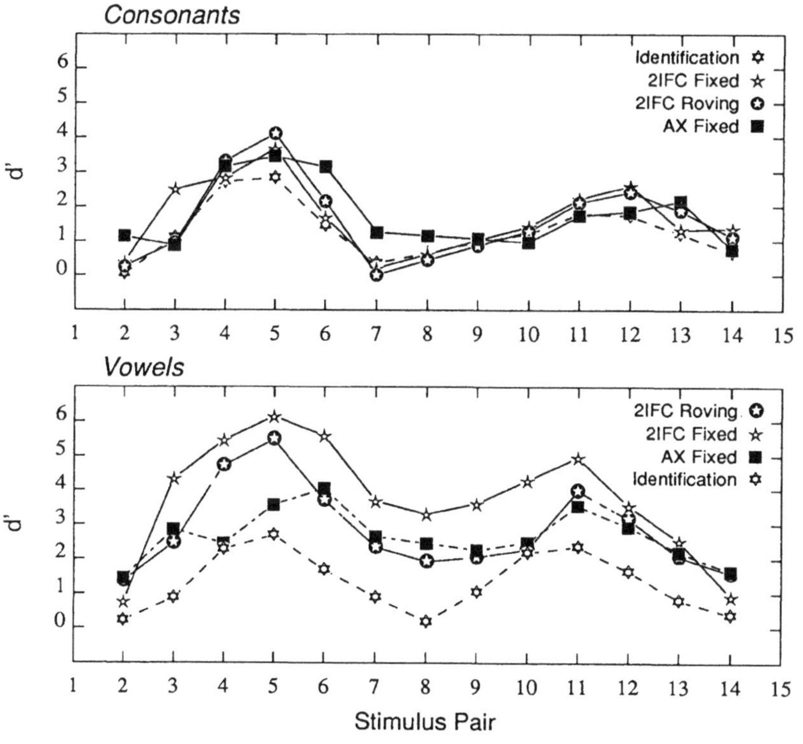

Fig. 4 2IFC Discrimination calculated according to alternative assumptions

Acknowledgements

The authors would like to thank Neil Macmillan and Dick Pastore for thoroughgoing discussions of the contents of this paper.
This research was supported by the Foundation for Linguistic Research, which is funded by the Netherlands Organization for Research, NWO.

References

Hessen, A.J. van (1988). A new speech modulation model based on sinusoidal representation, *Progress Report Institute of Phonetics Utrecht*, 13:2, 16-28.

Hessen, A.J. van and Schouten, M.E.H. (forthcoming). Modelling phoneme perception. Part 2 - a model of stop consonant discrimination, Submitted to *J. Acoust. Soc. Am.*

Macmillan, N.A., Kaplan, H.L., and Creelman, C.D. (1977). The psychophysics of categorical perception, *Psychol. Rev.*, 84, 452-471.

Auditory Metrics for Speech Perception

James R. Sawusch
Department of Psychology
State University of New York at Buffalo
Buffalo, New York 14260

One of the central problems of speech perception is the issue of how humans categorize the seemingly endless variation of the acoustic signal into a sequence of discrete linguistic units. Phonetic constancy seems to be achieved in spite of both variation in the tokens of an individual talker and variation across talkers. In their paper, Uchanski, Millier, Reed and Braida (this volume) deal with one part of this problem: token variability. Their central point is motivated by the observation that variation of tokens within a phonetic category occurs in natural speech. Consequently, the effects of this variation upon perception should be systematically investigated. Much like the research on the effects of talker variation (Mullennix, Pisoni & Martin, 1989), research on the perceptual consequences of token variation may lead to a better understanding of invariant attributes, normalization, and other processes designed to achieve perceptual constancy.

In addition to their data on the effects of token variation upon perception, Uchanski et al. also describe a quantitative model of perception that makes use of concepts from Signal Detection Theory and prototype models of perception. In what follows, I would like to build upon some of the issues about the dimensions of perception and the nature of auditory and phonetic coding that were raised and blend them with some new data to yield a more detailed picture of speech perception.

1. Token Variability

The main point of Uchanski et al. that the effects of token variability upon perception need to be explored and incorporated into perceptual models is well taken. Research on the acoustic properties of speech and the renewed search for invariant properties prompted by researchers such as Stevens and Blumstein (1978) has embodied this goal by using both multiple tokens from each talker and multiple talkers.

On the perceptual side, this question has not been systematically explored. The results of Uchanski et al., showing that the distances in perceptual space are reduced by token variation, are interesting. One would expect, then, that token variation might have other influences upon perception such as increased processing load, reduced memory accuracy, etc. If these effects of token variation could be shown to precisely parallel the effects of talker variation, then a single explanation for both might be possible. Alternatively, if there are distinct talker normalization processes in perception, we would expect both similarities and differences in the effects of talker and token variation across experimental tasks. It may very well be that the perceptual compensation for talker variation involves higher level processes that include the tuning of prototypes or some other linguistic representation, while the effects of token variation arise at an earlier point in processing (see Mullennix & Pisoni, 1990).

The invariant attributes that have been proposed by a number of researchers as the mediators between acoustic variability and phonetic constancy should play a key role in overcoming the effects of token variability. Conversely, much of the influence of token variability on perception may arise from the auditory coding processes that extract invariants or other dimensional information. For vowels, similar models have been recently proposed by Miller (1989) and Syrdal and Gopal (1986). Both models treat the frequency differences between adjacent peaks in the spectrum as the relevant dimensions for vowel categorization (see also Terhardt, this volume). Although neither model uses duration as a cue, we will, for the moment, add duration since perceptual studies show that it is used (see Dutton, 1990; Strange, 1989). If, as Uchanski et al. note, the primary acoustic cues left in their masked CVC syllables are F_0, F1 and duration, then a two-dimensional space might be expected with one dimension corresponding to F1-F_0 and the other to duration. In fact, these two dimensions seem to correspond quite well to the two dimensions derived from fitting their model to the human identification data.

This interpretation, however, is incomplete. The listeners in Uchanski et al.'s study were consistently able to identify the vowel /3^/ and did not confuse it with /ɛ/, /oɛ/ or /ae/. Since the F1 and F_0 of /3^/ cannot be used to distinguish it from these other categories, either the duration was the effective cue, which does not entirely match the fit of the model to the data, or another cue was present. The most distinctive aspect of the vowel /3^/ is the low-frequency F3. Put according to the model of Syrdal and Gopal, /3^/ is the only vowel for which F3-F2 would be under 3 barks, while F4 - F3 would be over 3 barks. However, if F2 and F3 information were present for /3^/, then such information might also have been present for a vowel such as /u/. In this case, listeners should not have confused /u/ and /i/ (or /I/ and /U/). These front-back confusions only make sense with the primary perceptual dimension being F1-F_0. Thus, the question is what information has remained in these tokens after the addition of the noise mask and whether this caused the listener to classify the vowels using acoustic correlates of vowel categories in a way other than in normal listening.

Perhaps some further insight can be gained by examining listeners' classification of other vowel tokens. Garrison and Sawusch (1987) presented single-formant vowels to listeners for classification. More recently, we followed up this earlier study with one where the stimuli were somewhat more comparable to those used here. Single formants were generated with two different durations. These stimuli spanned the range of F1, F2 and F3 for a male talker. Listeners were given twelve vowel labels to respond to these stimuli. They were reasonably consistent in their classification of the stimuli. There was a small effect of duration, with short stimuli producing more lax vowel responses. However, duration was at best a secondary cue since the dominant label never changed for a change in duration. As shown in Fig. 1, low frequencies were classified as /u/, /U/ and /o/, intermediate frequencies as /a/ and /ɔ/ then /ae/ and /ɛ/ with high frequencies as /e/, /I/ and /i/. There was no tendency to confuse front and back stimuli. There were also virtually no /3^/ responses by the 21 listeners.

These data provide both convergent evidence and new problems for a model based on differences between peaks. First, they demonstrate that listeners do not classify any F1-F_0 combination as /3^/. Some other acoustic cue(s) is required. Second, we found no evidence of front - back vowel confusions. Thus, there must be other cues present in either these single-formant stimuli, the stimuli of Uchanski et al., or both to explain the differences. One alternative, proposed by Miller (1989), is that a default value, based on averages from memory, could be supplied for any missing peak. If such defaults were used with isolated, single formants (in the F1 frequency region), it should lead to front - back vowel confusions such as confusion between /i/ and /u/. Since this was not found, the idea of filling in default values would not appear to be sufficient to explain the single-formant data.

It is also possible that the single-formant stimuli were classified according to both the F1-F_0 difference and their center of gravity (cf. Chistovich & Lublinskaya, 1979). The center of gravity could be computed as the weighted mean of the peaks in the spectrum. In addition, the moments about the mean (variance, skewness and kurtosis) would also be computed. Sawusch and Dutton (in press) have previously made a similar proposal and shown that the statistical moments of the spectrum can be used to distinguish front and back vowels reliably. Since front vowels have a higher center of gravity (mean) than back vowels, this approach predicts that listeners will not confuse single-formant /i/ and /u/. What I am proposing is that phonetic recognition is based upon a multidimensional space that involves the differences (or ratios) between adjacent peaks in the spectrum and the statistical moments computed over the peaks in the spectrum. If duration were added to this set, then we might have the potential to explain the identification data of Uchanski et al., our one formant vowel data, and vowel perception generally.

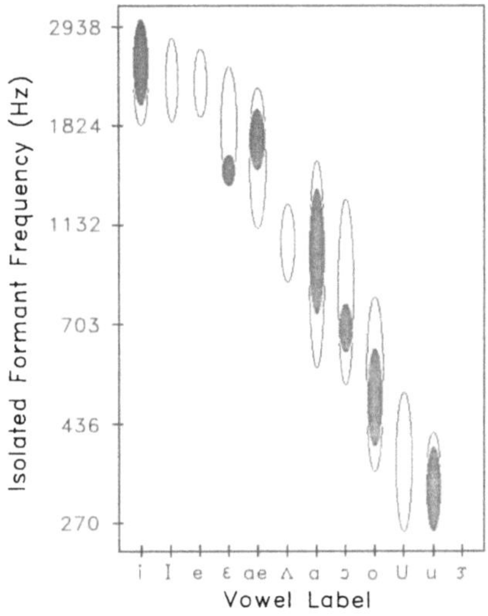

Fig. 1 Listener responses to single formant synthetic vowels. The most frequent response is represented by a dark region and other frequent responses are represented by light regions for the different single formants.

In the Uchanski et al. experiments with masked stimuli, vowel duration and F1-F_0 are the effective cues. The moments would be obscured by the masking noise which would make the extraction of all spectral peaks difficult and generally reduce the effectiveness of this cue. The /3^/ vowel, however, because of the close proximity of F2 and F3, might yield consistent estimates of F2 and F3. This would, in turn, produce values of F3-F2 which could be used to classify /3^/. What I am suggesting is that the noise masking of stimuli in Uchanski et al. reduces the dimensionality of the stimuli, but not uniformly for all of the vowels. Similarly, the use of single formants reduces the dimensionality of the stimuli but again not uniformly. The relatively smaller number of lax vowel responses, even with a duration cue, could reflect the fact that lax vowels generally show a low kurtosis moment value, while tense vowels and single formants show a higher kurtosis value (see Sawusch & Dutton, in press).

With a model that has a large number of perceptual dimensions, individual experiments, even with multiple tokens, may still be making idiosyncratic use of the larger perceptual space of human speech perception. Masking or the elimination of natural cues with reduced, synthetic speech may induce the listener to place a greater weight on dimensions such as duration or the kurtosis moment, which may not normally carry much weight in perception. This means that studies should not only use multiple tokens, but convergent paradigms and multiple sets of stimuli (masked and unmasked, natural and synthetic) to establish the role of token variation and yield a clear picture of the auditory dimensions of speech.

2. Phonetic Coding

A second main item in Uchanski et al.'s paper is the model and its use of phonetic prototypes. The use of phoneme or phonetic feature prototypes has been proposed by a number of researchers (e.g. Massaro, 1989; Samuel, 1982). The use of prototypes for categorization has a rich history (see Medin & Barsalou, 1987) and there is an extensive empirical literature supporting their role in perception and memory. Alternatives, such as exemplar-based models, have also been proposed (see Hintzman, 1986). Regardless, however, of whether a model uses prototypes or exemplars, one must still specify the unit of representation to which the prototype or exemplar corresponds. The feature, triphone, diphone, phoneme, and syllable have all been proposed. The choice of unit here is important since it will influence the nature of the invariant dimensions and values used to map onto the unit.

Gagnon and Sawusch (1990) ran a series of experiments designed to distinguish among alternative perceptual units such as context-sensitive allophones (triphones or Wickelphones), syllables, abstract phonemes and position-specific phonemes. The last alternative, the position-specific phoneme, is a phonetic unit that incorporates information about position within a syllable. This type of unit was proposed by Dell (1986), based upon production data from slips of the tongue. The experiments of Gagnon and Sawusch all used a priming paradigm in which a target syllable followed a prime syllable. Listeners were asked to name the target or make a lexical decision about the target. The phonetic overlap between prime and target was manipulated, as shown in Table I. By varying the vowel and the positions of the consonants between the prime and target, pairs were generated that contained different degrees of overlap, depending upon the representation chosen. Table II shows the degree of phonetic overlap between a reverse order prime and a target for the abstract phoneme, position-specific phoneme and context-sensitive allophone representations. Clearly a phoneme representation shows substantial overlap in perceptual units while an allophone representation shows no overlap. The position-specific phoneme is intermediate

Table I Examples of the various Prime-Target relations used in naming and lexical decision tasks.

Relation Type	Prime	Target
Identity	/tap/	/tap/
Change Vowel	/tIp/	/tap/
Reverse Order	/pat/	/tap/
Change Both	/pIt/	/tap/
Control	/lif/	/tap/

Table II Similarity between a Reverse Order Prime and Target according to Phoneme, Position-Specific Phoneme and Context-Sensitive Allophone representations. Corresponding units in the prime and target are connected by a line.

Representation	Reverse Order Prime	Target
Phoneme	/p/ /a/ /t/	/t/ /a/ /p/
Position-Specific	$/p_i/\ /a_m/\ /t_f/$	$/t_i/\ /a_m/\ /p_f/$
Allophone	$/{}_{\#}p_a/\ /{}_{p}a_t/\ /{}_{a}t_{\#}/$	$/{}_{\#}t_a/\ /{}_{t}a_p/\ /{}_{a}p_{\#}/$

in the predicted overlap. Table III illustrates the predictions for which prime-target conditions should be faster or slower for each of the possible units of representation. All of these predictions are based on the simple assumption that more perceptual overlap between prime and target leads to faster responding. For details of the predictions, see Gagnon and Sawusch (1990).

The results were quite clear cut and are shown in summary form at the bottom of Table III. For both naming and lexical decision, an identity match produced the fastest responses. Changing the vowel was the next fastest condition. The reverse order and change both (reverse order and change vowel) were not different from one another but were slower than the change vowel. Finally, the control condition was as slow or slower than the reverse order and change both conditions. This pattern is as predicted by the position-specific phoneme representation and cannot be accounted for by the other representations. Thus, it would appear that the language representation used in word recognition contains information about the positions of the features or phonemes within the syllable. This implies that one need not propose a single invariant attribute or region in perceptual space for both a syllable-initial and a syllable-final consonant. Rather, initial and final consonants are distinct entities (prototype or exemplar) which may be cued by distinct invariant attributes. This positional specificity has the added attraction of providing an indication of syllable boundaries and thus information about the potential locus of word onsets and offsets.

3. Summary

The proposal that has been described here involves the computation of nine cues or dimensions in vowel perception. In addition, there may also be an intermediate stage or level of processing between these cues and the vowel representation in memory that codes changes in these cues (cf. Nearey & Assmann, 1986). This large number of dimensions implies that perception is often overdetermined by the speech signal. However, in different experiments which expose listeners to different subsets of these cues, different patterns of results will be found. Consequently, it is important that we look for a pattern of results across tasks, tokens, talkers, speaking rates, and contexts to discover the auditory representation for phoneme recognition.

It is also important to consider the nature of the representation used to recognize words. Since the auditory cues must be mapped onto this language representation, a specification of the units from which words are built will constrain the possible forms of the auditory representation. A prototype representation, such as described by Uchanski et al. here, seems quite plausible. The data presented here simply add a qualifier to this proposal: The phonetic prototypes include a specification of the position of the phoneme within the syllable. Thus, the auditory cues need only specify an invariant region in the auditory space for a phoneme in a particular syllable position. The position-specific phoneme, in turn, provides additional information about lexical and syllabic boundaries for the process of word recognition.

Table III Predictions of relative RTs for each Prime-Target relation based upon the Phoneme, Position-Specific Phoneme and Allophone representations and the actual RT ordering from both lexical decision and naming tasks.

Representation	RT Ordering of Conditions
Phoneme	ID = RO < CV = CB < C
Position-Specific Phoneme	ID < CV < RO < CB = C
Allophone	ID < RO = CV = CB = C
Lexical Decision Data	ID < CV < RO = CB <= C
Naming Data	ID < CV < RO = CB = C

Acknowledgements

The research described here was supported by NIH grant R01-DC00219 to the State University of New York at Buffalo. I would like to thank Dawn L. Dutton, Deborah A. Gagnon, Laurie F. Garrison, Kevin H. Richardson and Carol A. Wannemacher for their comments and discussion.

References

Chistovich, L.A., & Lublinskaya, V.V. (1979). The 'center of gravity' effect in vowel spectra and critical distance between the formants: Psychophysical study of perception of vowel-like stimuli, *Hearing Research*, 1, 185-195.

Dell, G. S. (1986). A spreading-activation theory of retrieval in sentence production. *Psychological Review*, 93, 283-321.

Dutton, D. L. (1990, May). *The roles of three possible cues to dynamic vowel identity.* Paper presented at the 119th meeting of the Acoustical Society of America, State College, PA.

Gagnon, D. A. and Sawusch, J. R. (1990, November). *Priming and the perceptual units in auditory word recognition*, Presented at the 31st Annual Meeting of the Psychonomic Society, New Orleans, Louisiana.

Garrison, L. F. and Sawusch, J. R. (1987, May). *The perception of reduced vowel stimuli*, Paper presented at the 113th meeting of the Acoustical Society of America, Indianapolis, IN.

Hintzman, D. L. (1986). "Schema abstraction" in a multiple-trace memory model, *Psychological Review*, 93, 411-428.

Massaro, D. W. (1989). Testing between the TRACE model and the Fuzzy Logical model of speech perception, *Cognitive Psychology*, 21, 398-421.

Medin, D. L. and Barsalou, L. W. (1987). Categorization processes and categorical perception, in: S. Harnad (Ed.), *Categorical perception* (pp. 455 - 490). Cambridge: Cambridge University Press.

Miller, J. D. (1989). Auditory - perceptual interpretation of the vowel, *J. Acoust. Soc. Am.*, 85 (5), 2114-2134.

Mullennix, J. W. and Pisoni, D. B. (1990). Stimulus variability and processing dependencies in speech perception, *Perception & Psychophysics*, 47 (4), 379-390.

Mullennix, J. W., Pisoni, D. B., and Martin, C. S. (1989). Some effects of talker variability on spoken word recognition, *J. Acoust. Soc. Am.*, 85 (1), 365-378.

Nearey, T. M. and Assmann, P. (1986). Modeling the role of inherent spectral change in vowel identification, *J. Acoust. Soc. Am.*, 80, 1297-1308.

Samuel, A. G. (1982). Phonetic prototypes, *Perception & Psychophysics*, 31, 307-314.

Sawusch, J. R. and Dutton, D. L. (in press). Computational metrics for place of articulation information in consonants and vowels, in: Charles-Luce, J., Luce, P., and Sawusch, J.R. (eds.), *Theories in spoken language: Perception, production and development*. Norwood, NJ: Ablex.

Stevens, K. N. and Blumstein, S. E. (1978). Invariant cues for place of articulation in stop consonants, *J. Acoust. Soc. Am.*, 64 (5), 1358-68.

Strange, W. (1989). Dynamic specification of coarticulated vowels spoken in sentence context, *J. Acoust. Soc. Am.*, 85 (5), 2135-2153.

Syrdal, A. K. and Gopal, H. S. (1986). A perceptual model of vowel recognition based on the auditory representation of American English vowels, *J. Acoust. Soc. Am.*, 79 (4), 1086-1100.

Chapter 6
Word Perception and Beyond

The Interface Between Acoustic-Phonetic and Lexical Processing

Uli H. Frauenfelder
Max-Planck Institute for Psycholinguistics
Nijmegen
The Netherlands

1. Introduction to the Interface Problem

There has until recently been a rather clear division of labor between phoneticians and psycholinguists. Research in phonetics has focused on the acoustic-phonetic analysis of the speech signal and for the most part has not dealt with the problem of how this analysis relates to word recognition and sentence processing. Inversely, psycholinguists have generally concentrated on processing at the higher levels and have tended to neglect the complexities of the acoustic-phonetic input and its analysis. This approach to carving up the scientific problem space leaves cracks or neglected territory between the two disciplines. I want to argue along with others (Marslen-Wilson, 1984; Nooteboom, 1979) that this gray area, the interface between acoustic-phonetic and lexical processing, deserves more attention.

One unhappy outcome of this division of labor is the resultant ambiguity concerning the level at which the major problems in speech and word recognition need to be addressed. It is unclear, for example, to what extent the many-to-one mapping problem is to be dealt with by phoneticians, psycholinguists or both. Indeed we must determine where the language processing system handles both the phonetic and phonological variability that is intrinsic to the speech signal. Similar ambiguities arise in the study of the segmentation of the continuous speech input; does the continuous-to-discrete mapping take place at a phonetic or lexical level or both?

Given this state of affairs it is important to analyze the assumptions underlying this division of labor critically and to identify areas of common interest where cooperation is necessary to gain a deeper understanding of the mapping from sound to lexical representations. In the present paper, I begin by considering different hypotheses advanced in the psycholinguistic literature concerning the nature of this interface. I then consider the methodological challenge posed by evaluating these diverse proposals empirically and examine various sources of data that have been drawn upon to assess these proposals. Finally, I evaluate the proposals on the basis of a subset of these data coming from on-line experiments involving monitoring tasks.

2. Perspectives on the Interface

We can distinguish two general approaches to the interface problem. According to the first, one or more sublexical representations mediate the mapping between the signal and the mental lexicon. The second view holds that no sublexical representation is computed but that information extracted from the sensory input is mapped directly onto the lexicon.

2.1 Sublexical representations

The division of labor between phonetics and psycholinguistics is based essentially upon the assumed existence of sublexical representations where phonetic interests end and psycholinguistic ones begin (Marslen-Wilson and Frauenfelder, 1987). The postulation of such representations is more than simply a convenient line of demarcation between the disciplines, however. Sublexical representations are assumed to play a key role in solving the vexing mapping problem described above. For example, a phonetic or phonological representation provides a less variable and more abstract format for representing the information in the input and for accessing the lexicon. Further, the computation of sublexical units can simplify the segmentation process; either segment boundaries can be used as starting points for a lexical template matching process or the lexical hypotheses can be restricted to those matching certain sublexical units. Either way, wasteful matching of inappropriate lexical candidates can be avoided.

Although there is widespread agreement that sublexical representations play an important role in lexical processing, we find considerable variety in the proposals made to account for how they contribute. It is useful for the present purposes to oppose a unitary sublexical representation view with one in which multiple representations are computed or parsed during word recognition.

Unitary sublexical representation view

The most widely accepted view of the interface assumes a smooth transfer of information from the acoustic-phonetic to the lexical levels of processing via a single unitary level of sublexical representation. In this perspective,, the intermediary sublexical representation is defined in terms of some perceptual unit that represents the output of phonetic processing and the input to lexical processing. Two linguistic units have been the main contenders for the status of the perceptual units making up the sublexical representation: the phoneme and the syllable.

An example of a phoneme-based model can be found in the original cohort model (Marslen-Wilson and Welsh, 1978). Here a segmental representation is computed sequentially from the signal and mapped onto lexical representations. The lexical representations are themselves assumed to be made up of linearly concatenated segments. A similar model has also been defended by Pisoni and Luce (1987) who present a number of different arguments in favor of a segmental representation. The most explicit proposal for a unitary representation in terms of syllables has been made for the processing of French. It has been argued (Mehler, 1981; Segui, 1984; Segui, Frauenfelder, and Mehler, 1981) that the syllable constitutes the basic perceptual unit in French.

Multiple sublexical representations

The notion that the interface mediating between acoustic-phonetic and lexical processing is more complex than is assumed by the unitary perspective has been expressed in a number of recent models. A first major source of complexity lies in the characterization of perceptual units. It is possible to differentiate several different types of perceptual units: segmentation and classification units for analyzing speech and access units for making contact with the lexicon. Unlike the models assuming a unitary sublexical representations described above, there are others that distinguish between these different types of perceptual units.

Cutler and Norris (Cutler, 1989; Cutler and Norris, 1988; Norris and Cutler, 1985) have proposed a model in which the segmentation process operates quite independently from speech classification and lexical mapping. In their theory of word recognition for English, stressed syllables constitute the unit of lexical segmentation. Metrically strong syllables-roughly those not containing a reduced vowel - serve to locate word boundaries. When a syllable is identified as being strong, the set of lexical hypothesis beginning at the onset of this syllable is activated. However, these syllables do not serve as the unit of classification; instead classification is done in terms of some subsyllabic representations - perhaps phonemic - that serve also as the units for accessing the lexicon. We see here a more complex interplay between different types of units.

Other models incorporate more linguistic information in accounting for lexical recognition. Rather than assuming a simple mapping of the input onto sublexical representations and subsequent mapping of this representation onto the lexicon, these models use linguistic knowledge to construct highly structured sublexical representations. Church (1987) has developed a phonetic parser which takes as its input a phonetic representation. The allophonic information signaling the prosodic structure of the input is exploited along with phonotactic constraints to derive alternative syllabic segmentations of the input. Once this immediate constituent structure has been identified or parsed, the phonetic representation is "canonicalized" into a phonemic representation that is subsequently used to address the lexicon.

Finally, Frazier (1987) has criticized the unitary input representation approach and has sketched the outlines of a parser which actively uses phonological knowledge to structure the input. As in the parser of Church, Frazier's model exploits diverse types of information including phonetic cues, phonotactic constraints and prosodic regularities in analyzing the sensory input. The phonologically structured representations that are generated by the parser are then matched with the similarly structured lexical representations.

2.2 No intermediary sublexical representations

In contrast to the above models which assume that most of the hardest problems in speech and word recognition are handled in the mapping onto a sublexical representation, other models without a sublexical level of representation shift the burden to the lexical level. This is clearly the case for models like LAFS (Klatt, 1980, 1989), LAFF model (Stevens, 1986), and the revised cohort model (Lahiri and Marslen-Wilson, 1991) which all assume a deeper involvement of the lexicon.

The LAFS model assumes a direct mapping onto a lexical decoding network of spectral templates that are extracted from the signal. Word recognition involves computing a power spectrum of the sensory input every 10 ms and then comparing these spectra to spectral templates stored in a pre-compiled network. Words are recognized by tracing the best path through the network. The lexical decoding network is created so as to encode phonological processes that occur at word boundaries and therefore can deal with phonological variation especially at word boundaries.

Lahiri and Marslen-Wilson (1991) draw attention to the fact that lexical representations have been largely neglected in psycholinguistic circles. In their proposal these representations - drawn from current phonological theory- play a central role. The model assumes that featural information is extracted from the signal and mapped directly and immediately onto lexical representations (Warren and Marslen-Wilson, 1987, 1988). Not all featural information in the signal is used in the lexical mapping or represented in the lexicon. These authors claim that only featural information that is distinctive and non-predictable is included in the hierarchically organized lexical representation. The critical information varies across languages as a function of their phonological structure. This proposal is intended to deal with phonological variability and to explain how listeners recover the correct underlying form from its many surface manifestations.

Klatt (1980) has pointed out that the strategy of not making segmental decisions avoids introducing errors of classification and segmentation that can misdirect the lexical access process. Furthermore, these models explicitly address the phonological variability problem in the lexicon. However, the models must still account for how sublexical units like syllables and nonwords are perceived, perhaps as LAFS has done with a parallel phonetic analysis as in SCRIBER. In addition, the assumption that invariant features can be extracted reliably from the signal must be validated.

3. Methodological Approach

Many sources of evidence have been used to study the sublexical interface, including diachronic and synchronic facts described by linguistic theory, observational data of first and second language acquisition as well as slips of the tongue and ear, and finally experimental studies. We will concentrate here only on experimental research dealing with language perception.

The methodological challenge of deriving testable predictions from these distinct models and testing them experimentally is of course great. First, we are confronted with the chore of devising experimental procedures that tap into the mental processes and representations mapping the signal onto the lexicon. Second, in interpreting the results, we must extrapolate from subjects' experimental behavior elicited in these experiments to listeners' behavior in the course of normal conversation. This is difficult because most experimental procedures depend upon a secondary task to derive dependent measures. This secondary task necessarily requires some additional and possibly alternative processing. The variability observed in the results obtained with different experimental procedures and even with the same procedure (with minor experimental modifications) has forced researchers to be more prudent in drawing general conclusions about processing. These conclusions often take the form of information processing accounts for subjects' performance in specific tasks.

Diverse experimental tasks have been applied to the study of the interface. These include the gating task (Warren and Marslen-Wilson, 1987; Lahiri and Marslen-Wilson, 1991), ear switching (Huggins, 1964; Samuel, 1991), backward masking (Massaro, 1972) among others. For considerations of space, we will focus our discussion here upon only one technique, the so-called monitoring or detection procedure. Having served as the work-horse in the search for perceptual units, this technique already has a rich history since its invention more than two decades ago. In fact, it provides an excellent example of an experimental method for which specific theories or models have been developed.

3.1 The monitoring technique

Subjects performing in monitoring tasks are required to make speeded detection responses to previously specified targets (phonemes, syllables, etc.). For example, in the phoneme monitoring task, subjects must detect phoneme targets (generally stops consonants) in carrier items (e.g., words, nonsense syllables). To accomplish this task, subjects are assumed first to construct an internal representation of the target. This representation may vary as a function of the modality (visual or auditory) and/or the model (an example bearing the target) used to specify the target for the subjects. This representation is kept active while the listener analyzes the carrier items presented in lists or sentences. When this target representation matches the representation computed from the signal (sufficiently), the subject initiates a detection response. The detection latencies are taken to reflect the nature of the representation constructed from the input and the time-course of its computation.

A long history of controversy has surrounded the central question of which representations are exploited in the detection responses. The current consensus is that detection responses can depend either upon some sublexical representation(s) and/or upon the phonological representation stored in the lexicon. Which of these two representations makes the primary contribution to the detection response depends upon a number of details of the experimental procedure (Segui and Frauenfelder, 1986). To evaluate sublexical hypotheses, the detection procedure should, of course, tap into sublexical representations that are computed prelexically, that is before word recognition.

We can distinguish three related ways in which the monitoring task has been used to study sublexical representations and processing. In the first the properties of the target (in particular its size) are manipulated, while the carrier is maintained constant. According to the second approach, the properties of the carrier (e.g., phonological or prosodic) are varied, and the target is held constant. Finally, the relation between the target and carrier can be varied orthogonally in the same experiment. This distinction between approaches will serve to organize the following discussion.

Varying the nature of the target

Savin and Bever (1971) first exploited the monitoring procedure to study perceptual units. In a pioneering study they varied the target size and observed faster detection times for syllable than for phoneme targets. Their conclusion was that "phonemes are perceived only by an analysis of already perceived syllables (or at least already perceived consonant-vowel pairs)", p. 300. Foss and Swinney (1973) called this perceptual explanation into question on the basis of results showing that this inverse relation between the target size and detection latencies obtained even for word targets (i.e., RT words < RT syllables < RT phonemes). These data led the authors to conclude that the monitoring task does not tap into perceptual processes but rather into later-occurring identification processes. Both lines of reasoning were later criticized by Norris and Cutler (1988) who claimed that these monitoring studies as well as others comparing the detection of targets of different sizes (Segui, Frauenfelder and Mehler, 1981) were flawed. The RT advantage for larger over smaller targets, they argued, was purely artifactual. When no foils or catch trials were included among the filler items as was the case for these studies, subjects could respond to syllable (or word) targets on the basis of a partial match with the carrier before the sensory input corresponding to the entire target had been heard. Moreover, on experimental trials with larger targets subjects had a more informative target specification (e.g., the target specification /p/ versus /pa/) and presumably could make faster responses. When foils that forced subjects to conduct a more complete analysis of the carrier were included in the experimental lists, Norris and Cutler showed that the syllable advantage over phonemes was reversed.

These authors went on to test a strong version of the syllable hypothesis according to which the identification of the component parts of a syllable necessarily follows the segmentation of the entire syllable. For this test, they compared the detection latencies to English carrier syllables in separate lists with different types of foils. The location of the deviation between the target and the carrier foils was varied. For example, the targets mismatched the syllabic foils (e.g. "nap") either in their first (/*m*ap/) or the last (/na*t*/) phoneme. They obtained faster detection times for the lists containing early mismatching foils than for those with late mismatches. According to the syllabic hypothesis the location of the deviation of the foils should make no difference in the detection latencies since in both cases the entire syllable must be analyzed before a phoneme detection response can be made.

From this selective review of monitoring research comparing detection latencies to different-sized targets, we can already draw some tentative theoretical and methodological lessons. First, these results do not appear to support the discontinuous syllable hypothesis, at least for English. Subsyllabic units like the phoneme or syllabic constituents are better candidates, a possibility explored in the next section. These studies also illustrate the problems in drawing inferences about perceptual units on the basis of comparisons of detection latencies to targets of different sizes. Particularly problematic is determining the appropriate foils. Ideally, the foils should ensure that subjects respond neither earlier nor later than they would in the course of normal processing. Alternatively, however, it might be possible through careful manipulation of foils to induce variable delays in the detection responses and consequently to tap into different moments and levels of processing.

Varying the nature of the carriers

A second application of the detection task involves keeping the target constant and varying the properties of the carrier item such as its phonological structure (syllable structure, vowel length), prosodic structure (stress pattern) or lexical status (word-nonword). Most relevant for the discussion here is research which manipulated the phonological structure of the carrier. The first series of studies to be considered varied the syllabic structure of the carrier. When Treiman, Salasoo, Slowiaczek, and Pisoni (1982) compared RTs to the same phoneme targets in English nonsense syllables of different structure, they found faster latencies to targets that corresponded to the initial phoneme (C1) in carrier items with simple onsets (C1V, C1VC2) than those with complex onset clusters (C1C2V). The authors attributed the longer RTs for the latter condition to the additional processing required to segment the syllable onset into its phoneme constituents. This was taken to provide evidence that syllable onsets serve as units of speech perception.

A similar study (Cutler, Mehler, Norris and Segui, 1986) in English and French produced a comparable pattern of results. Subsequently, however, Cutler, Butterfield, and Williams (1987) proposed an alternative explanation for this RT advantage of carriers with simple onsets over those with complex ones. They attributed this effect to the match between the model (e.g., "Dan") used to specify the target to the subjects (i.e., the target is /d/ as in Dan) and the structure of the carrier items. In the above experiments, the target was generally modeled with words having simple onsets. When these authors varied the relation between subject's expectations based on the model (either CV, CVC, CCV model) and the carrier's structure, they observed faster detection times for models with syllable structures matching that of the carrier. However, a further experiment showed no influence of the manipulation of subjects' expectations at the phonemic level. These expectations were set up by varying the relation between the model and carriers - model and carrier matched in the first C, CV or CVC. The fact that the match between the model and carrier only played a role for complex and not simple syllable onsets led these authors to the same conclusion as Treiman et al. - the perceptual integrity of the onset - but on the basis of different data and reasoning.

More recently, Segui, Dupoux and Mehler (1990) evaluated the role of the carrier's syllabic structure while controlling the match between the model and carrier. Their results for French carrier stimuli replicated and extended the original findings of Treiman et al. (1982) by showing an advantage of simple CV carriers over those with complex onsets (CCV) and/or (complex) codas (CVCC). Dupoux (1990) analyzed these results in greater detail by opposing fast and slow subjects. His post-hoc analyses showed a clear effect of the complexity of the onset for both groups, but only an effect of the coda for the slow subjects. This difference across subject groups led him to abandon the discontinuous syllable hypothesis in favor of two phases of sublexical processing: first, the classification of the initial consonant(s) and the following vowel (i.e., the CV demi-syllable) and second the integration of this part with the information in the coda to construct a syllabic representation. The detection responses for the fast subjects were based upon a demi-syllable representation, whereas the slow detection responses were based upon a representation of the entire syllable whose computation was made possible by the additional processing time available. This suggests that subjects can respond in detection tasks using more than one type of sublexical representation.

The experiments presented in this section manipulated the phonological structure of the target-bearing carriers. Their results have been used to argue for subsyllabic units like the syllabic onset or the demi-syllable. The longer detection latencies to targets in complex onsets have been attributed to a process of decomposing the onset unit. This interpretation assumes that there are no acoustic-phonetic differences in the carriers being compared that explain the difference in detection latencies. However, it is probable that detection latencies depend upon the phonetic environment of the target. For example, a consonant is easier to process and/or detect when it is followed by a vowel than by another consonant (Cutler et al. 1986). The fact that the phonetic properties of the target and of its environment (see also Diehl, Kluender, Foss, Parker, and Gernsbacher, 1987) contribute to the detection latencies points to a problem of interpretation that arises in comparing the detection latencies to targets in different carriers. It is difficult to know whether the RT effects should be attributed to the higher order processes like the segmentation of complex onsets or to the bottom-up analysis of the phonetic segments.

It is, nonetheless, possible to vary the properties of the carrier while minimizing the contaminating influence of the target's local environment. An example of how this can be achieved is found in a phoneme monitoring experiment (Frauenfelder and Henstra, 1988). This experiment examined the role of the syllable in Dutch by manipulating the phonological structure and lexical status of the carrier. The basic assumption was that the lexical effect (RT advantage of word over nonword carriers) could be used to draw inferences concerning the efficacy of the syllable as an access unit. The experiment included three different conditions: baseline, syllabic match and syllabic mismatch. The baseline measure of lexical activation involved taking the difference in detection latencies to phoneme targets in matched monosyllabic words and nonwords (e.g., detection latency differences to the target /p/ in the Dutch word "loep" and the nonword "foep"). The stimuli in both syllabic match and mismatch conditions were created by embedding the baseline monosyllabic carriers initially in longer nonword sequences. For the match condition, CVC syllables were added to the baseline items to create matched pairs of bisyllabic nonwords ("loep.sem" and "foep.sem") in which the first syllable of the nonword carrier matched the baseline items. For the mismatch condition, we added VC syllables to generate pairs of bisyllabic nonwords ("loe.pem" vs "foe.pem") whose syllable structure mismatched the baseline monosyllabic items.

A comparison between the amount of lexical activation observed in the match and mismatch conditions provided us with an indirect way of estimating the contribution of syllabic structure to lexical activation. The bottom-up analysis required to detect the target phonemes was presumably identical in paired carriers within the three conditions since these targets were located in the same local phonemic environment. Consequently, any word advantage in reaction times can be interpreted in terms of lexical activation. If the syllabic unit participates in activating lexical representations, then more lexical activation should emerge when the syllabic input matches the lexical representation than when it mismatches.

The results for the three conditions are shown in Fig. 1. Mean RTs (measured from the onset of the target phoneme) showed significant effects of lexical status for each of the three different conditions, with no difference in the size of the lexical effect for the two embedded conditions.

These results provide no support for the claim that the syllable serves as the access unit in Dutch. If the syllable were an access unit, more lexical activation would have resulted in the syllable match condition than in the mismatch condition. In the latter condition, the second syllable would presumably have to be decomposed into its component parts to match the lexical entry. This additional operation should cost time and lead to less lexical activation,

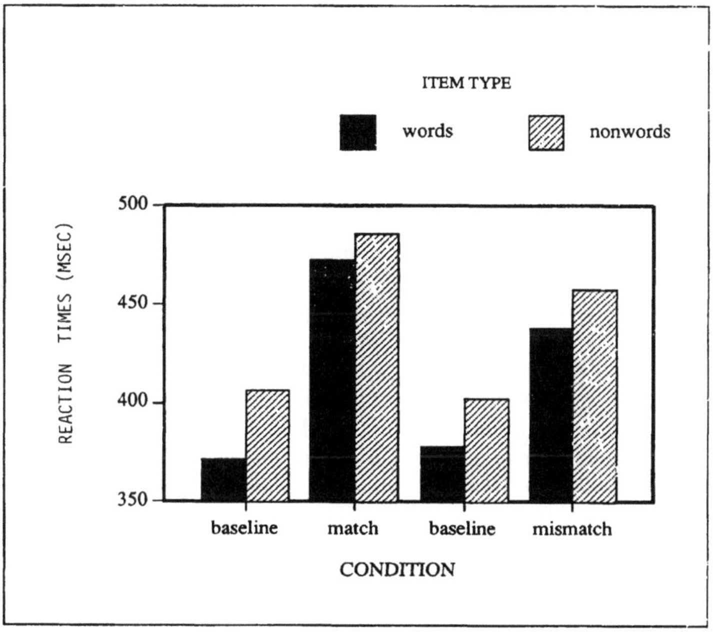

Fig. 1 Mean RTs (in msec.) for phoneme targets in the syllabic match and mismatch conditions and the corresponding base-line condition as a function of the lexical status of the (first) syllable.

a conclusion not supported by the data. This result suggests that some subsyllabic units - demi-syllables or phonemes -are involved in lexical activation. This failure to find evidence for the role of the undecomposed syllable as an access unit should not be surprising since mismatches between syllabic and lexical representations are extremely common in Dutch. For example, the plurals of many Dutch words contain syllables that straddle morpheme boundaries.

Varying the relation between target and carrier

The final monitoring approach to perceptual units to be considered here involves manipulating the relation between the target and the structure of the carrier. This approach avoids the problems associated with comparing detection latencies for targets of different sizes and for carriers with different acoustic properties. The original study adopting this approach (Mehler, Dommergues, Frauenfelder, and Segui, 1981) compared the detection latencies of CV (/pa/) and CVC (/pal/) targets in carriers whose first syllable was either CV ("pa.lace") or CVC ("pal.mier"). The findings for French showed faster detection times when the target matched the first syllable of the carrier word, independently of target size. This cross-over interaction between target and word type, the so-called syllable effect, was interpreted by the authors to show that French subjects segment the input into syllabic units.

In an important follow-up study, Cutler, Mehler, Norris, and Segui (1983, 1986) performed the same experiments but crossed the language of the stimulus materials and that of the subjects. Thus, English and French subjects received both English and French materials. The English subjects showed no syllable effects either in their native language or in French. The French subjects, in contrast, showed a syllable effect with both language materials. Cutler et al. (1986) ascribed this pattern of results to specific differences in the syllable structure between the two languages. Syllable boundaries in French are assumed to be "clear" and unambiguous, whereas in English they are not. French listeners exploit their knowledge of phonotactic constraints to segment the input into syllabic units which serve as the basis for their detection response. The absence of a syllabic effect in English is claimed to be due to the existence of ambisyllabicity in the language. Ambisyllabicity- where one segment belongs to two syllables - presumably makes syllabic segmentation difficult and unreliable, and therefore prevents English children from learning to syllabify the input and adults from using a syllabic segmentation strategy. Thus, listeners are assumed to bring the phonological knowledge of their native language to bear in the analysis of the carrier words.

Analogous monitoring experiments have been conducted in other languages including Spanish, Catalan, Portuguese and Dutch. The results from these studies have not yet produced a coherent picture. For example, syllable effects were obtained (Zwitserlood, Schriefers, Lahiri, and Van Donselaar, 1991) in Dutch which like English has ambisyllabic segments.This suggests that explanations based upon ambisyllabicity cannot be the whole story. Indeed, other phonological properties of the languages being compared - besides ambisyllabicity- have been advanced to explain the presence or absence of syllable effects in the monitoring task. These properties include the location of the stressed syllable, the size of the vowel and syllable inventories and the presence of vowel reduction (Sebastián-Gallés, Dupoux, Segui, and Mehler, 1991).

The evaluation of these diagnostic variables as predictors of subjects' monitoring performance cross-linguistically should help us better understand the syllable effect. However, it is equally important to understand how the phonetic properties of the carrier stimuli in a single language are influenced by the syllabic structure of the carrier and how this phonetic information could be used by listeners in detecting targets. Although the importance of phonetic information is generally recognized, one cannot escape the impression given by this monitoring research that the only relevant difference between the carrier words being compared lies in the location of the syllable boundary. The phonetic properties of the three initial segments (CVC) of the carrier words are generally not analyzed and thus not taken seriously in explaining the effect.

In monitoring experiments conducted in collaboration with T. Rietveld and A. van Til, we were interested precisely in the contribution of the durational and spectral phonetic cues to subjects' detection responses. It is well-established (Maddieson, 1984) that the duration of any given segment is inversely related to the number of other segments in the same syllable. This means that there are durational differences in the initial segments of the carrier items being compared that listeners might exploit to identify syllable structure. We (Rietveld and Frauenfelder, 1987) conducted a phonetic study that explored the effects of syllable boundaries on vowel and syllable durations. We varied not only the location of the syllable boundary but also the identity of the pivotal consonant, that is, the consonant serving either as the coda of the first syllable or the onset of the second in the matched carrier words (e.g., the /l/ in "palace" and "palmier"). Three classes of pivotal consonants were contrasted: liquids, nasals and fricatives. The size of the differences measured between the vowel durations in open and closed syllables varied as a function of the nature of the pivotal consonants. Liquids and nasal showed large durational differences, the fricatives none. In addition to these durational effects, spectral differences in the pivotal consonants potentially serve to identify the syllable structure. For example the listener could exploit the allophonic variants of the pivotal consonant (e.g., differences between front and back /l/'s).

In order to evaluate the contribution of these durational and spectral cues to syllabic segmentation, we tested whether syllable effects for Dutch vary as a function of the pivotal consonant. It is striking to note that the original French and English experiments (Mehler et al, 1981; Cutler et al., 1986) both employed exclusively stimuli with liquid pivotal consonants. Since these are the consonants for which the syllable structure is signaled clearly, it is of considerable interest to see whether the syllable effect generalizes to other consonants.

In this syllable monitoring experiment we employed word carriers with three different pivotal consonant classes: liquids (both /l/ and /r/), nasals, and stops. Examples of the stimuli pairs for these different pivotal consonants include: "polis" - "Poolse", "porie" - "poorten", "poker" - "pookte", and "steno" - "steentje". On each target trial subjects were first presented with an auditory specification of the target, then a warning signal and finally the carrier. The results for the four different pivotal consonants are shown in Fig. 2.

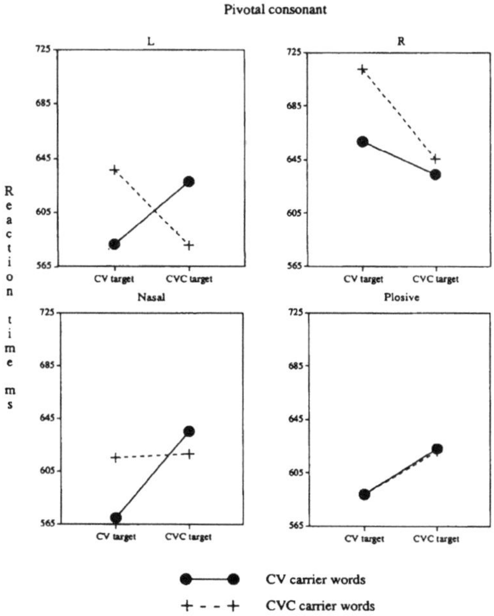

Fig. 2 Mean RTs (in msec.) for targets as a function of the syllabic structure of the Dutch carrier for four pivotal consonants types (Ls, Rs, nasals and stops).

The results revealed that the syllable effect - as reflected by an interaction between the two experimental factors - did not emerge for all pivotal consonants. An effect was obtained for the liquids (/l/ and /r/), a trend for nasals but no effect at all for the stop pivotal consonants. The experiment shows that the syllable effect does not generalize to all pivotal consonants but appears to be restricted primarily to stimuli with liquid pivotal consonants. As we pointed out above, these are the stimuli for which the clearest durational and spectral differences should be expected between carriers items. The Dutch subjects appear to exploit such phonetic information in making their detection response. However, when the information signalling syllable structure is weaker or absent, no effect emerges. This finding suggests that the syllable effect is at least in part phonetic and that the syllable does not constitute a general unit of speech processing in Dutch. Additional research manipulating the amount of phonetic information (e.g., with different pivotal consonants) is clearly required to test the generality of the syllable effect in languages like French in which these effects have been obtained. Furthermore, we also need to understand why no syllable effect has been found in languages like English despite the existence of allophonic cues to syllable structure. Such studies are clearly necessary to get a clearer picture of the phonetic contribution to the syllable effect.

4. Conclusion

In this paper I have presented three different perspectives on the interface between acoustic-phonetic and lexical processing. These differ in the way they view the involvement of sublexical representations in word recognition and in the methodology they adopt for studying these representations and processes. I have focused here upon three applications of the monitoring technique which are used to investigate these issues. This methodology is clearly geared to test the first two approaches which are based on the computation of sublexical representation(s) during word recognition. Indeed it is assumed that the detection latencies reflect the mental representations (units) and the processes responsible for the on-line processing of speech. Clearly, it must still be determined how the sublexical processing elicited by the detection task relates to normal speech processing (without this secondary detection task). If a direct correspondence is found, then it should also be possible to evaluate the third approach which denies the existence of sublexical representations.

Unfortunately, we are not yet in a position to specify the exact temporal and structural nature of sublexical processing during the process of target detection despite the wealth of monitoring data accumulated. However, there are signs that we are moving in the right direction. Some of the findings reviewed in this paper (especially Dupoux, 1990, and Norris and Culter, 1988) indicate that the detection task can be used to tap into different sublexical representations depending on the details of the experimental procedure. Various experimental factors (such as the nature of the foils/fillers, speed of subjects, etc.) influence the moment of the detection response and hence how far sublexical processing has progressed. A better understanding and careful manipulation of these factors should lead to new experimental results that produce a more coherent picture of sublexical processing. Research of this type should ultimately allow the further integration of phonetic and psycholinguistic approaches in the investigation of the acoustic-phonetic/lexical interface.

References

Church, K. (1987). Phonological parsing and lexical retrieval, *Cognition*, 25, 53-69.

Cutler, A. (1989). Auditory lexical access: Where do we start?, in: W.D. Marslen-Wilson (ed.), *Lexical representation and process*, MIT Press, Cambridge, MA.

Cutler, A., Butterfield, S., and Williams, J.N. (1987). The perceptual integrity of syllabic onsets, *Journal of Memory and Language*, 26, 406-418.

Cutler, A., Mehler, J., Norris, D., and Segui, J. (1986). The syllable's differing role in the segmentation of English and French, *Journal of Memory and Language*, 25, 385-400.

Cutler, A., Mehler, J., Norris. D., and Segui, J. (1987). Phoneme identification and the lexicon, *Cognitive Psychology*, 19, 144-177.

Cutler, A. and Norris, D. (1988). The role of the strong syllables in segmentation for lexical access, *J. of Exp. Psych. : Human Perception and Performance*, 14, 1, 113-121.

Cutler, A., Norris, D., and Williams, J.N. (1987). A note on phonological expectations in speech segmentation, *Journal of Memory and Language*, 26, 480-487.

Diehl, R.L., Kluender, K.R., Foss, D.J., Parker, E.M., and Gernsbacher, M.A. (?). Vowels as islands of reliability, *Journal of Memory and Language*, 26, 564-573.

Dupoux, E. (1989). *Identification des mots parlé: Détection de phonème et unité prelexicale*, unpublished doctoral dissertation, EHESS, Paris.

Foss, D.J. and Blank, M.A. (1980). Identifying the speech codes, *Cogn. Psychology*, 12, 1-31.

Foss, D.J. and Swinney, D.A. (1973). On the psychological reality of the phoneme: Perception, identification and consciousness, *Journal of Verbal Learning and Verbal Behavior*, 12, 246-257.

Frauenfelder, U.H., and Henstra, J. (1988). Lexical activation and deactivation of phonological representations, *Proc. of the Fourth International Phonology Conference, Krems, Austria.*

Frazier, L. (1987). Structure in auditory word recognition, *Cognition*, 25, 157-187.

Huggins A.W.F. (1964) Distortion of the temporal pattern of speech: Interruption and alternation. *J. Acoust. Soc. Am.*, 36, 1055-1064.

Klatt, D.H. (1980). Speech perception: A model of acoustic-phonetic analysis and lexical access, in: R.A. Cole (ed.), *Perception and production of fluent speech*, Hillsdale, N.J.: Lawrence Erlbaum Associates, 243-288.

Klatt, D.H. (1989). Review of selected models of speech perception, in: W.D. Marslen-Wilson (ed.), *Lexical representation and process*, MIT Press, Cambridge, MA.

Lahiri, A. and Marslen-Wilson, W.D. (1991). The mental representation of lexical form: A phonological approach to the recognition lexicon, *Cognition*, 38, 245-294.

Maddieson, I. (1984). Phonetic cues to syllabification, *UCLA working papers in Phon.*,59,101.

Marslen-Wilson, W.D. (1984). Perceiving speech and perceiving words, in: M.P.R. v.d. Broecke and A. Cohen (eds.) *The Proc. of the 10th International Phonetics Congress, Utrecht*, 99-104.

Marslen-Wilson, W.D. and Frauenfelder U.H. (1987). The interface between acoustic-phonetic and lexical processes, *Proc. of the 11th International Congress of Phonetic Sciences. Tallinn.*

Marslen-Wilson, W.D., and Welsh, A. (1978). Processing interactions and lexical access during word-recognition in continuous speech, *Cognitive Psychology*, 10, 29-63.

Massaro, D.W. (1972). Perceptual images, processing time, and perceptual units in auditory perception, *Psychological Review*, 79, 124-145.

Mehler, J. (1981). The role of the syllable in speech processing: Infant and adult data, *Philosophical Transactions of the Royal Society London*, B 295, 333-305.

Mehler, J., Dommergues, J., Frauenfelder, U., and Segui, J. (1981). The syllable's role in speech segmentation, *Journal of Verbal Learning and Verbal Behavior*, 20, 298-305.

Nooteboom, S.G. (1979). More attention for words in speech communication research?, in: B. Lindblom and S. Ohman (eds.), *Frontiers of speech communication research*, Academic Press, London.

Norris, D. and Cutler, A. (1985). Juncture detection, *Linguistics*, 23, 689-705.

Norris, D.J. and Cutler, A. (1988). The relative accessibility of phonemes and syllables, *Perception and Psychophysics*, 43, 541-550.

Pisoni, D.B. and Luce, P.A. (1987). Acoustic-phonetic representations in word recognition, *Cognition*, 25, 21-52.

Rietveld, T. and Frauenfelder, U.H. (1987) The effect of syllable structure on vowel duration, *Proc. of the 11th International Congress of Phonetic Sciences. Tallinn.*

Samuel, A.G. (1991) Perceptual degradation due to signal alternation: Implications for auditory pattern processing, *J. of Exp. Psych. : Human Perception and Performance*, 17, 2, 392.

Savin, H.B., and Bever, T.G. (1970). The non-perceptual reality of the phoneme, *Journal of Verbal Learning and Verbal Behavior*, 9, 295-302.

Sebastián-Gallès, N., Dupoux, E., Segui, J., and Mehler, J. (1991) Contrasting syllabic effects in Catalan and Spanish, *Journal of Memory and Language*, 31, 18-32.

Segui, J. (1984). The syllable: A basic perceptual unit in speech processing?, in: H. Bouma and D.G. Bouwhuis (eds.), *Attention and Performance X: Control of Language Processes*, Lawrence Erlbaum Associates, Hillsdale, N.J., 125-149.

Segui, J., Dupoux, E., and Melher, J. (1990). The syllable's role in speech segmentation, phoneme identification, and lexical access, in: G. Altmann (ed.), *Cognitive models of speech processing: Psycholinguistic and computational perspectives*, MIT Press, Cambridge, MA.

Segui, J., and Frauenfelder, U.H. (1986). The effects of lexical constraints upon speech perception, in: F. Klix and H. Hagendorf (eds.), *Human memory and cognitive capacities: Mechanisms and Performances*, Elsevier, North Holland.

Segui, J., Frauenfelder, U., and Mehler, J. (1981). Phoneme monitoring, syllable monitoring and lexical access, *British Journal of Psychology*, 72, 471-477.

Stevens, K.N. (1986). Models of phonetic recognition II: An approach to feature-based recognition, in P. Mermelstein (ed.), *Proceedings Montreal Satellite Symposium on Speech Recognition, Twelfth International Congress on Acoustics.*

Treiman, R., Salasoo, A., Slowiaczek, L.M., and Pisoni D. (1982). Effects of syllable structure on adults' monitoring performance, *Progress report No. 8 Indiana University Speech Lab Report.*

Warren, P. and Marslen-Wilson, W.D. (1987). Continuous uptake of acoustic cues in spoken word recognition, *Perception and Psychophysics*, 41(3), 262-275.

Warren, P. and Marslen-Wilson, W.D. (1988). Cues to lexical choice: discriminating place and voice, *Perception and Psychophysics*, 43, 21-30.

Zwitserlood, P., Schriefers. H., Lahiri, A., and Van Donselaar, W. (1991) On the role of the syllable in the perception of Dutch, manuscript.

Listening to Speech Through an Adaptive Window of Analysis

Howard C. Nusbaum and Anne S. Henly
Committee on Cognition and Communication
Department of Psychology
5848 South University Avenue
The University of Chicago
Chicago, IL 60637
USA

1. Speech Perception and Conceptual Categorization

How do we recognize spoken words? According to what has become the modal view in speech research (e.g., Marslen-Wilson and Welsh, 1978; McClelland and Elman, 1986), spoken word recognition is based on a mental lexicon that contains fixed, canonical (or perhaps prototypical) forms of word patterns (cf. Grosjean and Gee, 1987). As auditory information is processed from the speech waveform, properties of the stimulus pattern are compared to these canonical forms in the lexicon. The recognized word is the lexical form that provides, by some criterion, the closest match to the stimulus properties.

Given this particular perspective, several questions arise that are important for understanding speech perception. First, how are words represented in the mental lexicon? Second, what pattern properties are encoded from the speech waveform? Finally, how are these properties matched to words in the mental lexicon?

In many respects, this view of spoken word recognition is equivalent to traditional theories of categorization in cognitive psychology (cf. Smith and Medin, 1981; however see Medin and Barsalou, 1987, for a discussion of differences). Lexical forms are specified by a set of perceptual properties, just as a conceptual category such as *bird* can be specified by a set of properties such as *lays eggs*, or *has wings*. Making a conceptual classification of the kind *a robin is a bird*, is carried out by mapping properties from the category *robin* onto our conceptual representation of the category *bird*, much like mapping properties from a spoken stimulus onto our mental representations of words.

Just as there are structural similarities between the modal view of word recognition and traditional theories of categorization, there are similarities among the basic theoretical questions. How are conceptual categories represented (e.g., prototypes, exemplars, see Smith and Medin, 1981)? What information is encoded from a stimulus (Smith, 1989)? How are the encoded properties of a stimulus classified using the mental categories (e.g., Medin and Shaffer, 1978; Nosofsky, 1986)? In essence, the issues in both categorization and word recognition amount to understanding how we map information in the world onto mental structures.

Given that the theoretical issues are the same, it should not be surprising that the problems in developing theories of categorization and speech perception are the same. In particular, variability in mapping information onto mental representations poses a substantial problem in both domains. In speech perception, the effects of changing context and talker on recognition are well-established (Liberman, Cooper, Shankweiler, and Studdert-Kennedy, 1967). Similarly, changing context affects other forms of perceptual and conceptual categorization (e.g., Barsalou, 1982; Barsalou and Medin, 1987; Medin and Shaffer, 1978).

Within the domain of conceptual categorization, it is becoming clear that these effects of context and variability cannot be accounted for easily by positing fixed mental representations. Moreover, changing the nature of the fixed representation from a set of distinctive features to probabilistically weighted features or to defining any characteristic features does not solve these problems (Medin, 1989). In addition, research on *ad hoc* and goal-derived categories (e.g., Barsalou, 1983) has indicated that humans are extremely flexible in constructing categories to meet the needs of a particular task. Whatever theoretical form the mental representation of categories takes, it will have to be dynamic and adaptive.

Similarly, in speech perception, assuming a constant pattern specification for words may lead us to repeat some of the theoretical mistakes of cognitive psychology. The fundamental questions necessary to understanding spoken word perception should remain centered on the problem of how information in the speech signal is mapped onto the mental representation of words. However, in exploring these questions, it is not necessary to assume that words are represented in the lexicon with a static pattern structure, or that only one kind of sensory analysis is carried out to extract properties from the waveform, or even that there is one kind of process that maps these properties onto the lexicon.

2. An Adaptive Window of Perceptual Analysis

Much of the research in speech perception has been devoted to discovering *the* basic unit of perceptual analysis, with little regard for the higher-order task this analysis subserves -- recognizing words. The tacit assumption behind such an approach is that there exists a fixed unit of analysis which remains constant across tasks, even though the informational demands of the tasks may vary widely. Whether a subject is attempting to discriminate among members of the same phonemic class or different classes, whether monitoring for a phoneme, for a syllable, or for a word, the unit of perceptual analysis is assumed to be the same (although not the comparison process).

Conversely, work on word recognition has paid little attention to the unit of perceptual analysis, assuming that it must be a simple reflection of the units used to represent and recognize items in the lexicon. Although theoretical perspectives may differ quite a bit in the size of the units used to represent words, in most theories the unit of lexical representation and the unit of speech analysis are the same, and recognition decisions are based on a window of analysis equivalent to this unit (although this need not be the case, see Frauenfelder, this volume). For example, Klatt's (1980) model LAFS should make a word decision based on a single spectral template which is based on a 25.6 msec window of analysis computed every 10 msec. In the original version of Cohort theory, Marslen-Wilson and Welsh (1978) proposed that a single phoneme defined the smallest window of analysis, while Mehler and his colleagues (e.g., Mehler, Dommergues, Frauenfelder, and Segui, 1981) have argued for the syllable as the window of analysis.

Oddly, little consideration has been given to the possibility that the units of analysis, representation, and recognition may be dissociated. The smallest unit of sublexical representation in the lexicon only provides an indication of the minimal information necessary to discriminate one lexical form from another. However, properties encoded from the speech signal may take into account much more information than this minimal grain, effectively increasing the window of recognition analysis. Furthermore, the recognition decision could be based on one minimal, discriminating property (e.g., Marslen-Wilson, 1984), or much more information. Thus, the window of analysis of the waveform in any particular task will reflect the interaction of the canonical form of words in the lexicon, the encoding of properties in the speech signal, and the comparison process responsible for the recognition decision.

In spite of the diversity among theories, there is a common assumption. These theories assume that there is a single, unvarying window of analysis in word recognition that is intrinsically critical to understanding the process of word recognition. Unfortunately, this assumption is so deeply ingrained in the background of these theories that it has seldom been the focus of either analytic consideration or empirical investigation. Is such an assumption reasonable, and if reasonable, is there evidence to support it?

Obviously, the assumption of a fixed window of analysis holds if there is a fixed mental representation for words, a constant grain of analysis of the properties of the speech signal, and a single, invariant mechanism by which these properties are compared to the lexicon. But what if this is not the case? If words were to have various forms of representation, or the grain of perceptual analysis were to vary, or a number of different comparison processes were available, could we still assume a constant window of analysis for word recognition?

These questions are seldom raised explicitly simply because the assumption of a fixed window of analysis in speech perception is taken axiomatically in almost all empirical studies. Indeed, this was the starting point for several recent studies that we carried out to investigate the size of the window of analysis at a sublexical level (Nusbaum and DeGroot, 1991). We assumed, in addition, that listeners must represent phonetic information in order to recognize words, since this is the minimal linguistic distinction between words that is possible. However, we were interested in determining how this phonetic information is packaged for purposes of recognizing words. Do listeners encode and represent phonetic information in phonemes or whole syllables?

To investigate the window of analysis that is used to encode sound structure in speech, we used a speeded classification procedure. Following Garner (1974), all the information within a window of analysis should be perceptually integral; it should be difficult to selectively attend to one source of information within a window, ignoring others. On the other hand, information in adjacent windows should be perceptually separable; it should be easy to attend to information in one window and ignore information in another. Thus, two phonemes within a window of analysis should be perceptually integral, whereas phonemes in adjacent windows should be much more separable.

Previous research (e.g., Fowler and Smith, 1986; Shand, 1976; Tomiak, Mullennix, and Sawusch, 1987; Wood and Day, 1975) has shown that adjacent phonemes within a syllable are perceptually integral. For example, listeners cannot ignore variations in the vowel of a CV syllable when trying to classify the consonant (e.g., Wood and Day, 1975). These phonetic context effects argue that, within a syllable, adjacent segments are processed in the same window of analysis. These findings suggest that syllables are units of analysis rather than phonemes.

If this is true, then information within a syllable should be perceptually integral, and should be separable from information in adjacent syllables. To test this hypothesis we asked subjects to classify a target consonant while varying an adjacent vowel. In one set of stimuli, the adjacent vowel was in the same syllable as the target consonant, whereas in a second set of stimuli the adjacent vowel was in the preceding syllable. For each set of stimuli, subjects made phonetic classifications in both a unidimensional and an orthogonal condition. In the unidimensional condition, the consonant varied between /p/ and /t/ and the context was held constant. In the orthogonal condition, the consonant varied and the context vowel varied independently between /a/ and /æ/. The set of stimuli with context varying in the same syllable consisted of: [o'pʰa], [o'tʰa], [o'pʰæ], and [o'tʰæ]. The set with the context varying between syllables consisted of: [a'pʰo], [a'tʰo], [æ'pʰo], and [æ'tʰo]. In all the utterances the second syllable was stressed and the consonant aspirated, so that the consonant was perceived as the onset of the second syllable, rather than the coda of the first.

Subjects were extremely accurate in identifying the consonants in all conditions (over 98% correct). An examination of response times indicated that consonant classification was much slower when the context vowel varied (around 776 msec in the orthogonal condition) than when the context vowel was constant (around 719 msec in the unidimensional condition). Furthermore, there was as much integrality for segments in adjacent syllables as there was segments in the same syllable. Variation in the context vowel slowed consonant recognition as much when the target and context were in different syllables as it did when they were in the same syllable. These results indicate that in making phonetic decisions, the window of analysis is not constrained by syllable boundaries.

Another way of summarizing these results is that listeners make phonetic decisions using any coarticulatory information that could be useful, regardless of its distribution over intervening linguistic boundaries. This suggests that if words are represented in terms of phonetic structure, then the window of speech analysis might always be wide enough to include sufficient coarticulatory information to constrain phonetic identity. While this would not tell us how many of these windows would be needed to recognize a word, it would indicate the nature of the encoding process for segmental information prior to lexical matching.

Or that is the conclusion we might have drawn if we had stopped at this point. However, we took this research one step further. In a second experiment, we again asked a group of subjects to make phonetic decisions about a target consonant and either fixed or varied an adjacent context segment. As before, the adjacent segment was either in the same syllable as the target, or an adjacent syllable. However, this time the syllable boundary was also a word boundary. Our previous experiment indicated that phonetic decisions were not confined to information contained within a syllable. The question in this new experiment was whether a phonetic decision was more influenced by the context provided within a word than by phonetic context in an adjacent word.

Each stimulus consisted of two English words spoken without a pause between them. Each word pair contained a /g/ or /k/, which was the target phoneme, followed by an /r/ or /l/, which was the varying context. In the within-word stimulus set, the target velar stop and the context liquid were in the same word; the four within-word utterances were *paw grew*, *paw crew*, *paw glue*, and *paw clue*. In the between-word stimuli, the stop and liquid were in different words; the between-word stimuli were *hog root*, *hawk root*, *hog loot*, and *hawk loot*. To ensure that subjects heard the word boundary before the target stop in the within-word stimuli, and *between* the stop and liquid in the between-word stimuli, the words were chosen such that only one possible boundary location in each utterance would produce English words. Subjects classified the stop consonant when the context was constant (the unidimensional condition) and when the context varied independently from the target (the orthogonal condition). It is important to note that in another experiment we found that consonants in adjacent syllables are as perceptually integral as the consonants within a single onset (Nusbaum and De Groot, 1991).

Recognition accuracy for the consonants was over 98% correct across all conditions. As in the previous experiment, consonant recognition was faster when the context was constant (about 919 msec) than when it varied (973 msec). However, there was an interesting difference in the pattern of results. There was more integrality of phonetic information within words than there was between words. Consonant classification was 78 msec slower in the orthogonal condition than in the unidimensional condition when context varied within a word; when context varied in the adjacent word, classification was only 31 msec slower.

In many respects, these word stimuli are similar to the stimuli used in our other experiments in which we found equivalent integrality for context and target segments within syllables and between syllables. The primary difference between the earlier stimuli and the present stimuli is that the syllable boundary is also a word boundary. Although the results of our first study could be interpreted as evidence that the window of analysis for phonetic decisions is based on the distribution of useful coarticulatory information, these data argue against that conclusion. There is certainly as much useful coarticulatory information in an adjacent syllable that is a word as there is in one that is not a word. Taken together, the results of these two studies suggest that the window of analysis for phonetic decisions is somehow informed and modified by lexical status. The window of analysis for phonetic decisions seems to change based on the availability of different sources of information that could bear on the decision. Thus, there cannot be one fixed window of speech analysis at the segmental level.

3. The Window of Analysis at the Lexical Level

A similar conclusion can be drawn for spoken word recognition. A variety of different studies of word recognition have come to very different estimates of the size of the window of analysis. For example, Marslen-Wilson (1984; Warren and Marslen-Wilson, 1987) has argued for optimal efficiency in spoken word recognition. This means that listeners decide which word is spoken based on the earliest possible discriminating information. This implies a very narrow window of analysis for word recognition. However, other studies have suggested a much wider window of analysis. Taft and Hambly (1986) found that listeners use information after the optimal nonword point in a stimulus when making lexical decisions. Similarly, Luce (1991) has demonstrated that listeners are sensitive to the phonetic properties of a word even when they occur after the earliest, optimal discrimination point. However, the pattern of response times he observed suggests that the amount of signal used by listeners after this discrimination point seems to vary. Indeed, Luce concludes that there is a complex relationship between the nature of the information used in recognition and the size of the window of analysis. Across these different studies using isolated words, listeners appear to make decisions about words based on a range of sublexical window sizes from the smallest phonetic distinction to the entire pattern of a spoken word.

Of course, an isolated word has a well-defined beginning and ending. As a consequence, the window of analysis for isolated words cannot be greater than the word itself. Not only that, but in many cases by isolating a single word, the experimenter may indirectly suggest to the subject that the word is the optimal unit of analysis. Thus different experimental paradigms may constrain the size of the window of analysis. The picture changes radically when words are embedded in fluent speech. For example, Grosjean (1985) demonstrated that word recognition may depend on a substantial amount of segmental information after the end of a word. Thus, in fluent speech, the window of analysis can extend beyond the length of a spoken word, even including whole syllables of subsequent words.

This suggests that results regarding the window of analysis from studies using isolated words may not reflect the true scope of information needed for recognition. However, many studies employ isolated words because many models and theories assume that the window of analysis is contained within a word. In these models, recognizing a word embedded in fluent speech is no different than recognizing a word in isolation. Recognition is viewed as a simple sequential application of the same recognition process used for isolated words. By virtue of having recognized one word, the following word's onset can be located, and the recognition process repeated. In this way, each word is recognized in turn, one word after another, in the order in which they were produced. Although many models of word recognition rely on this strictly sequential process in order to segment the continuous waveform, this processing strategy should not be taken for granted. In fact, there has been little empirical support for the claim that identification of one word is completed before the next is begun. If words are not identified serially, the window of analysis becomes very difficult to interpret as a theoretical construct describing the distribution of information processing over the speech signal.

Recently, we carried out an experiment (Henly and Nusbaum, 1991) designed to test these simple assumptions: (1) words are recognized sequentially, and (2) the window of analysis for word recognition is contained within a word. Listeners were presented with target words 8 dB below a background of noise. The target words were generated by a CallText text-to-speech system in each of nine different conditions. Words were produced in isolation or with a preceding context syllable, a succeeding context syllable, or both. Half of the context syllables were words and half were nonwords. Ten targets were monosyllabic words and ten targets were trisyllabic words. All stimuli were produced in a monotone.

We were interested in finding out when the lexical status of the context syllables would affect recognition of the target. Subjects were instructed to identify any words they heard in the sequence of syllables. If word recognition is mediated by a sequential process with a fixed window of analysis equal to, or smaller than a word, we would expect better target recognition following a word than following a nonword since locating the onset of the target should be easier. However, after a target word is recognized, the lexical status of subsequent context should be irrelevant since the target would have been identified prior to moving the window of analysis onto the succeeding context item. If words are recognized one after another and the window of analysis is smaller than a word, context items after a word are outside the window and should not affect recognition performance.

The pattern of results did not support these predictions. It is interesting to note that there were essentially no reliable context effects for the trisyllabic targets. Context only affected identification of the monosyllabic targets. For these targets, across all following contexts, recognition accuracy was about 38% correct when the preceding context was a word and about 32% correct when it was a nonword. Thus, target identification was more accurate following a word than following a nonword, but only for monosyllabic target words. Although there was no main effect of lexical status for following contexts, under certain conditions, the lexical status of the following context affected target identification as well. When there was no preceding context item, identification of monosyllabic targets was better when the target was followed by a word (38% correct) than when followed by a nonword (33% correct).

It is difficult to interpret these results in terms of a fixed window of analysis for word recognition. The lexical status of context syllables reliably affects monosyllable identification and does not affect trisyllable identification. This suggests that listeners employ different windows for monosyllables and for trisyllables. Furthermore, under some conditions, the lexical status of a context that is presented after a word affects target recognition. Clearly, the window of analysis sometimes includes subsequent context and sometimes it does not. This suggests that there may not be an invariant window of analysis moving sequentially through the waveform, but rather an adaptive one which, driven by the information present in the context and the signal, may dynamically expand and contract depending on the location of the window and the need for more context.

Another way of looking at these results is that the internal structure of the trisyllables is sufficiently constraining that uncertainty about the onset and offset of the words does not impair recognition. For the monosyllables, locating the onset and offset of the target was more important to identification. These differences in the structural constraints provided by the target words appear to have affected the size of the window of analysis for word recognition. This means that the window of analysis for word recognition is informed by lexical structure. The window of analysis for words seems to be dynamic and is adjusted based on the informational requirements of the task, stimulus structure, and constraints provided by lexical knowledge.

4. Conclusions and Implications

Taken together, a variety of studies suggests that the window of analysis in speech perception cannot be characterized in any simple way either for segmental perception or word recognition. The idea that there is one fixed window of analysis depends on a set of assumptions about the recognition process that are being discarded in categorization research and perhaps should be rejected in speech research as well. These assumptions are: (1) the mental representation of a linguistic category, be it a phoneme or a word, consists of a fixed set of properties that specify its denotational structure; (2) a fixed set of properties are encoded from the speech waveform; and (3) an invariant recognition process compares the encoded properties to the linguistic categories looking for a close match.

It seems unlikely that our mental representation of words or phonemes can consist of a fixed set of concrete auditory or linguistic properties that are specified *a priori*. The acoustic specification of phonemes and words changes with the context and talker in so many ways that storing them all ahead of time seems impractical, if not impossible. Instead, linguistic categories need to be sufficiently abstract that they can provide a basis for generating these descriptions for any particular talker or context. Rather than represent a phoneme as a set of phonetic features, or a word as a sequence of auditory features or phonemes, it might be better to represent these categories as a kind of *theory* about each phoneme or word (see Medin, 1989; Murphy and Medin, 1985). Although this approach clearly begs the question of what constitutes a theory, in contrast with a more traditional view of category structure, it provides several advantages, even if viewed only as a metaphor.

To recognize a particular word, the listener must test a set of hypotheses derived from the theory of that word. The specific hypotheses that must be tested will depend on the constraints provided by the talker and context. To the extent that the set of word candidates is highly constrained by prior knowledge, the window of analysis may be very small and a single auditory property could be sufficient for a decision. If the constraints are much weaker, it is possible that more hypotheses are formed and evidence in favor of one word over another must be gathered over a longer window of analysis. Since the information needed for recognition can be specified as a function of contextual constraints, the analysis of the speech signal can be dynamically adjusted to meet the demands of the situation.

Viewing speech perception as a pattern recognition process encourages the assumptions that phonemes and words have fixed and specifiable pattern descriptions and that identifying the linguistic structure of speech is just a matter of comparing pattern properties in the world to these mental representations. The flexibility and adaptability of the perceptual process revealed in a number of experiments makes these assumptions questionable. Rather than attempt to characterize perceptual analysis as an invariant process carried out on fixed representations, it might be better to view speech perception as a process of constraint satisfaction. Listeners may establish a set of constraints on the linguistic interpretation of speech. Some of these constraints may come from an analysis of the speech signal and some may come from inferences using linguistic and pragmatic knowledge. When the talker is unknown and the domain of discourse is unknown, the set of possible messages is large. However, as speech is heard, talker characteristics are perceived that can constrain the set of segments that could correspond to the acoustic properties of the speech. This reduces the attentional demands on the listener (Nusbaum and Morin, 1991), permitting a shift of attention to other constraints such as those derived from the meaning of an utterance.

In summary then, it appears that it will be very difficult to characterize the window of analysis for speech at any level of representation. Regardless of the level of analysis, this window seems to be adaptive and dynamic. Moreover, it appears that the changes in the size of the window of analysis are informed by the linguistic knowledge of the listener. As a result, it may be more informative to investigate the principles that direct changes in this window and how listeners exploit linguistic structure to constrain the distribution of attention to the speech signal.

Acknowledgments

Preparation of this manuscript was supported, in part, by a grant from NIDCD, DC00601, to the University of Chicago.

References

Barsalou, L.W. (1982). Context-independent and context-dependent information in concepts, *Memory and Cognition*, 10, 82-93.

Barsalou, L.W. (1983). Ad hoc categories, *Memory and Cognition*, 11, 211-227.

Barsalou, L.W. and Medin, D.L. (1986). Concepts: Fixed definitions or dynamic context-dependent representations? *Cahiers de Psychologie Cognitive*, 6, 187-202.

Fowler, C.A. and Smith, M.R. (1986). Speech perception as "vector analysis": An approach to the problems of invariance and segmentation, In J. S. Perkell and D. H. Klatt (eds.), *Invariance and variability in speech processes*, Erlbaum, Hillsdale, NJ.

Garner, W.R. (1974). *The processing of information and structure*, Lawrence Erlbaum, Hillsdale, NJ.

Grosjean, F. (1985). The recognition of words after their acoustic offset: Evidence and implications, *Perception and Psychophysics*, 38, 299-310.

Grosjean, F. and Gee, J.P. (1987). Prosodic structure and spoken word recognition, *Cognition*, 25, 135-155.

Henly, A.S. and Nusbaum, H.C. (1991). The role of lexical status in the segmentation of fluent speech, *J. Acoust. Soc. Am.*, 89, 2011.

Klatt, D.H. (1980). Speech recognition: A model of acoustic-phonetic analysis and lexical access, in: R.A. Cole (ed.), *Perception and production of fluent speech*, LEA, Hillsdale.

Liberman, A.M., Cooper, F.S., Shankweiler, D.P., and Studdert-Kennedy, M. (1967). Perception of the speech code, *Psychological Review*, 74, 431-461.

Luce, P.A. (1991). Speeded comparisons of spoken words, *J. Acoust. Soc. Am.*, 89, 2010.

Marslen-Wilson, W.D. (1984). Function and process in spoken word-recognition, in: H. Bouma and D.G. Bouwhuis (Eds.), *Attention and performance X: Control of language processes*, LEA, Hillsdale, NJ.

Marslen-Wilson, W.D. and Welsh, A. (1978). Processing interactions and lexical access during word recognition in continuous speech, *Cognitive Psychology*, 10, 29-63.

McClelland, J.L. and Elman, J.L. (1986). The TRACE model of speech perception, *Cognitive Psychology*, 18, 1-86.

Medin, D.L. (1989). Concepts and conceptual structure, *American Psychologist*, 44, 1469-1481.

Medin, D.L. and Barsalou, L.W. (1987). Categorization processes and categorical perception, In S. Harnad (ed.), *Categorical perception*, Cambridge University Press, Cambridge.

Medin, D.L., and Shaffer, M.M. (1978). Context theory of classification, *Psychological Review*, 85, 207-238.

Mehler, J., Dommergues, J., Frauenfelder, U., and Segui, J. (1981). The syllable's role in speech segmentation, *Journal of Verbal Learning and Verbal Behavior*, 20, 298-305.

Murphy, G.L., and Medin, D.L. (1985). The role of theories in conceptual coherence, *Psychological Review*, 92, 289-316.

Nosofsky, R.M. (1986). Attention, similarity, and the identification-categorization relationship, *Journal of Experimental Psychology: General*, 115, 39-57.

Nusbaum, H.C., and DeGroot, J. (1991). The role of syllables in speech perception, in: Ziolkowski, M.S., Noske, M., and Deaton, K. (eds.). *Papers from the parasession on the syllable in phonetics and phonology*, Chicago Linguistic Society, Chicago.

Nusbaum, H.C., and Morin, T.M. (1991). Paying attention to differences among talkers, in: Y. Tohkura, Y. Sagisaka, and E. Vatikiotis-Bateson (eds.), *Speech perception, production, and linguistic structure*, OHM Publishing Company, Tokyo.

Shand, M.A. (1976). Syllabic vs segmental perception: On the inability to ignore "irrelevant" stimulus parameters, *Perception and Psychophysics*, 20, 430-432.

Smith, E.E., and Medin, D.L. (1981). *Categories and concepts*, Harvard University Press, Cambridge MA.

Smith, L.B. (1989). A model of perceptual classification in children and adults, *Psychological Review*, 96, 125-144.

Taft, M., and Hambly, G. (1986). Exploring the Cohort Model of spoken word recognition, *Cognition*, 22, 259-282.

Tomiak, G.R., Mullennix, J.W., and Sawusch, J.R. (1987). Integral processing of phonemes: Evidence for a phonetic mode of perception, *J. Acoust. Soc. Am.*, 81, 755-764.

Warren, P., and Marslen-Wilson, W.D. (1987). Continuous uptake of acoustic cues in spoken word recognition, *Perception and Psychophysics*, 41, 262-275.

Wood, C.C., and Day, R.S. (1975). Failure of selective attention to phonetic segments in consonant-vowel syllables, *Perception and Psychophysics*, 17, 346-350.

Integration of Acoustic-Phonetic Cues in Word Segmentation

Hugo Quené
Research Institute for Language and Speech
Rijksuniversiteit Utrecht
Trans 10
3512 JK Utrecht
The Netherlands

1. INTRODUCTION

In order to understand an utterance, a listener must identify the words which it contains. This task of word perception requires that listeners divide the continuous speech signal into chunks corresponding to separate words. This *word segmentation* can be achieved by means of several strategies.

First, word boundaries may be detected as a by-product of the word perception process. Words may be recognised well before their acoustic offset, especially in the case of long (polysyllabic) or contextually predictable words. If a word is successfully recognised before its offset, then its phonological specification becomes available. This enables the listener to anticipate at which point in the time signal the current word ends, and a new word begins. However, this *anticipation strategy* fails with shorter stimulus words not recognised before their offset (and with words-within-words, e.g. "cap\tain", Dutch "ban\k\et"; Frauenfelder 1985; Luce 1986).

Cutler and Norris (1988) propose a second perceptual strategy, where listeners use strong syllables as hypothetical word onsets. They argue that each strong (stressed or unreduced) syllable triggers a fresh lexical access, with the stressed syllable as a potential word onset. This *strong-syllable strategy* seems reasonable, if we consider the lexical data for Dutch in Table I. Only in the 10% of word tokens starting with a weak (unstressed, reducible) syllable does this strategy produce incorrect starting points for lexical access (e.g. *patrol*, Dutch *tomaat* "tomato", *elkaar* "each other").

However, this perceptual strategy is insufficient for correct word segmentation if the syllable division of the acoustic signal is ambiguous (due to insufficient phonotactic restrictions). When this happens, knowing that the syllable is word-initial is not enough: the exact boundary between the preceding and initial syllables, and hence the exact word onset, cannot be determined. Unfortunately, ambiguous syllable divisions are found quite regularly in normal speech, as shown by the following lexical data.

From a lexical database for Dutch (CELEX 1990), a list of all stressed syllables was generated (n=2169; excluding syllables only occurring with an ambisyllabic consonant, such as /ɑp/ as in /ɑpəl/). All possible segmentations of these strong syllables were generated, by deleting onset and coda consonants (e.g. /stur/ yielding /stu, tu, u, tur, ur/). This procedure yielded 902 segmentation alternatives which are identical to strong syllables in the original

Table I Numbers of lexical types and tokens derived from the CELEX database, broken down by number of syllables and stress pattern ("s": strong, stressed, not reducible; "w": weak, unstressed, reducible).

nr. sylls	stress pattern	nr. types	nr. tokens
1	s	4 713	24 269 023
2	sw	11 658	4 753 446
	ws	3 372	1 481 539
3	sww	5 083	710 826
	wsw	5 582	1 003 460
	wws	1 849	257 398
4	swww	1 008	80 600
	wsww	1 583	118 438
	wwsw	3 155	229 714
	wwws	853	55 342
5 and >	swwww?	108	5 146
	wswww?	110	5 777
	wwsww?	680	40 557
	wwwsw?	1 292	55 133
	wwwws?	504	18 065
	(other)	41	669
	total s?	22 570 (54.3%)	29 819 041 (90.1%)
	total w?	19 021 (45.7%)	3 266 092 (9.9%)
	grand total	41 591	33 085 133

list (e.g. /tur/). This means that roughly 42% of all strong syllables have an ambiguous boundary. If we limit ourselves to ambiguity at syllable onset only, there are still 304 (14%) alternative segmentations yielding existing syllables. Hence, even if a word starts with a strong syllable, its exact onset location is ambiguous in 14% of all strong syllables.

Thirdly, word boundaries are usually correctly detected in phonetically ambiguous fragments, such as the following (1):

(1a)	ice cream	i scream	(Lehiste 1960)
(1b)	lettuce	let us	(Taft 1984)
(1c)	dearest you	dear stew	(Koster 1987)
(1d)	divan "couch"	die van "that one of"	
(1e)	tegenzet "counter-move"	thee gezet "tea made"	

The above problems with knowledge-driven strategies for word segmentation suggest that word segmentation also depends on *sensory* word boundary information. In other words, phonetic correlates of the intended word boundary probably contribute to listeners' perceived word segmentation. Two types of acoustic-phonetic correlates of word boundaries are generally observed:

(1) spectral word boundary phenomena, e.g. glottal stop, vocal fry, laryngealisation (Lehiste 1960; Gårding 1967; Nakatani and Dukes 1977; Cohen 1987), blocking of coarticulation (Su, Daniloff and Hammarberg 1975; Lewis, Daniloff and Hammarberg 1975);
(2) temporal word boundary phenomena, e.g. word-initial consonant lengthening (Lehiste 1960; Gårding 1967; Oller 1973; Nakatani and Schaffer 1978; Nooteboom 1972; Quené 1992), onset lengthening of word-initial vowels (Lehiste 1972; Oller 1973; Klatt 1976; Quené 1992).

The fact that these phenomena are correlated with contrastive word boundary positions does not imply that they are also relevant from a perceptual viewpoint. The experiment reported here investigates primarily whether the temporal cues mentioned above are indeed perceptually relevant for word segmentation. This is done by observing subjects' perceived word segmentation of two-word combinations, in which the durations of the appropriate speech fragments are manipulated.

Second, the experimental manipulation of durational parameters enables us to adress the issue of 'direct mapping' between acoustic signal and the mental lexicon (Luce, Pisoni and Goldinger 1990; Marslen-Wilson 1989). We assume that spectral cues contribute to word segmentation (since they do not contribute directly to word recognition). If the 'direct mapping' hypothesis is true, i.e. entries in the mental lexicon are accessed directly through the acoustic signal, without an intermediate representation in phonetic or phonological segments, then we arrive at the following prediction. Since spectral and temporal word boundary cues are integrated across a time window, an interaction between the two types of cues should be observed. If both spectral and temporal boundary cues are perceptually relevant, they should 'reinforce' each other: temporal cues should be more effective if they 'coincide' with the original spectral cues. Conversely, if the 'direct mapping' hypothesis is false, we arrive at the opposite prediction. Since spectral and temporal boundary cues are processed separately, their perceptual effects should be additive. Temporal cues contribute equally to perceived word segmentation, irrespective of the original spectral cues. In summary, the following experiment also investigates whether there is an interaction between spectral cues (as determined by the intended boundary position) and temporal boundary cues.

2. Experimental Method

2.1 Stimulus material

Stimuli were constructed by combining two meaningful Dutch monosyllables sharing a pivotal consonant. Only monomorphematic words were used, and function words were avoided. Three types of boundary ambiguity were introduced, depending on the number of intervocalic consonants and the possible boundary positions (see Table II). However, type-3 word combinations with a sonorant pivotal consonant are not allowed in Dutch. For each of the 3+3+2 remaining cells, 3 combinations of meaningful words were constructed. Accent position was balanced between the two words, and approximately balanced across consonant categories and ambiguity types. In addition, 10 filler combinations were constructed, which were identical to the stimuli in all relevant aspects.

Table II Three types of boundary ambiguity. "#X#" indicates that a word boundary can occur either before or after the /X/ segment.

	nr.cons.	ambiguity	example
type 1	1	V #C# V	/te#n#aj/
type 2	2	VC#C# V	/vɛr#x#ɑl/
type 3	3	V #C#CV	/me#t#rup/

2.2 Speech material

Both contrasting versions of the 24 combinations were embedded in a disambiguating sentence, in which only one stimulus segmentation was allowed. Corresponding sentences were as similar as possible with respect to number of syllables and words, stimulus position in sentence, etc. No important prosodic or syntactic break occurred within or immediately before or after the two-word sequence. In 9 out of 24 cases, it was necessary to extend the second of the two relevant words (in both versions) with a suffix, in order to fulfill these requirements. The following example demonstrates the ambiguous combinations and their carrier sentences:

word combination:	/max/ + /xaut/	
ambiguity:	/max#aut/ "stomach old"	/ma#xaut/ "mom gold"
carrier sentences:	als je *maag oud* wordt...	als je *ma goud* geeft...
	"if your stomach old gets..."	"if you mom gold give..."

All 2x24 stimulus sentences and 2x10 filler sentences were read twice by a professional speaker of Standard Dutch, and recorded on audio tape using high-quality equipment. Each stimulus was digitized (at 20 kHz, 9 kHz LPF, 12 bits) and excised from the carrier sentence (usually the second realisation, unless affected by pausing, hesitation, mispronunciation, etc.). The excerpted stimuli sounded natural, and did not suffer from 'clicks' at their onset or offset. They were LPC-analysed (30 filter poles, window 25 ms, shift 10 ms), and their source type (voiced or unvoiced) and F0 were established with a program using sub-harmonic summation. Filler combinations were digitised, excerpted and processed identically.

2.3 Experimental conditions

The analysis frames corresponding to (a) *pivotal consonant* and (b) *post-boundary vowel onset* were established, by means of a segmentation program with visual and auditory feedback. Vowel onset segments stretch from the first vowel frame to the frame with amplitude over 90% of the vowel peak amplitude (logarithmic).

The durations of these speech fragments were shortened (67%) or lengthened (134%) with respect to their original duration. Manipulations were done by changing the number of samples for the appropriate frames. The (4x2x24=196) stimuli were re-synthesised, and recorded in pseudo-random order on DAT with 2.0 s ISI (preceded and followed by 10 fillers).

2.4 Subjects and procedure

The stimulus tape was presented to 80 native Dutch subjects. Most of them were language students; none of them reported hearing defects. Subjects listened individually to the tapes over binaural headphones in a sound-treated booth. Their response sheet gave two possible contrastive segmentations (excluding segmentations involving geminate consonants), from which a forced choice had to be made. Orthographic contrasts between response alternatives were to be ignored.

2.5 Results

The percentages of responses corresponding to the initial pivotal consonant are given in Table III below. These proportions (calculated for each item, across 80 subjects) were converted to rationalised arcsine data (Studebaker 1985). These were fed into an analysis of variance with the following factors: (a) manipulated duration of pivotal consonant, (b) manipulated duration of post-boundary vowel onset, (c) intended boundary position, (d) stimulus cell [depending on pivotal consonant type and ambiguity type, see section 3.1], (e) stimulus combination [nested under (d)]. All factors except (e) were treated as fixed.

Table III Percentage of "initial pivotal consonant" responses, for two contrastive (intended) boundary positions, and four manipulation conditions. Each data point is based on 1920 responses (80 subjects x 24 items).

	pivot.cons.:	long	long	short	short
	vowel onset:	long	short	long	short
intended	/C#/	16.2	20.5	15.1	19.5
bound.position	/#C/	62.7	65.4	52.0	50.7

These results show that both temporal word boundary markers are indeed perceptually relevant: manipulation affects subjects' perceived responses [(a) $F_{1,16}$=29.2, p<.001; (b) $F_{1,16}$=8.3, p<.05]. However, subjects' perceived word segmentation is far more strongly affected by (c) the intended position of the word boundary [18% vs 58%; $F_{1,16}$=95.6, p<.001]. The scoring differences between contrastive boundary positions are far larger than those between manipulation conditions, as shown by Table III.

In addition, the effects of temporal manipulations and intended boundary position interact. Both of the manipulated temporal boundary cues influence subjects' perceived segmentation, but *only* if the 'carrier' segment occurs in word-*initial* position. Varying the duration of the *pivotal consonant* affects subjects' responses if this consonant is word-initial (64% vs 51%;

Table III, bottom line); these variations are ineffective if the consonant is word-final. Similarly, varying the duration of the *post-boundary vowel* onset has the strongest perceptual effect if this vowel is intended as word-initial (16% vs 20%; Table III, top line); no difference is observed if the vowel is preceded by an onset consonant within the same word. These observations are supported by significant interaction effects in the analysis of variance [(ac) $F_{1,16}$=13.3, p<.01; (bc) $F_{1,16}$=10.1, p<.01].

3. DISCUSSION

Subjects' perceived word segmentation depends most on the unmanipulated *spectral* boundary cues corresponding to the intended boundary position. In addition, both *temporal* boundary markers contribute to word segmentation: manipulations of these markers yield significant differences in the perceived position of the word boundary. In general, it seems that phonetic cues can contribute to the perceptual division of the speech signal into separate words, although they are insufficient means to achieve this end. Otherwise, one would expect perfect segmentation scores (viz. 0% and 100% for /C#/ and /#C/ stimuli, respectively) for those conditions where all available temporal and spectral cues indicate the same intended segmentation. The invalidity of this prediction (viz. 15% and 65%, respectively) shows that phonetic cues have only a limited influence on word segmentation. Nevertheless, listeners are sensitive to spectral and temporal cues that may indicate the intended word segmentation, when phonotactic and other higher-order cues are ineffective (as in the experiment described here). This finding converges with Frauenfelder's conclusion (this volume) with regard to perceived syllable constituency: "the Dutch listener appears to be sensitive to allophonic cues in carrier words that can signal the [syllable] structure of the words."

Subjects' responses also indicated that the manipulated temporal boundary markers are particularly effective if they are carried by a word-initial speech segment. This result is compatible with a *'direct-mapping'* model (Luce, Pisoni and Goldinger 1990; Marslen-Wilson 1989), if spectral cues are carried primarily by word-initial segments. Independent evidence for this 'word-initiality' of spectral cues is provided by Gårding (1967) for Swedish, by Nakatani and Dukes (1977) for American English, and by Cohen (1987) for Dutch.

According to the 'direct-mapping' model, acoustic information from a given time window is perceptually integrated: all acoustic parameters, both spectral and temporal, are processed simultaneously and in parallel. Therefore, 'coinciding' cues (indicating the same segmentation) may perceptually reinforce each other. Such an interaction was indeed observed in the present experiment. The relevant time window for word segmentation purposes need not be longer than one or two speech segments, in order to account for the above results.

In conclusion, it seems that Dutch listeners are sensitive to sub-phonemic cues for word segmentation. The observed interaction between spectral and temporal boundary cues can be explained adequately by a 'direct-mapping' model for word perception. All acoustic cues within a given time window are integrated, contributing simultaneously to both word perception and word segmentation.

References

Celex (1990). CELEX Dutch Database, release N 3.1. computer software. Centre for Lexical Information, Nijmegen.

Cohen, A. (1987). Juncture revisited, in: R. Channon and L. Shockey (eds.), *In honour of Ilse Lehiste*, Foris, Dordrecht, 7-18.

Cutler, A. and Norris, D. (1988). The role of strong syllables in segmentation for lexical access, *J. Experimental Psychology: Human Perception and Performance*, 14, 113-21.

Frauenfelder, U.H. (1985). Cross-linguistic approaches to lexical segmentation, *Linguistics*, 23, 669-687.

Gårding, E. (1967). ***Internal juncture in Swedish.*** Gleerup, Lund. Travaux de l'Institute de Phonétique de Lund; 6.

Klatt, D.H. (1976). Linguistic uses of segmental duration in English: acoustic and perceptual evidence, *J. Acoust. Soc. Am.*, 59, 1208-21.

Koster, C.J. (1987). *Word Recognition in Foreign and Native Language: Effects of Context and Assimilation*, dissertation Universiteit van Amsterdam.

Lehiste, I. (1960). An acoustic-phonetic study of internal open juncture, *Phonetica*, 5, supplement.

Lehiste, I. (1972). The timing of utterances and linguistic boundaries, *J. Acoust. Soc. Am.*, 51, 2018-24.

Lewis, J., Daniloff, R. and Hammarberg, R. (1975). Apical coarticulation at juncture boundaries, *J. Phonetics*, 3, 1-7.

Luce, P.A. (1986). A computational analysis of uniqueness points in auditory word recognition, *Perception and Psychophysics*, 39, 155-59.

Luce, P.A., Pisoni, D.B. and Goldinger, S.D. (1990). Similarity neighborhoods of spoken words, in: G. Altmann (ed.), *Cognitive Models of Speech Processing: Psycholinguistic and Computational Perspectives*, MIT Press, Cambridge.

Marslen-Wilson, W.D. (1989). Access and integration: Projecting sound onto meaning, in: W.D. Marslen-Wilson (ed.), *Lexical Representation and Process*, MIT Press, Cambridge.

Nakatani, L.H. and Dukes, K.D. (1977). Locus of segmental cues for word juncture, *J. Acoust. Soc. Am.*, 62, 714-19.

Nakatani, L.H. and Schaffer, J.A. (1978). Hearing 'words' without words: prosodic cues for word perception, *J. Acoust. Soc. Am.*, 63, 234-45.

Nooteboom, S.G. (1972). *Production and Perception of Vowel Duration: a Study of Durational Properties of Vowels in Dutch*, dissertation Rijksuniversiteit Utrecht.

Oller, D.K. (1973). The effect of position in utterance on speech-segment duration in English, *J. Acoust. Soc. Am.*, 54, 1235-47.

Quené, H. (1992). Acoustic-phonetic cues for word segmentation. To appear in *J. Phonetics*.
Studebaker, G.A. (1985). A "rationalized" arcsine transform, *J. Speech and Hearing Research*, 28, 455-62.
Su, L.-S., Daniloff, R. and Hammarberg, R. (1975). Variation in lingual coarticulation at certain juncture boundaries, *Phonetica*, 32, 254-63.
Taft, L. (1984). *Prosodic Constraints and Lexical Parsing Strategies*, PhD thesis University of Massachusetts.

Relations between Phoneme Scores and Syllable Scores for Normal-Hearing and Hearing-Impaired Subjects

Arjan Bosman, Guido F. Smoorenburg

Laboratory of Experimental Audiology
Department of Otorhinolaryngology
University Hospital Utrecht
Heidelberglaan 100
NL-3584 CX Utrecht
The Netherlands

Adelbert W. Bronkhorst

TNO Institute for Perception
Kampweg 5
NL-3769 DE Soesterberg
The Netherlands

1. Introduction

The intelligibility of a speech item does not only depend on its inherent acoustical/phonetical characteristics but also on the context in which it occurs. For instance, coarticulation and phonological rules provide context for adjacent phonemes, whereas linguistic, syntactic and semantic rules may provide additional context within syllables. The effects of context on speech intelligibility are stronger for items embedded in larger speech fragments, like phonemes in sentences, than for items within smaller fragments, like phonemes in isolated syllables, as more contextual cues are available for larger fragments. Within the scope of this study all interactions among a target phoneme and its surroundings will be denoted as context.

In auditory speech perception listeners may use contextual cues to fill in ill-perceived speech fragments. Under adverse listening conditions they have to rely on contextual information, as in this case not all auditory information will be available, and missing elements have to be filled in. In the hearing impaired less of the acoustical information will be available in comparison to normal-hearing listeners. This is especially the case for those hearing impaired having a so-called discrimination loss (i.e. maximum phoneme identification score below 100% at any presentation level). In order to compensate cognitively for the lack of auditory information, hearing-impaired listeners may make relatively more use of contextual cues than normal-hearing listeners. Therefore, we want to study whether the scores based on various speech elements are different for hearing-impaired and for normal-hearing listeners.

In this paper the effect of context will be estimated from the relations between the percentages of phonemes and syllables identified correctly (phoneme score and syllable score, respectively), using a simple statistical model. In this model the effect of an increase of context will show itself as a decrease in the number of statistically independent elements per item.

A reference group of young normal-hearing listeners and three groups of hearing-impaired listeners were used. The syllable material consisted of meaningful (sense) and meaningless (nonsense) syllables of the consonant-vowel-consonant type (CVC syllables). The CVC syllables were presented in quiet and in noise.

2. Analysis of Data

In general, context effects may result in higher whole-item identification scores than might be expected from an estimation on the basis of independent perception of its constituent elements (phonemes). If all elements behave statistically independently, the whole-item score can be simply expressed as a product of scores found for its elements (element scores). Assuming equal intelligibility for all elements results in a power relationship between whole-item score and element scores. According to Fletcher (1953), the effect of context can be quantified by a lowering of the exponent. So, the relationship between whole-item scores (p_w) and element scores (p_e) can be expressed as (Smoorenburg, 1985; Boothroyd and Nittrouer, 1988; Bosman, 1989):

$$p_w = p_e^j, \ 1 \leq j \leq n \tag{1}$$

in which n is the number of (linguistic) elements per item and j the number of statistically independent elements per item. Parameter j follows from eq. (1) by taking the logarithm of p_w and p_e. In the case of nonsense CVC-syllables, j will be about three if contextual effects like coarticulation are negligible, and for sense CVC syllables j will be less than three, due to syllable meaning. So, the j-factor provides a measure of the overall context effect.

Recently, a different approach to the quantification of context effects was proposed by Bronkhorst (1991). In this approach parameters are introduced representing chances of filling in ('guessing') ill-perceived elements. Predictors are given, not only of the wole-item scores and element scores, but also of scores for partially correct items. Preliminary results show that this approach yields a more detailed insight into the nature of context effects than eq. (1).

3. Materials and Methods

The speech material consisted of meaningful (sense) and meaningless (nonsense) CVC syllables (Bosman, 1989) and of sentences of 8 or 9 syllables (Plomp and Mimpen, 1979). The speech material was uttered by a female speaker and presented in quiet and in noise. The noise consisted of gaussian noise shaped to the long-term average spectrum of the speaker.

A reference group and three groups of hearing-impaired subjects were used: young normal-hearing university students (YNH), subjects with noise-induced hearing loss (NIHL), elderly subjects with presbycusis (PRES) and subjects with Ménière's disease (MEN). All groups consisted of 20 subjects. The pure-tone audiograms showing the threshold of hearing as a function of frequency are shown in Fig. 1 for YNH, NIHL, PRES and MEN subjects, respectively.

Both types of CVC syllables were presented at levels relative to the speech reception threshold (SRT) for sentences. For all subjects the CVC syllables were presented in 5 dB steps around each individual's SRT for sentences. The level of the noise was set halfway each subject's dynamic range. The sentences were also presented around the SRT, but with a smaller stepsize of 2 dB. Only presentation levels relative to sentence SRT were used to avoid floor and ceiling effects in view of the considerable spread in hearing loss among our subjects.

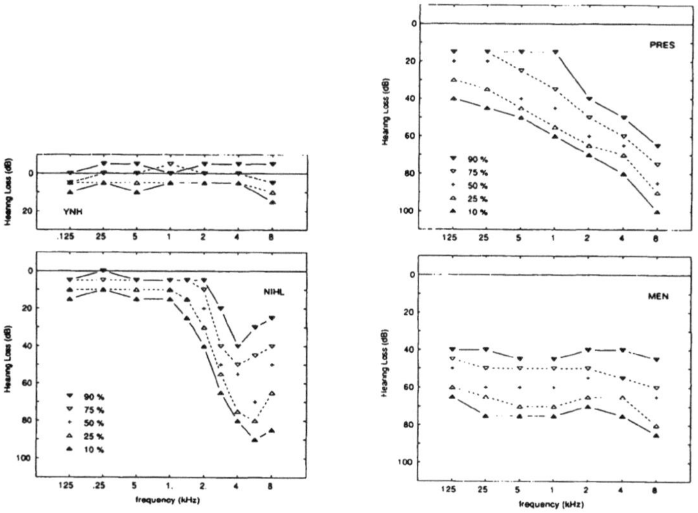

Fig. 1 The pure-tone audiograms for YNH, NIHL, PRES, and MEN subjects. The distribution of the thresholds is expressed in 10%, 25%, 50%, 75%, and 90% percentiles.

4. Results

The phoneme scores and syllable scores for sense and nonsense CVC syllables are shown in Fig. 2 for YNH, NIHL, PRES, and MEN subjects, respectively (see also Bosman and Smoorenburg, 1991). Fig. 2 clearly shows that the effect of syllable meaning (sense vs. nonsense) is much larger for syllable scores than for phoneme scores. Apparently, syllable scores are much more sensitive to context effects than phoneme scores.

To illustrate the approach proposed in Sect. 2, whole-syllable scores for sense and nonsense syllables are plotted as a function of phoneme score in Fig. 3 for the YNH subjects. The average phoneme score at each syllable score is presented by a triangle. The dashed curves correspond to values for the j-parameter of 2.5 (left curve) and of 3.0 (right curve). The average values of j for syllable scores in the range from 25% to 75% are presented in Table I. This table shows that for all groups of subjects j is in the order of 3.0 for nonsense syllables, whereas it is reduced to about 2.5 for sense syllables. The

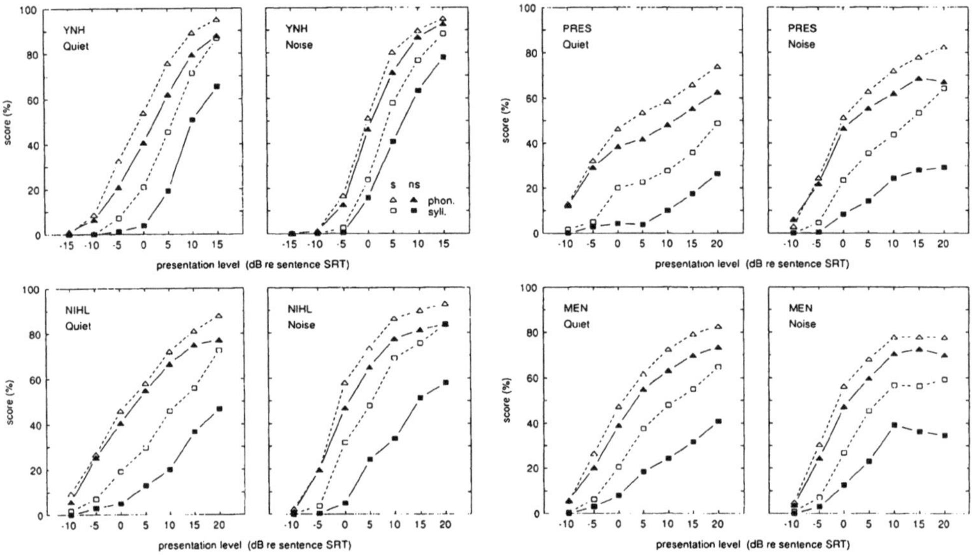

Fig. 2 Average phoneme and syllable scores for sense and nonsense CVC syllables as a function of presentation level for YNH, NIHL, PRES and MEN subjects. Phoneme scores and syllable scores are denoted by triangles and squares, respectively. Sense (s) and nonsense (ns) scores are denoted by open and filled symbols. Left frame: quiet; right frame: noise.

number of independent elements is about three in both the quiet and the noise conditions for nonsense syllables. For sense syllables in noise there is a tendency to have fewer independent elements than in quiet. The slightly reduced effect of context in quiet might be due to the threshold of hearing, which selectively limits the audibility of spectral components in quiet, whereas in noise spectral information is mainly determined by the noise spectrum. In other words: in quiet, parts of the speech spectrum are filtered by the threshold of hearing, especially for those listeners with high-frequency hearing loss. Consequently, not all contextual cues may be available in quiet.

The usefulness of this simple model can be further illustrated by relating whole-sentence scores to syllables scores (for sentences). The values of parameter j are presented in Table II. This table clearly shows that the sentences are highly redundant, as the sentences contain only about 2.5 independent elements (syllables). Again, there is not much variation among subject groups. The j-values for NIHL and PRES subjects are somewhat lower than for the other subjects, indicating that these listeners may make more use of context than YNH and MEN listeners.

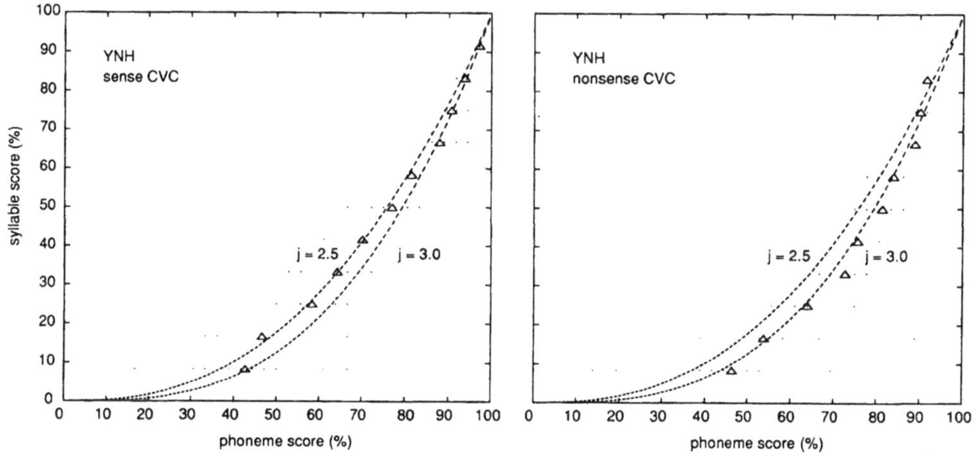

Fig. 3 Syllable scores as a function of phoneme scores for YNH subjects with sense syllables (left frame) and with nonsense syllables (right frame). The dashed curves correspond to j values of 2.5 and 3.

Table I. The number of statistically independent phonemes estimated with eq. (1) for sense and nonsense CVC-syllables presented in quiet and in noise. Values of j were averaged across syllable scores of between 25% and 75%.

	Quiet		Noise	
Group	sense	nonsense	sense	nonsense
YNH	2.7	3.2	2.4	3.1
NIHL	2.5	3.0	2.4	3.1
PRES	2.7	2.8	2.3	2.9
MEN	2.4	3.1	2.3	2.9

5. Discusssion and Conclusions

The effect of syllable meaning on the perception of individual phonemes was roughly the same for all groups of subjects. This suggests that there is not a substantial effect of hearing loss on the use of context information for CVC syllables. In short stimuli, like

CVC syllables, there is not much context information available. This may suppress differences in behavior among normal-hearing and hearing-impaired listeners. At low levels of performance (syllable scores below 20%), some of the hearing-impaired subjects responded either in full syllables or not at all. Apparently, a response was given only when they felt sufficiently confident about the perceived syllable. This behavior of responding either 'all' or 'nothing' had only a limited effect on the values of j, as we included only data from syllable scores between 25% and 75%. When looking at the perception of phonemic features, the PRES subjects tend to pay more attention to the feature of glide suggesting increased attention for phoneme transitions compared to the other listeners (Bosman, 1989). However, this appears to have hardly any effect on phoneme scores.

Table II The number of statistically independent syllables estimated with eq. (1) for sentences presented in quiet and in noise. Values of j were averaged across sentence scores of between 23% and 77%.

Group	Quiet	Noise
YNH	2.4	3.0
NIHL	2.1	2.5
PRES	2.5	2.6
MEN	2.9	2.8

In longer speech fragments, like sentences, more context is available. For sentences the NIHL and PRES subjects with gradually acquired hearing loss tend to show lower values of j, implying more use of context information, than normal-hearing listeners or listeners with a history of fluctuating loss (MEN subjects). This latter finding is in favor of the hypothesis that hearing-impaired listeners may try to compensate cognitively for their hearing deficits by paying more attention to contextual cues than normal-hearing listeners.

References

Boothroyd, A. and Nittrouer, S. (1988). Mathematical treatment of context effects in phoneme and word recognition, *J. Acoust. Soc. Am.*, 84, 101-114.

Bosman, A.J. (1989). *Speech perception by the hearing impaired*, Doctoral Thesis, University of Utrecht.

Bosman, A.J., and Smoorenburg, G.F. (1991). The intelligibility of CVC syllables and sentences presented in quiet and in noise to normal-hearing subjects and to subjects with three types of hearing impairment, Submitted to *Audiology*.

Bronkhorst, A.W. (1991). *Voorspelling van spraakverstaan in fluctuerend lawaai. Toepassing van een statistische beschrijving van contexteffecten*, Internal report TNO-IZF, Soesterberg.

Fletcher, H. (1953). *Speech and Hearing in Communication*, Van Nostrand, New York.

Plomp, R. and Mimpen, A.M. (1979). Improving the reliability of testing the speech reception threshold for sentences, *Audiology*, 18, 43-52.

Smoorenburg, G.F. (1985). Het spraakaudiogram in relatie tot de gebruikte meetmethode, in: *Spraakaudiometrie*, Nederlandse Vereniging voor Audiologie.

From Speech to Language: On Auditory Information Processing

E. Terhardt
Electroacoustics and Audiocommunication
Technische Universität München
POB 202420, D-8000 München 2

1. Introduction

When discussing the perception of speech, we are seldom really concerned about perception of speech alone, but in fact about essential aspects of *language* as well. What we most urgently wish to understand is this: What are the principles and "mechanisms" by which the acoustic speech signal is abstracted into linguistic objects such as phonemes, syllables, words, clauses, sentences, paragraphs, etc. - let alone "meaning". In other words: How does the auditory system strip off *information* from the speech signal?

The present paper discusses that question from a basic and general point of view, i.e., in terms of a number of notions on sensory information acquisition. As speech is an "artificial" type of signal that is specific to man, it is not *a priori* apparent to what extent such general principles will apply. It is, however, obvious that an understanding of general principles of sensory information acquisition is indispensable for understanding what is special about the perception of speech and language.

The approach, some implications of which shall be analyzed in more detail, is entirely based on the theory of biological evolution, and has been suggested by Lorenz (1959, 1973), Popper (1962), Campbell (1966), MacKay (1967), and others. The approach may be outlined as follows:

Sensory systems - and so the auditory system - have evolved according to Darwin's principle of natural selection. This is equivalent to phylogenetic *adaption* of organisms to the physical conditions of the environment. Phylogenetic adaptation in turn is equivalent to *learning by trial and error*. In this process, an enormous amount of *knowledge* on the environmental conditions that are relevant for survival has been acquired and is included in the structures and basic functions of sensory systems. That knowledge is a "mirror image" of the external world - i.e., of those aspects that under given long-term conditions are relevant for survival of species.

The following three main sections present an attempt to learn from the above approach one or two lessons relevant for understanding of "how speech gets abstracted into language". Section 2 is concerned with the concept of information and its implications for sensory systems. Section 3 discusses a general model of sensory information processing systems and its implications for speech perception. Section 4 includes a few signal- and system-theoretical considerations on the physical conditions of audio communication.

2. Information in Sensory Systems

Information is neither a physical nor a sensory entity; it is a theoretical concept - such as, e.g., mathematics. In principle, one can get along without employing the concept of information, that is, describe any technical and biological process - such as the functions of the human brain and of a digital computer - in terms of physico-chemical relationships, i.e., transmission and interaction of physical signals. What makes the concept of information useful and, in fact, indispensable, is that it makes description of certain highly complex aspects of physico-chemical interactions manageable, i.e., by abstraction from irrelevant physical details.

2.1 Information is characterized by involvement of categories and conditioned decisions

Information is characterized by selection between a number of alternative categories, i.e., objects. Physically, objects - such as, e.g., a phoneme - are always represented by signals such as the pertinent sound wave. When one and the same object appears at different occasions, the pertinent signals are never exactly identical; this is true both of external signals, and of physiological signals in the human brain. So an object emerges as a result of abstraction from certain structural details of the pertinent signal. Abstraction is achieved by *conditioned decision*. Phenomenologically, information is characterized by involvement of discrete objects, and information *processing* is characterized by conditioned decisions, i.e., discontinuous operations on signals.

These notions merely describe in general terms what happens in a digital computer; they are a basis of the mathematical theory of information. In the latter, binary decisions are - somewhat arbitrarily - employed as a means of measuring the quantitative aspect of information, i.e., the number of bits necessary to represent a particular message. To see the relevance and implications of the concept of information for sensory processes such as speech perception, it is important to notice that it is involvement of discrete objects and conditioned decisions that are the basic, general, and essential *qualitative* features of information and information processing.

2.2 Information is reflected by conditioned (re)action

Every living organism incessantly interacts with the external world; its survival (both as an individual and as a species) is dependent on its ability to optimally respond to external events, by immediate, appropriate interpretation of incoming sensory signals. The physical response of a living system to a stimulus, i.e. its behavior, exhibits the aforementioned features of information and information processing: conditioned decision in favour of one of several or many alternative (re)actions.

The (re)action of a very simple (e.g. monocellular) organism is dependent on a relatively small number of internal physico-chemical processes; the number of alternative types of action is limited (though on an absolute scale, even monocellular organisms are enormously complex). For a highly developed organism such as man, physical actions depend on a process of much higher complexity, namely neural processing; the number of types of action available is much greater. One of the most complex types of action that man is capable of is the production of speech. Yet for any organism the principle is one and the same: both physical action and physical response to a stimulus are dependent on conditioned decisions that in turn are dependent on stored knowledge which in turn is provided partly genetically (by evolution), partly by learning (in the widest sense of the term) of the individual. Any physical action of any living organism can be seen as the ultimate result of a chain of knowledge-based conditioned decisions. As the hierarchy of conditioned decisions corresponds to ascending levels of abstraction, the physical response to a stimulus reflects ultimate abstraction.

In the light of these notions, the processing of a stimulus in the sensory system of a highly developed organism must be regarded as the starting phase of conditioned physical response. In other words: what we ordinarily view as "signal processing" or "information processing", can as well be seen as a significant and essential part of conditioned physical response. It is thus apparent that information processing is an extremely practical phenomenon.

2.3 Sensory information processing is universal and prevalent

As information processing in this sense is decisive for evolu
apparent that any living organism by nature is a "decision m
its lifetime and is adapted to the physical requirement
Abstraction by conditioned decisions, and conditioned evalu
is one of the most natural and prevalent phenomena in living
should see the pronounced tendency to *categorize* sensory
music. The composition of language of phonemes, words etc
music of pitch- and pitch-interval categories, are just highly
a universal and prevalent phenomenon.

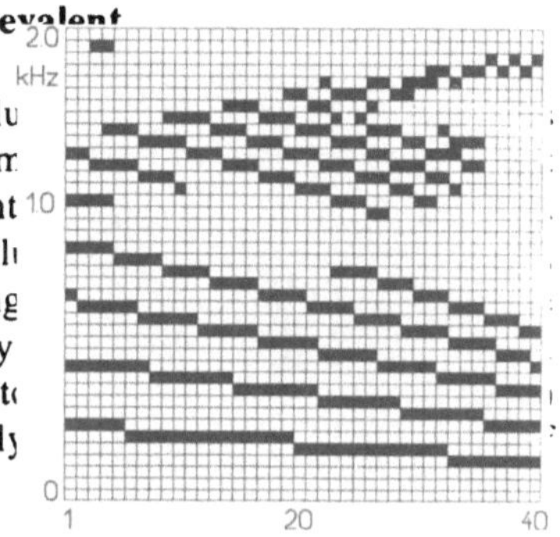

2.4 Sensory information processing begins at the utmost periphery

The evolutionary principle implies that a sensory system will neither waste time nor effort on processes that do not efficiently contribute to survival-relevant abstraction. From this point of view, the discontinuous nature of neural signals (action potentials) gets particular significance with respect to the sensory periphery. If one conceives the pulse-interval modulated pattern of action potentials in the auditory nerve just as a peculiar (somewhat awkward) neural representation of the stimulus signal, one probably misses the point. The nerve impulses should indeed be regarded as discontinuous signals that on the primary auditory level represent discrete auditory objects. In other words: Abstraction by conditioned decision begins already in the cochlea. The hair cells of the organ of Corti must be seen as the very first mechanism of abstraction that we meet when we ascend the auditory pathway - rather than as just signal transducers. Somewhat provokingly, one may be inclined to say that auditory cognition begins in the cochlea (and, likewise, visual cognition in the retina).

2.5 Contourization: the first step of abstraction

What is the *psychophysical* evidence for these conclusions, i.e., what is the evidence from the domain of subjective sensations? According to the above notions on the basic features of information, pertinent psychophysical phenonema must be of a discontinuous nature and must be dependent on conditioned decisions. Such a phenomenon indeed exists at the lowest level of the sensory hierarchy; it is labeled *contour.*

While the meaning of that term is most readily apparent from vision - i.e., a shape in the geometric-spatial domain - it can in a generalized sense be applied to the time domain as well: the instant of time at which a perceptual "event" occurs, such as a syllable of speech. To understand the implications of the contour concept, it is helpful to recall the most significant characteristics of visual spatial contour.

2.6 Characteristics of the visual spatial contour

The primary visual spatial contour may be conceived of as a one-dimensional "virtual line" in a two-dimensional space such as the eye's retina. The following characteristics should be

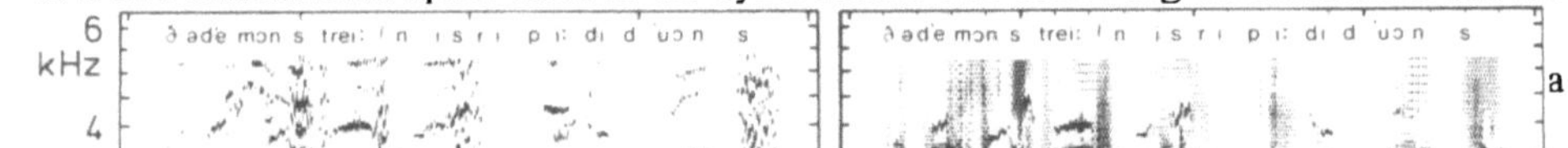

a of
loes
the
l by
less
m a
s of
om-
iges
tion
ir at

the outer periphery provides what is rigorously enforced by evolution: rapid, robust comprehension of what goes on in the environment, as an indispensable precondition for an adequate response.

2.7 Spectral pitch as a primary auditory spatial contour

On the basis of the above notions it is not too difficult to see what is the auditory equivalent of visual spatial contour: it is *spectral pitch,* i.e. the pitch of sinusoidal Fourier components of sound (cf. Terhardt, 1987; more arguments on this notion are included in section 4). When one takes into account that the auditory "geometry" has only one dimension, the low-high continuum, it is apparent that a "contour" in that "space" must be "null-dimensional", marking just a point on the low-high scale. In all other respects, spectral pitch turns out to be analogous to visual spatial contour; it exhibits to a striking extent the features a-g listed in sec. 2.6:

- Spectral pitch is a discrete phenomenon (a).
- By "analytic listening" it can be heard as a primitive auditory object (b).
- It is not completely defined by the audio signal's instantaneous short-term Fourier spectrum but must be extracted from it by a decision process, for example, peak detection (c).
- It is monotonically dependent on the frequency of a pertinent part tone, and robust with respect to variations of amplitude, phase, and presence of more spectral components (d). It is independently created by each of the two ears in a remarkably rigid manner (e); cf., - Van den Brink (1975a).
- As the frequencies of part tones emitted by a source are little or not at all affected by sound transmission, spectral pitch is a highly reliable clue to a particular sound source (f); cf. sec. 4.
- Finally, spectral pitch as a sensory phenomenon exhibits contrast-effects (enhancement), after-tone, and shift "illusions" (g); See e.g. Terhardt (1989, 1991), Viemeister (1980), Wilson (1970), Zwicker (1964).

2.8 The spectral-pitch pattern as a binary number

In vision, a *Gestalt* is essentially defined by a set of contours, including the position of the latter within the sensory continuum. This is entirely analogous to the information represented by a binary number (a "word") in a computer: its meaning is dependent on the presence or absence of bits at predefined positions. For the *auditory* continuum, which is just one-dimensional, the analogy is perfect: The spectral pitches evoked by an audio signal will appear at positions on the low-high continuum that are robustly specified by the pertinent frequencies of part tones. So within a short interval of time, any set of spectral pitches specifies a "binary word". As the part-tone frequencies are governed by the sound source - as opposed to the transmission path (cf. sec. 4.3) - successive "bit patterns" of that kind include a lot of information on the source.

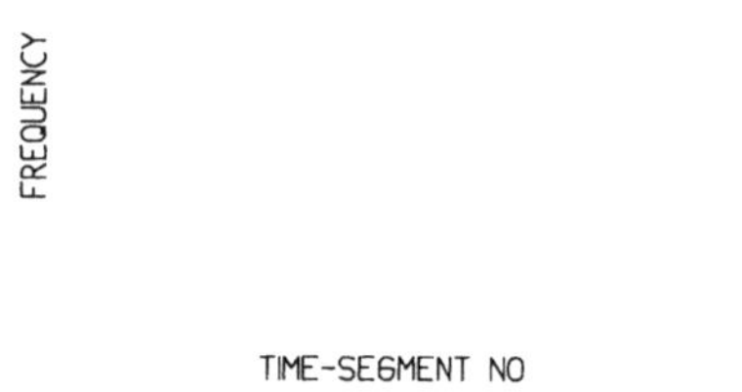

Fig. 1 Simulated spectral-pitch-time-pattern of the diphthong /a-ε/. Both the frequency region 0-2 kHz and the time interval shown are represented by 40 samples. Frequency (ordinate) is scaled in terms of critical-band rate. Fundamental frequency descends linearly with time from 200 to 100 Hz. F_1 moves from 750 to 500 Hz; F_2 from 1200 to 1800 Hz; F_3 from 2500 to 2700 Hz; F_4=3500 Hz. Suprathreshold prominence of spectral pitches is indicated by black squares. Each black square represents a primitive auditory object, i.e. a primary auditory contour, i.e., a spectral pitch. Frequency corresponds to place.

This is illustrated in Fig. 1, where a sequence of 40 discrete spectral-pitch patterns is shown, each including 40 discrete frequency frames. As a signal, a diphthong /a-ε/ was constructed with a fundamental frequency that descended linearly with time from 200 Hz to 100 Hz. The spectral-pitch patterns were calculated by an algorithm described earlier (Terhardt, 1979). To make the discrete nature of the patterns apparent, only 40 discrete frequency samples in the range 0-2 kHz were chosen (Actually, the low-high continuum covering the entire auditory frequency range should include a number of frequency samples on the order of 10^3). So in each time-segment the information is included in a "40-bit-word": black squares indicate that a spectral pitch with corresponding frequency has occurred with suprathreshold salience. One can see that the sequence of 40 binary patterns - which can be conceived to include a time span of 200 ms - indeed carries a great deal of information on the diphthong: it is visually apparent that the fundamental frequency descends, while the formant pattern changes according to the transition from /a/ to /ε/.

One can see in Fig. 1 a series of "inter-formant" spectral pitches, between 1 and 1.5 kHz. We have found this phenomenon earlier (Terhardt, 1979). Its significance for vowel perception remains to be examined.

TIME ——→

Fig. 2 Part-tone-time-pattern (left), and texture-pattern (right) of the utterance "The demonstration is repeated once". The vertical width of the lines represents part-tone amplitude. Note that while the part-tone pattern is contourized only in the frequency domain, the texture-pattern is contourized both in the frequency- and time-domains. Both types of pattern include the information to synthesize a speech signal that is aurally almost indistinguishable from the original one.

The simple type of binary spectral-pitch representation shown in Fig. 1 is not meant to include each and every aspect of the audio signal. For example, it is evident that loudness is not included. Indeed, here applies the distinction made by Stevens and Galanter (1957), between sensory attributes that include the aspect of "how much" (prothetic continua), and those carrying the aspect of "what and where" (metathetic continua). It is the latter type that accounts for the organizational and categorical aspects of sound; the above pattern of "binary words" illustrates this.

2.9 The part-tone-time-pattern and its temporal contourization

A variant of the spectral-pitch pattern which turns out to be very useful for aurally adequate speech analysis is the so-called part-tone-pattern (Heinbach, 1988). The latter differs from the former by including the absolute amplitudes of part-tones instead of only their relative prominence. As was demonstrated by Heinbach (1988), the part-tone-pattern as a function of time includes practically all aurally relevant information.

Recently, Mummert (1990) has worked out an approach to include temporal contours, i.e., cues that emphasize significant temporal events such as plosives. In this way, speech can be represented by a two-dimensionally contourized pattern termed "texture pattern". Fig. 2 shows examples of a part-tone-time-pattern (left) and a texture pattern (right) of the utterance "The demonstration is repeated once" (male speaker).

2.10 Virtual contour

A phenomenon that strongly supports the above notions on contourization as a key principle to sensory information processing is virtual contour (also labeled "subjective contour", "illusory contour"). Both in visual scene analysis and in the visual arts, virtual contours play a very important role. It is indeed obvious that visual virtual contours are "induced" by primary contours; the former can be regarded as a product of knowlege-based processing on a low level of the sensory hierarchy.

The auditory equivalent of visual virtual contour is *virtual pitch* (cf. Terhardt, 1987, 1989, 1991). Although for virtual pitch the intimate relationship between primary and virtual contour does not suggest itself so readily, it has early been conceptualized, i.e., in the virtual-pitch theory (Terhardt, 1970; 1972). That concept has indeed proved to be successful. The dependence of virtual pitch on spectral pitch was challenged - and confirmed - by a considerable variety of experiments (e.g., van den Brink, 1975a,b, 1977; Houtsma, 1981; Houtsma and Rossing, 1987; Moore et al., 1985; Terhardt, 1971, 1975, 1983; Terhardt and Grubert, 1987; Walliser, 1969).

2.11 Temporal auditory contour

As the ear has only one "spatial" dimension, i.e. "low-high", temporal organization and contourization are of particular significance. One finds psychophysical evidence for peripheral temporal contourization - segmentation of a sound stream into primitive objects - in the smallest type of temporally distinct object that can be found in conscious auditory sensation: the individual "rattles" of which a "rattling" or "rough" or "fluttering" sound is composed.

The highest "flutter frequency" that can be perceived is about 300 Hz. This limit corresponds well with the upper limit of the steady-state pulse rate on a fiber of the auditory nerve (Pickles, 1982). Auditory flutter (roughness, rattling) is most pronounced for flutter frequencies of about 50-80 Hz. These numbers suggest that the temporal position of a primitive auditory object is resolved with a precision in the order of 1 ms, while its temporal extension (length) typically is 10-20 ms.

The latter figures approach the length of phonetically significant time intervals such as voice-onset time and the length of a plosive. It is not without significance that in this respect the gap is filled between auditory attributes and linguistic categories. This can be illustrated by the following notion. If we regard 15 ms as the typical length (temporal extension) of a primitive auditory object, the chain that relates speech to language is outlined by the following "one-to-five hierarchy":

- The majority of phonemes comprise 1-5 primitive auditory objects.
- The majority of syllables comprise 1-5 phonemes.
- The majority of words comprise 1-5 syllables.
- The majority of clauses comprise 1-5 words.
- The majority of sentences comprise 1-5 clauses.
- The majority of paragraphs comprise 1-5 sentences.

And so on.

Whatever may be the deeper implications of this list, at least it suggests that the "no-man's land" between the domain of acoustic-sensory signals and that of linguistic units actually is remarkably small.

After having discussed the *concept* of information with respect to sensory systems and speech perception, let us now turn to some implications of sensory information *processing*.

3. Implications of Sensory Information Processing

3.1 Evidence for hierarchical sensory processing

With regard to cognitive processes, there is no doubt about hierarchical organization of sensory information acquisition. Both in vision and audition one finds numerous examples for the general principle that a *Gestalt* is, on a lower hierarchical level, composed of "sub-gestalts", each of which in turn is composed of "sub-sub-gestalts", and so on. In perception of speech and language, the hierarchical organization - and perception - on the phonemic, syllable, word, clause, etc. levels is commonplace.

What as yet tends to be overlooked is that knowledge-based, hierarchical processing of information begins right at the periphery - so that composition of sensory objects into sub-objects extends down into the hierarchy to its contourized input. It is not without significance that one often finds the term *contour* used both in the narrow sense of a visual shape, and in a metaphorical sense such as in the phrase "In the story, Mr. Smith hardly takes on any contours". Indeed, the narrow and the metaphorical sense of the term contour have in common that they both represent the aspect of information; they merely refer to different levels of abstraction.

An example of the significance of hierarchical perception at low levels is the perception of pitch. Traditionally, one tends to conceive of the relationship between stimulus parameters and perceived pitch as a straightforward input-output relationship (in an extremely simplicistic approach, as a kind of synonymity of pitch and frequency). This approach has turned out to be one of the most serious obstacles in understanding pitch perception. From many everyday observations it can be made apparent that the pitch of perceived "tonal objects" is *multiple*, both "horizontally" (within one hierarchical level), and - most significantly - "vertically" (across levels).

As an example, consider the sound of a note played on a pipe organ in a mixture register. Pressing the pertinent key will cause several pipes to sound simultaneously with oscillation frequencies that are nearly in ratios of small integers. On a moderately high level of abstraction - to which attention normally is pre-set - one indeed hears a single note, just as intended by both the composer and the organ player. If one switches attention to the next lower level (i.e., listens more "analytically"), one can hear the individual pitches of the various pipes. So what at a higher level is heard as one single object, is at a lower level perceived as a set of sub-objects. At yet another level below, one may even hear some of the sinusoidal part tones of which each of the pipe-sounds is (theoretically) composed - i.e., sub-sub-objects of the musical note. The same hierarchical relationship exists between virtual pitch and spectral pitch - as it does, in vision, between virtual and primary contour. Indeed, pitch is multiple both "horizontally" and "vertically".

Both in vision and audition on can find many examples of horizontal and vertical multiplicity. Ordinary acoustic examples are the cocktail-party situation and polyphonic music. Possibly such phenomena as "duplex perception" can be more adequately interpreted and understood in the framework of a hierarchical model (cf. the discussion and comparative examples given by Bregman, 1987). While listening to monophonic speech, the "observing self" addresses different levels of the hierarchy, depending on whether one pays attention to, e.g., the linguistic content, the melodiousness or sonority of the voice, the speaker's sex and age, etc. It is significant in this respect that at any instant of time one can either recognize who is talking, or what he or she is saying - but not both at the same time (see the discussion by Bregman, 1987, on his "rule of disjoint allocation").

It will appear that in fact there does not exist any case of perception that can be understood in terms of a simple input-output concept, i.e., without explicitly taking account of hierarchical organization (cf. Ohman, 1975).

3.2 Hierarchical information processing and types of memory

To facilitate the discussion, the hierarchical model of sensory information processing shown in Figure 3 was worked out. Although it is fairly general and leaves many aspects and details undefined, it includes a number of features that are sufficiently well-defined to be challenged by comparison with observations and experimental data.

At all levels a set of sensory objects is converted by a knowledge-based process (PROC) into another - more comprehensive - set of objects. The new set of objects provides the input to the next process, and so on. The objects that may reside at the lowest level, the most primitive sensory objects, are primary spatial and temporal contours.

A process in general operates on a certain number of *successive* sets of objects; in the model this is accounted for by "object buffers" (OBJ BUF). The object buffers represent a kind of short-term memory, while the knowledge implied in the processing algorithms is long-term, i.e., on a short-term time scale unaffected by the input.

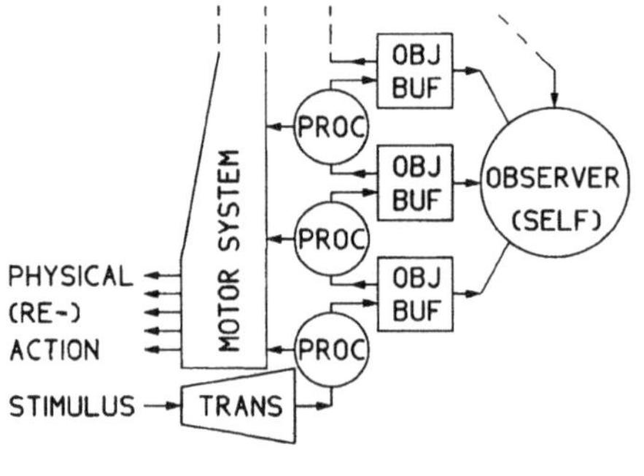

Fig. 3 Outline of a general model of hierarchical sensory information processing. TRANS: Transfer-organ, e.g., outer, middle, and inner ear, including primary contourization. PROC: Autonomous processors. OBJ BUF: Buffers for sensory objects ("short-term memory").

If it is assumed that the number of successive sets of objects that the system can take advantage of at any level is the same - as suggested by the above "one-to-five rule" - the length of the time-interval actually included in the "short-term memories" or object buffers, grows geometrically with ascending level. So for high-level objects of speech and language, the time period actually covered by the contents of an object buffer may be as long as hours, days, or years. It is thus apparent that in such a hierarchical system the labels long-term memory and short-term memory must not be prematurely associated with functional aspects of the pertinent memories. With regard to the functional aspects, it is important to make a distinction between information stored in object buffers, and the knowledge included in processing algorithms. While the latter evidently is "long-term" at any level, the former is "short-term" at low levels but "long-term" at high levels. Many observations even suggest that the long-term knowledge included in the processes is "more long-term" - i.e., rigid - at low levels, and "less long-term" - i.e., more flexible - at high levels.

3.3 Open-endedness, distributed knowledge, autonomy, and distributed recognition

The chain of information-processing operations - including recognition of speech - does not have a definite end, i.e., output; it is "open-ended". This is the most drastic difference from a simple input-output model. Both the knowledge employed for appropriate processing, and the level at which "meaning" is extracted from a stimulus, are *distributed* in the hierarchy. This in turn implies that the processing units essentially are *autonomous,* so that processing through ascending levels is unidirectional, i.e., does not depend on inter-level feedback. As at a particular level conversion of a set of objects into another set is equivalent to a recognition process, another implication of the model is that recognition is distributed as well.

For speech and language this implies that there is no such thing as "the" meaning of an utterance, but rather a hierarchical chain of abstractions ("meanings") that in principle is endless. Consequently, physical (motoric) response may be induced from any level - although not with full autonomy. It appears reasonable to assume that levels compete with respect to inducing motoric responses. This aspect has however not as yet been explicitly worked out; it is hidden in the box labeled "motor system".

It is evident that stripping off information from the speech signal, i.e., abstraction, requires knowledge that is adequate for that purpose, i.e., speech-specific. If we take the concept of hierarchical processing seriously, we can hardly avoid the conclusion that the speech-specific knowledge employed for processing must be *distributed* in the auditory hierarchy - including low levels.

3.4 Introspection

The features of the model addressed so far are - at least in principle - sufficient to account for the responses to sensory information, i.e., the behavioristic aspect. For that purpose it is not necessary to include "subjective" phenomena. However, the latter type of phenomenon provides an invaluable additional source of knowledge on perceptual processes - i.e., by introspection; and as human observers we could hardly ignore it, even if we wished to.

Therefore, the model explicitly includes the "oberserving self". The latter is by definition presumed to participate in the processes in a most restricted manner, i.e., confined to *observation*. This implies that, by switching attention, the "self" has observational access to objects at any level - without being able to change anything.

In the light of this model, phenomena such as horizontal and vertical multiplicity of sensory objects, ambiguity, and "illusions" can be accounted for. For example, consider an "illusory contour" or an "illusory figure" (for a survey see Parks, 1984). Although at a higher level of perception one usually notices that the "illusory" figure is - in a sense - not "real", one is unable to change the percept. This is a striking proof of the unidirectional, autonomous operation of the sensory system, and of the notion that the "self" is confined to observation. The hierarchical approach to sensory information processing, if taken seriously, reveals that it is a misconception to call such phenomena "illusory". They are no more illusory than anything else that the "self" can observe.

4. On the Physical Conditions of Audio Communication

The model of sensory information processing discussed above is general, i.e., incomplete in many details. In particular, it does not include specifications of the algorithms and knowledge employed by the processing units (PROC in Figure 3). Exploration of those specifications is by far the bigger portion of research that needs to be done. From the notion that any sensory system is a "mirror image" of its ordinary physical environment, it follows that it is of particular importance to analyze in some depth the physical conditions of sensory perception.

In the following sections, a brief and sketchy attempt is made to theoretically verify some of the physical conditions that are essential for the present model, in particular with respect to speech communication.

4.1 Multiplicity of sources and corruption of audio signals

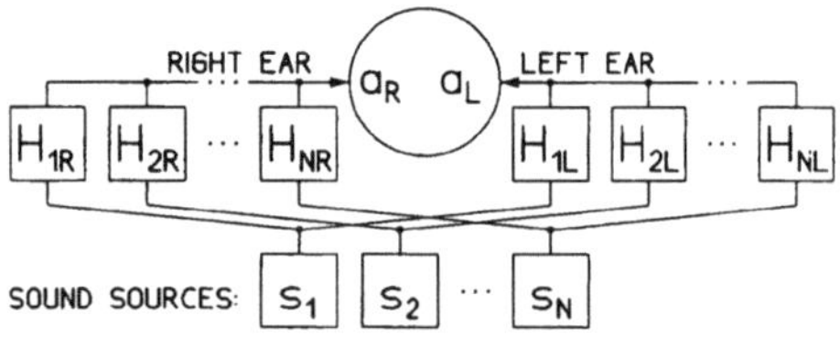

Fig. 4 Schematic illustration of the typical listening conditions. s_1...s_N: source signals. H_1..H_N: Transfer functions of linear, generally time-variant transmission paths. a_R, a_L: Audio signals (at the eardrums).

One of the most remarkable features of auditory perception in general - and speech perception in particular - is its robustness with respect to corruption of the audio signals that enter the outer ear canals. The typical and ordinary listening condition is schematically illustrated in Figure 4.

A number N of sound sources is simultaneously present, emitting the signals $s_1(t)...s_N(t)$. Ordinarily, the transmission paths of sound waves are linear systems, so they can be accounted for by complex transfer functions $H(f)$ which in general are dependent on the distance and direction of the sources relative to each of the two ears. As indicated in Figure 4, generally the transfer functions pertinent to the paths from any source to the two ears are different. So either source contributes to either of the two audio signals $a_R(t)$, $a_L(t)$ with a signal that can be determined by convolution of the source signal with the pertinent impulse response - provided that the impulse responses (i.e., transfer functions) are constant. Rigorously, the latter is usually not the case, as both the sources and the listener may move.

Auditory analysis of the environmental acoustical "scene", and perception of the information emitted by the sources, are entirely dependent on the two scalar audio signals $a_R(t)$, $a_L(t)$ at the eardrums. As evidently the auditory system is very efficient in analyzing what in any respect "is going on" in the acoustic environment, there must exist certain physical signal parameters that can be employed for, e.g., making a distinction between sources, and between contributions of sources and contributions of the transmission paths; and, of course, it is evident that the perpheral auditory system actually does take advantage of those parameters.

4.2 Coding of information in source signals

With respect to transmission of information from a single "sender" - e.g., a human speaker, or a musical instrument - to a "receiver", i.e., one single ear of a listener, the situation can be schematically described as in Figure 5. The audio signal $a(t)$ at the eardrum is typically dependent on:

a. A primary source signal produced by an oscillator (OSC), such as the glottis, jet turbulence, or a bowed string.
b. A time-variant linear transmission path with the transfer function $H_S(f,t)$ such as the vocal tract, and the string-bridge-body system of a violin, including the directional characteristics of sound emission (which in turn is controlled by the sender, as well); this yields the ultimate source signal $s(t)$.
c. A time-invariant linear transmission path with the transfer function $H_T(f)$, such as the sound field in a room.

d. A time-variant linear transmission path with the transfer function $H_R(f,t)$, i.e., typically the contribution by diffraction of sound at the listener's body, head, and pinna; it is controlled by the receiver, i.e., by movement.

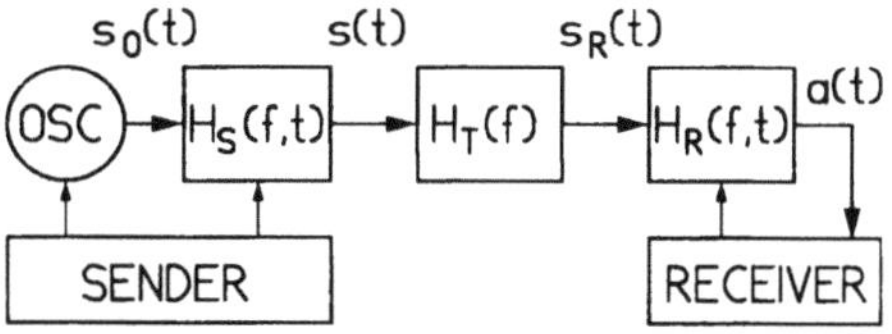

Fig. 5 Essential aspects of information transfer from a sender (e.g., speaker, musician) to a receiver (one ear of the listener). OSC: Oscillator, e.g., glottis. $H_S(f,t)$: Time-variant linear transmission system, e.g., vocal tract. $H_T(f)$: Time-invariant linear system, e.g., sound field. $H_R(f,t)$: Time-variant portion of linear transmission system. OSC and $H_S(f,t)$ are controlled by the sender; $H_R(f,t)$ by the receiver. In the audio signal $a(t)$, all those influences are superimposed.

With respect to speech communication, the problem of stripping off information from the audio signal can be described by saying that the receiver must infer from $a(t)$ the sender's control actions on both the oscillator(s) and the pertinent time-variant transmission function $H_S(f,t)$. It is apparent that this includes a kind of compensation of what is contributed by both $H_T(f)$ and $H_R(f,t)$. In the ordinary multiple-source, binaural-listening situation (Fig. 4), 2N communication channels of the type shown in Figure 5 must be taken into consideration.

With regard to these conditions, the evident efficacy of auditory information acquisition is conceivable only by assuming that

- the receiver must possess knowledge on how oscillators and time-variant transmission paths ordinarily behave;
- the audio signal $a(t)$ must include robust primary clues to making a distinction between characteristics of sound oscillators and transmission paths.

It is apparent that the information available to the auditory system is to a very large extent dependent on the *temporal behavior* of the pertinent units, i.e., oscillators and time-variant linear systems.

4.3 Description of transferred signals by discrete time-variant Fourier-components

An intuitive approach to account for these notions is included in several recent concepts such as those discussed by Bregman (1990), Darwin and Gardner (1987), Hartmann (1988), McAdams (1989), Scheffers (1983), Singh (1987), Summerfield and Assmann (1990), and Zwicker (1984). That approach is largely consistent with the present concept of primary auditory contourization, i.e., the notion that it is the frequency of discrete Fourier components (spectral frequency) that provides robust information on external sources, and that spectral frequency on the primary auditory level is represented as spectral pitch.

Somewhat naïvely and prematurely, the arguments are as follows. Any source signal can be described by a number n of discrete cosine components, the frequencies and amplitudes of which are time-variant:

$$s(t) = \sum_{\nu=1}^{n} \hat{s}_\nu(t) \cos[2\pi f_\nu(t)t + \psi_\nu] \tag{1}$$

where $\hat{s}_\nu(t)$ and $f_\nu(t)$ are the instantaneous amplitude and frequency of the ν-th component, while ψ_ν are constant starting phases. As by specification of $\hat{s}_\nu(t)$ and $f_\nu(t)$ any type of signal can be represented with any number n of components, the approach of Eq. (1) as such is, in a sense, redundant. It gets however sensible if one assumes that the time-variance of both $\hat{s}_\nu(t)$ and $f_\nu(t)$ is "reasonably slow", compared to the part-tone period. If it is moreover assumed that the time-variance of transfer functions is "relatively slow" as well - this will be specified more precisely below - one can with some approximation describe the audio signal $a(t)$ by:

$$a(t) \approx \sum_{\nu=1}^{n} s_\nu(t) |H(f_\nu,t)| \cos[2\pi f_\nu(t)t + \psi_\nu + \phi(f_\nu,t)] \tag{2}$$

where $|H(f,t)|$ and $\phi(f,t)$ denote the absolute magnitude and phase at frequency f of the entire complex transfer function, i.e., with respect to Figure 5,

$$H(f,t) = H_S(f,t)H_T(f)H_R(f,t) \tag{3}$$

Eq. (2) implies that the audio signal $a(t)$ is composed of "the same" discrete Fourier components as the oscillator signal $s(t)$, i.e., part tones with the same instantaneous frequencies, while the amplitudes and phases are different. This makes it apparent that the time-variant part-tone frequencies are robust clues to the oscillator signal - provided that Eq. (2) is true with sufficient approximation.

The decisive criterion for validity of Eq. (2) is the effective length of the transmission path's "memory", i.e., impulse response. If neither the part-tone amplitudes and frequencies, nor the transfer functions change significantly within the effective length of the impulse response, Eq. (2) is correct with reasonable approximation. That condition indeed is fulfilled for many types of transmission path, such as a free sound field, and a typical electroacoustic transmission line. It is not fulfilled in a reverberant room. (Application of the approach to reverberant transmission paths requires taking account of some additional arguments which are omitted here.)

As an example, consider the vocal tract. The length of its impulse response can be assessed from formant bandwidth. As the formants correspond to the natural frequencies of the vocal tract, the effective length of the latter's impulse response can be represented by the decay-time-constant that corresponds to the smallest formant bandwidth. The latter is about 50 Hz, which corresponds to a decay-time-constant of 6.4 ms. If neither the voice-source parameters nor the vocal-tract transfer function change appreciably within that time interval, Eq. (2) can be employed. It will appear that in many cases this condition is fulfilled with sufficient approximation.

It is apparent that the above somewhat "naïve" approach is valid and useful for getting more insight into the information-relevant aspects of audio signals. The above evaluations reveal that - within certain limits - it is the time-variant frequencies of discrete Fourier-components that carry reliable information on sound sources. The part-tone-frequency time-patterns can be conceived of as most effective cues for both segregation of simultaneous source signals and identification of any source's type and instantaneous state. This is illustrated in Fig. 6 with three schematic frequency-time patterns.

What finally remains to be considered is the extent to which the approach is compatible with peripheral auditory signal analysis.

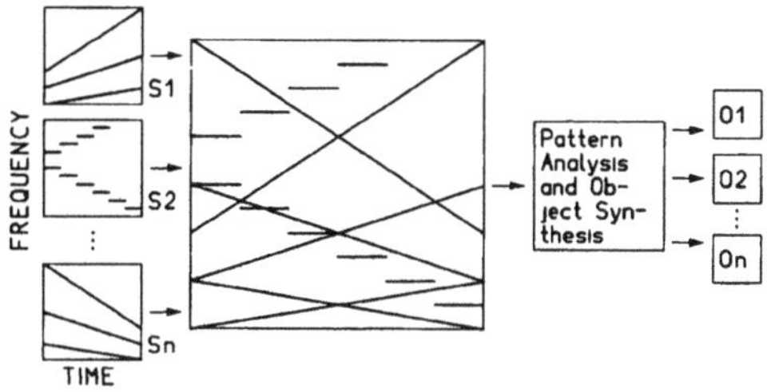

Fig. 6 Schematic part-tone-frequency time-patterns of source signals $s_1...s_n$ (left) are, at the lowest auditory level represented by a compound spectral-pitch time-pattern (middle). The latter provides the basis for active, knowledge-based interpretation, yielding auditory representation of sources (right).

4.4 Auditory relevance of the discrete time-variant Fourier-synthesis model

As suggested above, a mathematical description of a signal in terms of discrete cosine components or part tones, is arbitrary. It makes little sense to say that any signal "objectively" is composed of such components. What gives part tones a kind of reality is the fact that under certain conditions we can hear them, with pertinent spectral pitches. The latter fact is indeed remarkable. It indicates that the peripheral auditory system actually takes advantage of the fact outlined above, that the time-variant frequencies of part-tones are robust carriers of information on external sources. What are the conditions and limits for hearing discrete time-variant part tones, i.e., spectral pitches?

The essential aspects of monaural auditory spectrum analysis can be described by the transformation

$$A(f,t) = \left| \int_{t-T_A}^{t} a(\tau) w(f,t-\tau) e^{-j2\pi f\tau} d\tau \right|, \tag{4}$$

where *A(f,t)* denotes the time-variant absolute magnitude spectral function termed the "audio spectrum"; *a(t)* is the audio signal; and *w(f,t)* is a window function that "cuts out" an interval of length T_A from the audio signal, the *analysis interval.*

Eq. (4) makes it clear that the audio spectrum pertinent to the instant *t* includes information only on that portion of *a(t)* that is within the analysis interval. If that portion of the audio signal is composed of discrete cosine components with constant frequencies, and if the frequencies are sufficiently apart, they will be reflected in the instantaneous magnitude spectrum by peaks (note that the short-term magnitude Fourier spectrum is a *continuous* function of both time and frequency). A "contourization" mechanism such as a peak detector can determine the frequencies and amplitudes of those "primitive auditory objects". In other words, if the amplitudes and frequencies of the cosine components of the Fourier-synthesis representation Eq. (2) do not appreciably change within the analysis interval T_A, they can -

within certain limits - be discovered by the analyzer, i.e., represented by frequency and amplitude as a function of time.

Appropriate auditory representation of time-variant part tones is thus dependent on how fast their amplitudes and frequencies change as *compared to the effective time-window length* T_A of the analyzer. If those variations are slow enough, the time-variant Fourier-synthesis model indeed is significant with respect to the peripheral auditory representation of the essential time-variant audio-signal parameters.

Table I. Effective window length (analysis interval) T_A of the auditory frequency analyzer, as a function of frequency.

f/kHz	0.1	0.5	1	2	4	8
T_A/ms	24	22	16	8	2.7	0.74

The length of the analysis interval, T_A, as a function of analysis frequency can be assessed from data on auditory time- and frequency-resolution. Table I gives numerical values that we have found typical (see also Flanagan, 1972, chapters 4 and 5). It is apparent from the table that the analysis window is short enough for temporal parameter changes of both speech and music within the window in most cases to remain small - as is necessary for the emergence of pronounced spectral peaks.

If the window length at medium and low frequencies were significantly shorter, the pertinent analysis bandwidth would be proportionally wider, and frequency resolution of part tones would suffer. Reversely, if the window were longer, time resolution would suffer. It will thus appear that, if one had to design a short-term Fourier analyzer for the purpose of extracting spectral pitches as primary auditory contours from speech and music, one probably would arrive at window parameters that differ not very much from those shown in Table I. In this sense, and with regard to the physical conditions mentioned, the most peripheral auditory mechanism, i.e., the short-term Fourier analyzer, appears indeed to be well adapted to the conditions of the external physical world (see also Huggins, 1952).

It is in the light of the above signal-theoretical considerations that one can understand that the part-tone-time-pattern extracted from any type of real audio signal includes practically all the aurally relevant information (cf. sec. 2.9).

5. Conclusion

With respect to the topic of central processes in perception of speech, the main conclusion from the present considerations may be condensed to the notion that "central processing" in fact is just not central. It is distributed over all levels of the auditory system, and significant steps of abstraction are carried out at low levels.

Acknowledgments

I am grateful to Markus Mummert for preparing the part-tone- and texture-patterns, Fig. 2. This work was carried out in the *Sonderforschungsbereich 204 "Gehör", München*, supported by the Deutsche Forschungsgemeinschaft.

References

Assmann, P.F. and Summerfield, Q. (1990). *J. Acoust. Soc. Am.*, 88, 680-697.

Bregman, A.S. (1987) in: Schouten (1987), 95-111.

Bregman, A.S. (1990). *Auditory Scene Analysis*, MIT Press, Cambridge, Mass.

Brink, G. van den (1975a). *Acustica*, 32, 160-165.

Brink, G. van den (1975b). *Acustica*, 32, 166-173.

Brink, G. van den (1977) in: E.F. Evans and J.P. Wilson (eds.), *Psychophysics and Physiology of Hearing*, Academic Press, London, 373-379.

Campbell, D.T. (1966). Evolutionary Epistemology, in: P.A. Schilpp, (ed.) *The Philosophy of Karl R. Popper*, Open Court Publ., La Salle.

Darwin, C.J., and Gardner, R.B. (1987) in: Schouten (1987), 112-124.

Flanagan, J.L. (1972). *Speech Analysis, Synthesis, and Perception*, Springer, Heidelberg/New York.

Hartmann, W.M. (1988) in: G.M. Edelmann, W.E. Hall, and W.M. Cowan (eds.), *Auditory Function*, Wiley, New York, 623-645.

Heinbach, W. (1988). *Acustica*, 67, 113-121.

Houtsma, A.J.M. (1981). *J. Acoust. Soc. Am.*, 70, 1661-1668.

Houtsma, A.J.M., and Rossing, T.D. (1987). *J. Acoust. Soc. Am.*, 81, 439-444.

Huggins, W.H. (1952). *J. Acoust. Soc. Am.*, 24, 582-589.

Lorenz, K. (1959). *Zeitschr. f. exp. und angew. Psychol.*, 4, 127-162.

Lorenz, K. (1973). *Die Rückseite des Spiegels*, Piper, München.

MacKay, D.M. (1967). *Freedom of Action in a Mechanistic Universe*, University Press, Cambridge.

McAdams, S. (1989). *J. Acoust. Soc. Am.*, 86, 2148-2159.

Moore, B.C.J., Glasberg, B.R., and Peters, R.W. (1985). *J. Acoust. Soc. Am.*, 77, 1853-1860.

Mummert, M. (1990) in: *Fortschritte der Akustik (DAGA 90)*, Bad Honnef-Wien, 1047--1050.

Ohman, S. (1975) in: A. Cohen and S.G. Nooteboom (eds.), *Structure and Process in Speech Perception*, Springer, Heidelberg, 36-47.

Parks, T.E. (1984). *Psychol. Bull.*, 95, 282-300.

Pickles, J.O. (1982). *An Introduction to the Physiology of Hearing*, Academic Press, London.

Popper, K.R. (1962). *The Logic of Scientific Discovery*, Harper & Row, New York.

Scheffers, M.T.M. (1983). *Sifting Vowels: Auditory Pitch Analysis and Sound Segregation*, Ph.D. Thesis, Rijksuniversiteit Groningen, The Netherlands.

Schouten, M.E.H. (ed.) (1987). *The Psychophysics of Speech Perception*, Nijhoff, Dordrecht, The Netherlands.

Singh, P.G. (1987). *J. Acoust. Soc. Am.*, 82, 886-899.

Stevens, S.S., and Galanter (1957). *J. Exp. Psychol.*, 54, 377-411.
Terhardt, E. (1970) in: R. Plomp and G.F. Smoorenburg (eds.), *Frequency Analysis and Periodicity Detection in Hearing*, Sijthoff, Leiden, The Netherlands, 278-290.
Terhardt, E. (1971). *Acustica*, 24, 126-136.
Terhardt, E. (1972). *Acustica*, 26, 173-199.
Terhardt, E. (1975). *Acustica*, 33, 344-348.
Terhardt, E. (1979). *Hearing Research*, 1, 155-182.
Terhardt, E. (1983). *J. Acoust. Soc. Am.*, 73, 1069-1070.
Terhardt, E. (1987) in: Schouten (1987), 271-283.
Terhardt, E. (1991). *Music Perception*, 8, 215-238.
Terhardt, E., and Grubert, A. (1987). *Perception & Psychophysics*, 42, 511-514.
Viemeister, N.F. (1980) in: G. van den Brink and F.A. Bilsen, (eds.), *Psychophysical, Physiological, and Behavioural Studies in Hearing*, Delft University Press, Delft, The Netherlands, 190-199.
Walliser, K. (1969). *Acustica*, 21, 319-329.
Wilson, J.P. (1970) in: R. Plomp and G.F. Smoorenburg (eds.) *Frequency Analalysis and Periodicity Detection in Hearing*, Sijthoff, Leiden, The Netherlands, 303-315.
Zwicker, E. (1964). *J. Acoust. Soc. Am.*, 36, 2413-2415.
Zwicker, U.T. (1984). *Speech Communication*, 3, 265-277.

Bei Fragen zur Produktsicherheit wenden Sie sich bitte an:
If you have any questions regarding product safety,
please contact:

Walter de Gruyter GmbH
Genthiner Straße 13
10785 Berlin
productsafety@degruyterbrill.com